ELK GROVE VILLAGE PUBLIC LIBRARY
3 1250 01052 589
P9-CCM-483

Praise for *Malignant*

"An extraordinary work of disciplined observation and astonishing precision, *Malignant* reveals how the common course of cancer has worked its way into the American imaginary."
—Jonathan Simon, Adrian A. Kragen Professor of Law, UC Berkeley School of Law

"In my nineteen years as a cancer survivor I have never read a book that was so spot-on when it comes to understanding the inadequacy of our current plan of attack in the war on cancer, which we have been fighting for over thirty years."
—Natalie Conforti, three-time young adult cancer survivor and advocate

"Lochlann Jain is the rare academic whose writing is as beautiful as her ideas."
—Carl Elliott, author of *White Coat, Black Hat: Adventures on the Dark Side of Medicine*

"In this alternately galvanizing and moving report, Jain offers both a queer patient's–eye view and an astute scholar's analysis. *Malignant* extends the scholarship and activism surrounding HIV/AIDS to alert us that, in the case of cancer, ubiquity = death."
—Lisa Duggan, author of *The Twilight of Equality? Neoliberalism, Cultural Politics, and the Attack on Democracy*

"As cancer increasingly becomes a metaphor for our lives, what do we do about the growing evidence of the role of the environment in cancer causation? Jain's complex and nuanced picture challenges the reader to dig down for our own conclusions. *Malignant* will be of enormous value."
—Judy Norsigian, Executive Director, Our Bodies Ourselves

"Lochlann Jain offers a fresh and profound set of insights about the total social fact of cancer in the United States. Patients and cancer prevention advocates will benefit enormously from reading this fascinating book."
—Richard Clapp, Professor Emeritus, Boston University School of Public Health

"How is it possible, S. Lochlann Jain asks in this moving, brutally honest book, for cancer to 'be inside so many people and remain outside society'? This searing exploration . . . helps us understand why government, corporate, and military leaders are so reluctant to embrace cancer as a public issue and how their failure to do so affects our understanding of the disease."
—Gerald Markowitz, coauthor of *Deceit and Denial: The Deadly Politics of Industrial Pollution*

"Both extremely personal and highly analytic, *Malignant* offers an idiosyncratic, irreverent, and probing mash-up of cancer in the U.S. today. The cancer that emerges is untidy, more a set of relationships than a thing. While highly critical of standard claims to authority and expert knowledge, suppressed politics, misplaced priorities, and victim blaming, Jain retains empathy and humor."
—Robert A. Aronowitz, author of *Unnatural History: Breast Cancer and American Society*

"Jain takes an anthropologist's approach to exploring the intricacies of an experience on a shared cultural stage. This book brings new insights into the lived struggle of a patient, activist, and academic in understanding the full complexity of cancer."
—Karuna Jagger, Executive Director, Breast Cancer Action

"Lochlann Jain's brilliant memoir/documentary offers us a thoroughly uncomfortable, provocative, and enticing read. We are led, step by meticulously researched step, into the abyss of the cancer culture, all the while being invited into the intimacy of Jain's own cancer story as a young adult. *Malignant* is a necessary read for our time, a remarkable achievement."
—Janie Brown, Executive Director, Callanish Society

"From the minute you start reading the first pages of this book, to the moment (hours later) when you arrive at its last pages, Lochlann Jain manages to grip you and hold you captive. The writing is marvelous, and the scholarship is incredible—but you aren't prepared for the disarming humor, or the delicate dissection of the psyche that Jain achieves. I could not stop reading this book. In the end, found myself enriched and wiser for it."
—Siddhartha Mukherjee, author *Emperor of All Maladies: A Biography of Cancer* (Pulitzer Prize winner)

"Malignant is a brilliant piece of medical anthropology, a beautifully poetic fusion of the personal and the political."
—Robert N. Proctor, author of *Golden Holocaust: Origins of the Cigarette Catastrophe and the Case for Abolition*

Malignant

The publisher gratefully acknowledges the generous support of the General Endowment Fund of the University of California Press Foundation.

Malignant

How Cancer Becomes Us

S. Lochlann Jain

UNIVERSITY OF CALIFORNIA PRESS
Berkeley · Los Angeles · London

University of California Press, one of the most distinguished university presses in the United States, enriches lives around the world by advancing scholarship in the humanities, social sciences, and natural sciences. Its activities are supported by the UC Press Foundation and by philanthropic contributions from individuals and institutions. For more information, visit www.ucpress.edu.

University of California Press
Berkeley and Los Angeles, California

University of California Press, Ltd.
London, England

Library of Congress Cataloging-in-Publication Data

Jain, Sarah S. Lochlann, 1967–
Malignant : how cancer becomes us / S. Lochlann Jain.
pages cm
Includes bibliographical references and index.
ISBN 978-0-520-27656-7 (hardback) — ISBN 978-0-520-27657-4 (paper) — ISBN 978-0-520-95682-7 (ebook)
1. Cancer—Government policy—United States.
2. Cancer—Research—United States. 3. Cancer—Risk factors—Government policy—United States.
4. Carcinogens—Government policy—United States.
I. Title.
RC276.J35 2013
362.19699'4—dc23
2013018303

Manufactured in the United States of America

22 21 20 19 18 17 16 15 14 13
10 9 8 7 6 5 4 3 2 1

In keeping with a commitment to support environmentally responsible and sustainable printing practices, UC Press has printed this book on Rolland Enviro100, a 100% post-consumer fiber paper that is FSC certified, deinked, processed chlorine-free, and manufactured with renewable biogas energy. It is acid-free and EcoLogo certified.

To my family:
Chosen, who let me in.
Blood, whom I would have chosen.

Contents

Introduction

We Just Don't Know It Yet

I knew a woman who went to medical school because she wanted to be with people at critical, life-changing moments; she imagined that sharing dire information would create an intense mutual experience.

My own decidedly undramatic life-changing moment took place in a tiny, somewhat battered office. The doctor flipped back and forth and back again among the three pages of the report she had received from my radiologist. As she fidgeted, I surveyed the posters on her office wall of Banff National Park, in the Canadian Rockies, where I had been hiking the previous day as I wound up a visit with my parents before flying back to my job in California.

As my eyes wandered, I could tell the doctor really, really didn't want to look at me. Finally, she glanced up and, in a last-ditch effort to avoid her part in the vaunted Bad News Experience, asked if I already knew what the report said. I shook my head.

A few minutes later, as we drove away from the curling-edged posters in that office and toward the surgeon's office to see how soon I could get the cancer out, my mother called my dad and asked him to look after the kids for another couple of hours. Meanwhile, I looked at more pictures—this time, those in the brochure the nurse had given me. I speculated on what "invasive" meant. Half of all Americans will be forced to consider this word at some point, and half of those will die wondering why the billions of research dollars thrown at the word haven't exterminated it from the English language.

Cancer can kill: this fact makes it concrete. Americans collect data on it, write histories and memoirs about it, blog about it. Still, it's a devious knave. Cancer takes some people within days of diagnosis, while other people spend years waiting for a final outcome. While one sleeps it may clump into hard or soft tumors, or it may eddy into lymph fluid or lodge in the crook of one's liver or lung to initiate new colonies. Often the treatment, not the cancer, ties one to the sofa. At diagnosis, I knew I was in trouble not because of how I felt, but by the look on my mother's face.

Too wily to be tethered to a solid noun, the conundrums of cancer match its craftiness. Despite news articles promising a cure since 1907 (albeit by putting patients into the ice box),[1] scientists continue to furiously debate how cancer arises, whether it should be studied as one disease or hundreds, whether mice provide adequate research models, and who might benefit from the arsenal of commonplace, if dangerous, cancer treatments such as chemotherapy and radiation. Policymakers and political lobbyists discuss (or don't) how to test and regulate the thousands of carcinogens in our environment and the significance of cancer clusters. And despite some of the shiniest, priciest, most marble-staircased hospitals in the country, treatments remain only partially effective for most cancers. The word's tangibility dissolves in sheer bafflement, for doctors and patients alike, over what, exactly, it describes.

A week after my diagnosis, following the first of several operations, my surgeon presented me with my pathology report. Abbreviated as "path report," this description of the removed tissue joins other morsels of cancer lingo, such as the conversion of stomach-wrenching chemotherapy into the too-familiar "chemo," the more manageable "mets" or "hotspots" for life-threatening metastases. His meeting with me and my mom was especially awkward because my mother had been a student of his in a medical school class that had petitioned against his use of pornographic slides in his lectures. A clearly nervous medical student joined the quartet.

Dr. Slideshow had surely had similar interactions hundreds of times—the patient's questions hastily scrawled on slips of paper, based on half-understood newspaper articles summarizing medical trials; the uneasy smiles; the vague attempts at reassurance. The physician's role in going over the path report must get tedious; despite the shock and horror for the patient, cancer treatments are fairly rote, based on ludicrously few variables.

My path report began with a description of the original tissue: "In the fresh state, the specimen weighs 683 g." *(Fresh! Specimen!)* I pictured the lump of flesh on a Weight Watchers scale ready for dissection. From the description of what had been my tissue, the report rapidly narrowed into a series of inscrutable markings and scores. It indicated how many nodes contained cancer and how many and what size the tumors were. At that time, I had only the vaguest notion of cancer—so far in my brief cancer-life it had been a conglomeration of humiliation, shame, a thing that threatened my shot at tenure, and random concerns about artificial sweeteners and nonstick pans. The path report, in contrast, represented cancer as a set of numbers. The image of a computer converting lines of poetry into zeros and ones flashed through my mind.

The path report rendered my flesh into data points comparable to other people's flesh, and from there into a mountain of evidence about various treatments. By the time treatment ended, the "specimen" would be far from "fresh," so the mobile path report came in handy. I took it to the members of my cancer circle—the many specialists who could translate the numbers into their expert languages—and later, in considering a medical malpractice suit for three years of missed diagnoses, to my attorneys. The report became a vector connecting me to all the bureaucracies each represented. My flesh had *become* the pathology report—portioned, sliced, flattened onto slides, observed, categorized, and finally rendered into this emailable document.[2]

I couldn't see a way to admit that the three pieces of paper so utterly wrecked me and at the same time audition for a strong character role within the medical performance (surely the patient should be a respectable, full-fledged member of the team, not merely a victim of circumstance?). In truth, I didn't know the least thing about my new role. I could more or less enact curiosity-driven researcher, loving girlfriend, stern teacher, doting Mima, dependable big sister, cash-strapped daughter, fun-loving chum, polite dinner guest, competent student, active teammate . . . but sick patient? Not in my repertoire.

The italicized type and banal officiousness of the path report served as my portal to an entirely new world, one Susan Sontag lavishly described as "the kingdom of the ill."[3] My journey to this kingdom differed from the romantic tradition of my discipline, anthropology, whose research trips require years of language preparation and mythic days floating down pristine rivers in dugout canoes. The moat I crossed to take up my new residence was more like a silty, crocodile-filled gorge, with no paddle in sight.

I had previously thought of cancer as a straightforward enough, if unwanted, thing embedded in a well-oiled institution that closely monitored its flock in pursuit of the knowledge that would shortly result in a cure. The histories of cancer that I'd read generally told a story of progress, from the use of primitive treatments (ground puppy bones, sandalwood, turpentine) to more effective ones (x-rays and vaccines.)[4] Even the bleakest of histories assume that a cancer (part cell division, part social history) can be described within the context of the history of medicine and the evolution of research strategies, treatments, and activism.[5]

In that moment of my postdiagnostic, post-first-surgery encounter with the *doctor-resident/path report/mom-gown-bandages/possible micro-metastases/white coat/tiny room,* I realized that no well-managed organization watches over cancer. Cancer, in all its nounishness, refers to everything . . . and nothing. Cancer pervaded the office, residing in each of these objects and people and the relations among them, but nowhere could it be specified as a thing. The main tumors were gone: *cancer* had only just begun.[6] What on earth, then, do we mean when we refer to this concept, cancer?

Bitter debates, driven by jostling participants, rage around basic questions. Should premalignant lesions count as cancer when it comes to gathering statistics and deciding on treatment? Should insurance cover the costs of not exactly medically necessary reconstructive surgery? What about experimental treatments? Where and how should we even be looking for cancer? In each of these issues, the stakes are enormous, yet hardly anyone seems to challenge the terms and intersections of the debates. Anything *but* an objective thing, cancer can be better understood as a set of relationships—economic, sentimental, medical, personal, ethical, institutional, statistical.

Given the billions spent and made in developing treatments and the magnitude of the destruction of bodies and the social fabric, we desperately need new ways of understanding cancer—not as a disease awaiting a cure, but as a constitutive aspect of American social life, economics, and science. *Malignant* builds on this idea, presenting cancer as a process and as a social field, while also exploring its brutal effects at the level of individual experience.

I read personal, medical, economic, cultural, and epistemological together. These realms have—in often entirely obvious but complexly discounted ways—misleadingly separated the fact of cancer from its all-too-human interpretations. My mash-up includes the peculiar authority of the socio-sexual psychopathologies of body parts; the uneven effects of expertise and power; the possibly cancerous consequences of donating eggs to a girlfriend desperate to have a baby; the huge industrial investments that manifest themselves as bone-cold testing rooms; and the teeth-grittingly jovial efforts to smear makeup and wigs over the whole messy problem of bodies spiraling into pain and decay.

The quest to discern the interests behind how and when cancer is named can also diagnose the interests that produce and treat the disease. *Malignant* seeks the places at which these reciprocating diagnoses most paradoxically intersect, such as prognoses, research trials, legal battles, and screening debates. Unraveling the guiding logics of these institutions enables us to better understand who claims knowledge about cancer, and how—through methods as varied as statistics gathering or lay experience. While my argument will hopefully be useful in considering other diseases, a focus on our affair with this fundamentally unknown illness uniquely shines light on the institutions and perspectives that constitute illness in America.

PERFECT STORM

If you look up *cancer* in a medical dictionary, you will read that cancer begins when an injured cell speeds up the normal process of division. Eventually these quickly dividing cells may form a tumor, which then may build its own set of blood vessels in order to feed itself in a process called angiogenesis. (Blood cancers, or liquid tumors, don't form static tumors in quite the same way.) Some cells may break off from a localized tumor and move to a different part of the body, colonizing a vital organ or bone. For most cancers, once this metastasis happens, you are probably sunk (a term one will not find in medical journals but that nonetheless feels accurate). These distinguishing features describe at least several hundred diseases that flutter under the cancer banner.

A more truthful account of cancer would require a full-blown epic movie series, for cancer has become a central, silent, ubiquitous player in twentieth- and twenty-first-century America. One would watch images of our greatness fading in and out to a heart-swelling orchestral score. Each of America's iconic industries—agriculture, oil and gas, cosmetics, plastics, pesticides, tobacco, medicine, construction, military —has undoubtedly led to tens of millions of cancer deaths. The unique way in which cancer presents, decades after exposures, makes it central to the growth of both the industries and the illness, in short, to the existence of the United States as we know it.

If I were to direct such a movie, I would start by examining how cancer has become a potent metaphor for anything evil or scary. As a result, cancer—or at least the fight against it—provides a moral ground for anyone taking a stand against something bad, something that indeed might "metastasize" or spread, whether guns, fascism, or gay people. If the disease itself provides the archetype of malevolence such that "curing cancer" offers an equivalent to "saving the world" in all kinds of thought experiments, the stereotype of the diseased victim that one treats with kid gloves can be useful, too. Witness Tour de France winner (or ex-winner, since he has now been stripped of his seven victories) Lance Armstrong's use of his year in treatment to at once explain his greatness and divert attention from his performance-enhancing drug use.

Tobacco's relation to cancer has been well rehearsed. But for good measure my production crew would run footage from the 1970s, describing how the cigarette industry brains shifted the demographics of lung cancer with the jingle "You've come a long way, baby" for their special feminist cigarette, Virginia Slims. By sponsoring women's tennis and advertising specifically to African Americans when no one else would, cancer incidentally joined progressive causes. The tobacco industry's role in cancer does not end with the millions of lung cancer deaths. The industry inadvertently enabled the rise of the field that became epidemiology as a result of controversial attempts to link lung cancer to smoking. My blockbuster would describe how cancer also provided opportunities for major public health campaigns and philanthropic endeavors, shaping the form of both of those areas of the American Experience. In one ironic twist, the widow of the ad executive behind the 1930s advertising campaign "Reach for a Lucky Instead of a Sweet" became one of the main activists promoting the War on Cancer, launched in 1971. Cancer giveth fortunes and taketh them away.

Another thread of the documentary would focus on notable Americans prematurely lost to the disease: from Steve Jobs to James Baldwin, from Humphrey Bogart to Judi Bari. A full section would detail the life of Rachel Carson, the scientist who initiated the modern environmental movement with her book *Silent Spring* before her own name was added to the list of brilliant people—people we needed—dead of cancer. I'd include a section titled "The Celluloid Send-Off," which would review a century of film and the star appearances of cancer as a sentimental storytelling trope.

I would wrap my producer's blood pressure cuff around the military technologies that pumped the lifeblood of an American Century. The development of chemotherapy resulted from the autopsies of soldiers who had been killed by nitrogen mustard gas in World War I; it was found that the gas eradicated white blood cells from bone marrow and lymphatic tissue. Although the use of radiation as an experimental therapy for cancer patients began before World War II, the increased focus on its development coincided neatly with the government's attempt to represent the "friendly" potential of nuclear technology. *(Sure, radiation killed all those Japanese people, but it can do good things too!)* Both of these cancer treatments led to the creation of a massive, powerful, and lucrative infrastructure even amid controversy about their efficacy. The military and cancer have enabled one another in ways that have yet to be understood.

Midcentury cancer experts adopted industrial research methods—often those developed by the automobile industry—in which multidisciplinary teams worked together.[7] Meanwhile, the use of cancer patients for medical experiments during the early and mid–twentieth century led directly to the development of the human subjects protocols in 1978 that now protect patients and guide all manner of research. At least half an episode of my film would be devoted to the first treatments for the HIV/AIDS epidemic, which were initially developed as experimental cancer treatments in the 1960s.

We would have to figure out a way to trace the forces at play in the appearances and disappearances of the corroding bodies that lie at the center of each of so many conflicting projects.

None of these facets of cancer-in-action are in the dictionary—but they would be in my documentary. So would the growth trajectory of the pharmaceutical industry, along a crucial vector starting with Jonas Salk's 1955 claim that patenting the polio vaccine would be like patenting the sun and extending to Genentech's proclamation in 2008 that it would charge the highest market rates for its cancer drug Avastin. (And it did so for three years, until the Food and Drug Administration [FDA] withdrew Avastin from the market as a breast cancer treatment, since it did nothing to improve survival rates.)[8]

The documentary would not, however, attempt the impossible project of unscrambling the too-quickly dividing cells from American history. Much as we might want to render cancer an external threat to be battled, it just is not so. Cancer *is* our history. Cancer has become us. Manifest within individual bodies—many, *many* bodies—it is also embedded within this country's key industries, medicine not least among them.

The combination of a for-profit medical system, the rise of trials and institutionalized industrial methods of cancer research and treatment, and the enormous investments required for radiation and chemotherapy have created the perfect storm, turning the once-backwater specialty of oncology into a major economic force that ties together treatment, pharmaceuticals, insurance, law, and research. Cancer has the highest per capita price of the nation's medical conditions.

In the last five decades, cancer has gained traction as a multibillion dollar business. The National Cancer Institute's budget alone totaled $5.3 billion in the fiscal year 2011–2012; other federal agencies (including the FDA, Centers for Disease Control [CDC], and Department of Defense [DOD]) chip in a further $670 million for cancer research; and nonprofits, industry, and the state contribute several hundred million more.[9] The National Cancer Institute (NCI) reports that the medical costs of cancer care add up to some $125 billion, with a projected 39 percent increase, to $173 billion, by 2020,[10] while the National Institutes of Health (NIH) doubles that with an estimate for 2010 of $263.8 billion. Their accounting includes $102.8 billion in direct medical costs (or health expenditures), $20.9 billion for indirect morbidity costs (lost productivity due to illness); and $140.1 billion for indirect mortality costs (lost productivity due to premature death).[11]

While some methods of calculation find that cancer and its patients take up *too* many resources, from another angle, cancer patients are cash cows. Each cancer patient generates millions of dollars in revenues. If one wonders why we would extend the life of a pancreatic patient for a dozen days with a $16,000 drug, let's remember that this money does not evaporate after twelve days; it continues to circulate in stock prices, salaries, and smaller crumbs of an infinitely profitable cancer pie.[12] Just as the demon of communism justified the proliferation of a lucrative nuclear industry, so cancer fills the core of so many economies that if a cure were to be found, the economy might just crash.[13]

The medical industry has found a way to align (or perhaps it emerged from the alignment of) just enough ducks to be able to tart up a coercive economy in market terms. Putting a market value on health makes this possible. If you wanted my money, the best way to get it would certainly not be to rob me (I have only $43 in my pocket) or to take me to court (my insurance will offer you only $1 million if you slip on a banana peel in my apartment). Nor would it be to take me to the collection agency, offer me a mortgage, or get access to my life insurance. The best way to get my money would be to offer me many rounds of treatment for a deadly illness and make sure my insurance pays for them. For medical care—more than housing, childcare, education, food, fashion, transportation, or gym fees—an insured person can pay much, much more than his own worth. She can pay much more than any free market would bear. This economic skew creates a health bubble in which anyone with insurance, and especially anyone with both cancer and insurance, is a gift that just keeps on giving to those who can provide what he needs.[14]

The resulting distortion affects consequential definitions of health. My financial advisor, for example, might recommend that I take pills with a co-pay of $35 a month, rather than pay a gym membership fee of $99 a month. Costs remain high even for tests and treatments that have not significantly improved in the last decade, such as magnetic resonance imaging. It's no surprise, then, that healthcare has become the most profitable industry in the economy.[15] And most people will pay anything for a small chance at living longer. As one young man put it, "If they told me to eat pinecones, well, I would do it." If oncologists started prescribing them, and insurance covered the cost, pinecones would become more and more expensive. One in five dollars in the economy goes toward this haphazard version of "health."[16]

As many commentators have noted, a privately funded, for-profit medical system does not create the most likely scenario for the shattering of scientific frontiers. The pharmaceutical industry offers a case in point. With the cost of bringing a drug to market in excess of $800 million and low FDA approval rates for new cancer drugs, any investment in new drugs is highly risky. Simple math confirms that drugs with expandable markets will bring more profits than drugs for targeted illnesses impacting smaller populations. The annual top-ten list of most profitable drugs in the United States typically includes drugs with elastic definitions of diagnosis—depression, anxiety, insomnia, high cholesterol, sexual dysfunction: all markets that have been steadily increasing.

This market force disinclines private industry from working on subcategories of cancer. Various problems result. First, drugs are often tested on large and diverse subject groups in order to capture the largest populations. The results of such studies make it impossible for doctors to extrapolate just which individuals would benefit from any given treatment. Second, little incentive exists to produce generic drugs, which bring low profits. For this reason, for example, mechlorethamine, or nitrogen mustard, one of the original chemotherapy drugs tested in the 1960s in the treatment of childhood leukemia, has been in short supply. A recent study on the impact of the shortage found that the substitute drug significantly reduced survival, having "devastating effects on [children] with [otherwise curable] cancer."[17]

Several common cancers, therefore, come under the purview of rare diseases, which the Orphan Disease Act of 2002 describes as affecting "more than 200,000 in the United States and for which there is no reasonable expectation that the cost of developing and making available in the United States a drug for such disease or condition will be recovered from sales in the United States of such drug."[18] This remains generally the case even with the rise of a few "boutique" drugs, in which extremely expensive drugs are profitable at the cost of excluding many from access.[19] Ironically, what makes for good science makes for poor economics; subsets shrink markets, thus reducing the chances that companies will develop more specific treatments.

Thus, health resists market quantification. Putting health in market terms somehow crushes the notions of choice that undergird true market actors and give them an intimidating tinge (sure, you *could* refuse this $100,000-a-week incubator for your sick child). Such systematic market and health forces have nothing per se to do with ill intent. (I'm not saying that anyone is evil.) No one necessarily wants corporate interests to trump human well-being or important scientific research. But the chances that a sector whose binding legal concern is stockholder profit will lead to adequate research and better public health are slim. When the question becomes one of math, anyone can do it.

While insured people can "afford" much more than we are worth, the expenses that remain, such as co-pays, deductibles, or costs after certain coverage ceilings, can be crushing. When I moved from Canada to the United States to go back to work after my treatment (yes, I ended up staying in Canada for treatment), my insurance covered only 80 percent of my follow-up medical care. The bills from the Stanford Cancer Center for the remaining 20 percent added up to hundreds and then thousands of dollars (much more than I was told when I called in advance to find out how much it would cost, and more than half of that total resulting from an accounting error). The bills came weekly, not monthly—no matter how many hours I spent on the phone explaining the mistake. Soon enough I felt trapped inside a snow globe with endlessly generated medical bills spilling down around me, creating ghastly drifts of white envelopes with that Stanford crest that came to mean "do not open this." Collection agencies call 46 percent of cancer patients in the United States; I was one of them.[20] Experts often attribute over 60 percent of personal bankruptcies in the United States to the catastrophic financial burden of illness, with little mention of the skewed economy that distributes not just enormous wealth but also enormous debt. Even if you enter the illness casino with a few coins jangling in your pocket, seeking healthcare is a gamble in which the house enjoys vastly superior odds.

To add to the built-in paradox of the for-profit healthcare system, money made from treating cancer aligns a little too comfortably with the profits made from causing cancer. In the FDA's first attempt to bring cigarettes under their regulatory purview as a drug (nicotine) delivery device, the Supreme Court in 2000 weighed economic and physical health and, in the final opinion, explicitly noted that the tobacco industry played too important a role in the U.S. economy to be regulated by the FDA—even as it recognized that nicotine was an addictive drug whose dose tobacco companies intentionally manipulated.[21]

Here is another example that demonstrates the tightly linked interests that both cause and treat cancer. In 1978, Imperial Chemical Industries (ICI), one of the largest companies in the world, specializing in agrochemicals and pharmaceuticals, developed the cancer drug tamoxifen. In 1985, along with the American Cancer Society, ICI founded the National Breast Cancer Awareness Month with the aim of promoting mammography as the most effective tool against breast cancer. In 1990 Imperial Chemical Industries was accused of dumping DDT and PCBs, known carcinogens, into the Long Beach and Los Angeles harbors.[22] Zeneca, producer of tamoxifen, demerged from ICI in 1993, and later merged with Astra AB in 1999 to form AstraZeneca. Astra AB had developed the herbicide acetochlor, classified by the EPA as a probable carcinogen.[23] In 1997 Zeneca purchased Salick Health Care, a chain of for-profit outpatient cancer clinics. Subsequently AstraZeneca launched a major publicity campaign encouraging women to assess their risk factors for breast cancer, downplaying the dangers of tamoxifen in order to create a market for its prophylactic, or chemopreventative, use and, more recently, for the breast cancer drug Arimidex (anastrozole), approved in 2002 and used as an alternative to tamoxifen (Arimidex went off patent in 2010).[24]

Dr. Samuel Epstein, a professor emeritus of occupational and environmental health at the University of Illinois School of Public Health, commented on this situation: "You've got a company that's a spinoff of one of the world's biggest manufacturers of carcinogenic chemicals, they've got control of breast cancer treatment, they've got control of the chemoprevention [studies], and now they have control of cancer treatment in eleven centers—which are clearly going to be prescribing the drugs they manufacture."[25] AstraZeneca has been successfully sued by several states for illegal price inflation of tamoxifen. Among other such cases, AstraZeneca settled one in Idaho and lost another on appeal in Massachusetts when the court upheld a $12.9 million fine.[26]

Similarly, even while General Electric and DuPont sell millions of dollars' worth of mammography machines and film annually, they have also poured tons of toxic waste into the air and water, creating high numbers of Superfund sites (abandoned hazardous waste sites so designated by the Environmental Protection Agency).[27]

In such a climate, the focus on awareness and screening does not bring us any closer to understanding the ways that key aspects of the economy involve both causing and treating cancer. (All of us who drive, buy strawberries, live in homes, wear PJs coated with flame retardant, and receive purchase receipts covered in carcinogens take part in that.) Yet even if one believes in the legitimacy of causing and curing cancer as market opportunities, cancer cannot be understood solely through an analysis of economic interests.

Susan Sontag believed that one must free illness of its metaphors in order to truly see it, and she dug up the history of derogation surrounding the proverbial emperor of maladies.[28] I suggest, on the contrary, that the key lies not in undressing the emperor, but in examining the costumes. Cancer appears *only* at the nexus of our ways of thinking about it. I don't mean to argue that "it" doesn't exist, or that it doesn't maim and kill people. But it can't carry meaning outside of the meshy nets we use to locate and describe it. The history that Sontag identified, as well as many other histories that she didn't, offers clues about cancer's role in America.

Cancer, as a chimera, gains different registers of meaning in different places. It envelops and is an effect of oncologists, insurance provisions, support groups, survivor workshops, and medical research. Cancer is

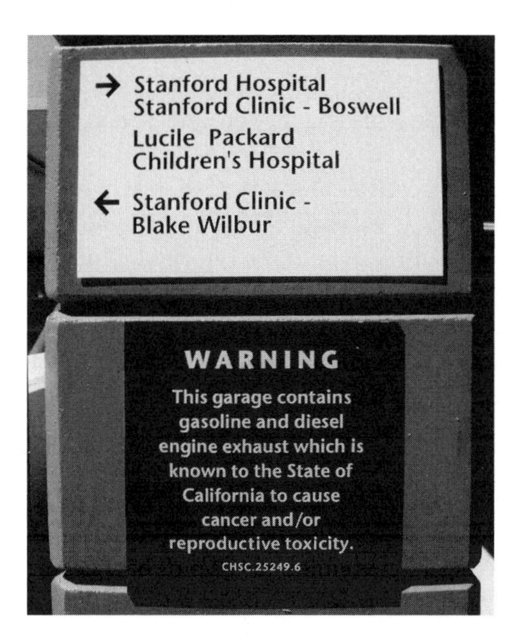

FIGURE 1. California Proposition 65, passed in 1986 through a ballot measure, requires businesses to post warning signs when exposing customers or bystanders to specific levels of chemicals listed on a twenty-two-page roster of known, legal carcinogens. The business must determine any likely exposure that will result from a chemical. The signs are posted everywhere in California, like flags of surrender. (Photo by author, Stanford Cancer Center parking lot)

stacks of *Reader's Digest*s, furtive glances and hasty conversations in waiting rooms. It is evenings spent working out complicated medical bills and long phone calls with befuddled insurance bureaucrats. It is cracking the code of how to play your "cancer card" and what value, versus what backlash, it might have. It is wondering if anyone would come to your funeral. Would you look like a big dork if you died in the summer while everyone was on vacation?

In a renowned 1923 analysis of gift exchange in different cultures, the French anthropologist Marcel Mauss unpacked connections he found in a ritual that had previously been understood as the purely benevolent act of offering and receiving. In so doing, he coined a term, *total social fact,* for a practice whose effects both connect and fissure through seemingly distinct areas of life, thus weaving them together. In a legendary passage, Mauss explains the total social fact (I substitute *cancers* here for practices of gifting that he describes): "These phenomena are at once legal, economic, religious, aesthetic, morphological and so on. [Cancers] are legal in that they concern individual and collective rights, organized and diffuse morality; they may be entirely obligatory, or subject simply to praise or disapproval. [Cancers] are at once political and domestic, being of interest both to classes and to clans and families. They are religious; they concern true religion, animism, magic and diffuse religious mentality. [Cancers] are economic, for the notions of value, utility, interest, luxury, wealth, acquisition, accumulation, consumption and liberal and sumptuous expenditure are all present."[29]

Like a Maussian gift, cancer has entered our collective imaginations at all of these levels. Not only does it work through the metaphors of metastasis, recurrence, and remission, but it is also at one moment a paper trail and at another an identity, at one place a statistic and at another a bankruptcy; here, a scientific quandary, there, a transcendent image of a cell. One person's losses offer another a chance to leave a mark on humanity. A body image taken offers another to be found. The project of making cancer—as plural as it is singular, as vast as it is microscopic, as diffuse and discrepant as it is descriptive—resonates under one word. The simple noun *cancer* consolidates this collective achievement.

Cancer in all its complexity is not solely a biological phenomenon, but a politics with which to engage and struggle. Why does metastatic breast cancer receive only 3 percent of research dollars when the tens of thousands of people who die of breast cancer will die of metastatic cancer? Who suffers the effects of the recent court decision to disallow graphic warnings on cigarette packages? How are cost and benefit determined in screening debates? Who should pay for inevitable surgical errors? Who considers, and who suffers from, the unintended consequences of institutional blind spots? The questions framed in various expert and lay areas, and the forms that the answers take, provide clues about the values that underpin our understandings of cancer, just as crude oil oozing from a pipeline onto the Arctic snow discloses the dominant values of the society that laid the pipe. My book is not only about how the framings of cancer affect psychic, medical, and institutional experiences, but also about how understandings of cancer reflect back onto the cultures that have defined it.[30]

Astrologists and scientists alike derive meaning from the set of dividing cells and its namesake, the constellation in the zodiac. The configuration we dimly recognize as a crab, suspended between its brighter siblings Gemini and Leo, takes shape through a specific alignment of stars, some of which we see as they were hundreds of millions of years ago. Cancer's earthy doppelganger, also, threatens to disintegrate with each shift in perspective.[31] The pathology report, the prognoses, the scars, the data and graphs, the looks on parents' faces, the shiny hospitals with their infusion rooms and IV drips, the marches and fundraising translate the uncertainty at the center of what we call cancer into a thing that we *can* call cancer. But just barely.

LAY YOUR BODY DOWN

After my first surgery, Dr. Slideshow wanted to see my new scar. He turned away as I changed into the hospital gown. With the clumsy gestures of my stripping and him turning, we joined a centuries-old pageant. One gown and one stethoscope-in-relation-to-gown—these rituals and costumes make the prodding, cutting, digging, and stitching correspond to an otherwise unthinkable etiquette.

I hold enormous respect for the expertise that doctors gain through their years of tough physical and intellectual training. No denigration of that skill comes with the observation that white coat and hospital gown divide those who define the bureaucratic and medical realm of illness from the one who necessarily, if perhaps not wholly, comes to be defined by it. Recognizing how that dynamic operates might be of service to everyone, since as doctors and/or as patients, we all play roles in this script.

Forms of cancer-knowledge tend to push each participant to identify with one side of the equation (objective, scientific, "neutral") or the other (subjective, emotional, "biased").[32] As a patient, you can't forget for an instant that the data do not fully describe your life. But researchers and scholars tend to frame the disease in the abstract, as if it could exist outside of the actual people who manifest it. Because of that propensity, it takes an effort to consciously remember—*really remember*—that people's lives are more than just data, that actual people play critical roles in the very existence of the disease and how we understand it.

No matter how sympathetically told, medical history *necessarily* goes on to tell of the ultimate "triumph" of the treatments.[33] In the 1960s, for example, hematologists began testing the effects of high and low doses of chemotherapy on children with leukemia. Yet the temporal horizon of the children stretches not over decades, but over months, days, minutes. Their stories do not move on to the next, better version of chemotherapy. Some of these children abide a horrible illness and die; some live with continued health issues, missing school, losing and gaining friends. Whatever the details, cancer creates for these children a new kind of story of their lives, and it's not an abstracted story of medical progress.

A pairing of articles can further demonstrate the stakes in this clash between the modes of thinking ascribed to the patient (subjective etc.) and to the doctor (objective etc.). Rose Kushner, a well-known journalist in the 1970s, worked to bring cancer out of the closet at a time when many people were still not told of their diagnosis, let alone expected to take an active role in treatment decisions. After her cancer recurrence, Kushner wrote about the then-new treatment of chemotherapy in an article titled "Is Aggressive Adjuvant Chemotherapy the Radical Halsted of the '80s?" For the reasons she cites, she opted against taking the chemotherapy.[34]

Like many cancer patients, Kushner acquired an encyclopedic knowledge of the scientific research on her disease. A procedure of her time, referred to simply as "the Halsted," consisted of a ghastly mastectomy that removed muscle, tissue, and sometimes bone in order to clear huge margins around the tumor, based on the surgeon William Halsted's theory that cancer spreads outward from the initial tumor. Shortly before Kushner wrote her article, surgeons abandoned the radical mastectomy after nearly a century of use; trials found it no more likely to stop cancer from recurring than excision of the tumor alone followed by radiation. Thus, Kushner highlights a key point: people with cancer, and especially women, have suffered severe consequences of treatments later found to be at best ineffective, and at worst, profoundly injurious.

In 2007, long after Kushner's death from metastatic breast cancer, the noted cancer historian and physician Barron Lerner wrote his own commentary on her piece as part of his larger research into the illnesses of celebrities.[35] Although in a 2003 history of breast cancer he, too, acknowledged the gender imbalance in cancer treatments,[36] Lerner's reading of Kushner's article makes clear an irony. Because she had to lay her body on the altar of medical expertise, he suggests, Kushner could not help but be biased in her analysis of the debates about chemotherapy. "Rose Kushner's award-winning article," he concludes, ". . . provides a cautionary tale about individuals who function simultaneously as patients and spokespeople."[37] Astonishingly, he thinks she had *too much* at stake—not because she was a journalist, but because she was a patient—to have truly understood the data.

Kushner observed that the trials for chemotherapy did not include categories for stage and age at diagnosis, thus impairing the ability of oncologists to determine the efficacy of the treatment for specific individuals. Early trial results demonstrated an improved survival rate of only 3 percent, and Kushner graphically listed side-effects of chemotherapy that many physicians discounted: "baldness, nausea and vomiting, diarrhea, clogged veins, financial problems, broken marriages, disturbed children, loss of libido, loss of self-esteem, and [impaired] body image."[38] Despite billions of dollars invested in research and hundreds of trials showing fractional differences in survival rates, the particular cocktail of drugs that Kushner writes about has not significantly changed since its introduction in the 1970s. Neither has the dim likelihood of it working. Indeed, the debate continues—Is it ethical to give thousands of people such a dangerous treatment for the potential benefit of a few?—though chemotherapy has settled into such a standard of care that to refuse it seems like an irrational death wish.

The journalist and patient saw cancer and its medical management as enmeshed in institutional relationships with uncertain pay-offs. On the patient side, chemotherapy offers more than a treatment. A life filled with boring and painful details includes wondering if the phlebotomist will be gentle; hearing the nurse trying to insert the IV needle say, "If I can't get it in three tries, I'll find someone else"; imposing on friends and family for a ride home from the hospital. Whether chemotherapy would have saved Kushner's life cannot be known. The point of her article is clear, however: for some people, the math of risk and chance requires different kinds of accounting in conditions of such deep uncertainty and hazy research results.

Debates about efficacy aside, in suggesting that Kushner *should* have done chemotherapy Lerner misses an opportunity to understand the inescapably physical experience of a human undergoing an invasive procedure. In his very inability to grasp this, his article underscores how medical history so often elides the stories and experiences created by, and necessary for, the science. He can do this through a logic that is central to the reality of cancer treatments to this day: chemotherapy may or may not work for your future survival if you take it, but it definitely won't work if you don't take it.

The difference in perspective made evident in the Kushner-Lerner pairing emerges as a dynamic in thinking about which kinds of evidence gain stature: the interpretation of one who has much at stake by virtue of literally embodying the disease, or the understanding of someone for whom a tightly specified set of research data offers no more than a professional tool. Institutions support the separation and even mutual inscrutability of these forms of knowledge.[39] In the hospital, individual bodies take up their roles in a system buoyed by a threat even in its aim to cure: either undergoing or not undergoing what medicine has to offer can hurt you. In the hospital, you know exactly where you stand in relation to those roles: which doors you can use; how your body should be clothed; who can flirt with whom; and which people will be referred to in the third person, even when they are lying right there on the bed. The very design of the place demands certain behaviors and supports certain hierarchies.

Or so I was thinking as I drove down Alpine Road adjacent to Stanford University, where some of the richest, most educated cyclists in the United States find that the narrow cycling path drops them into the middle of a car-infested junction. No matter how high-tech the cars, motorcycles, or racing bicycles in the intersection, nor how brainy or well connected the riders and drivers, they inhabit a system of crisscrossing roads that limits communication among the participants. Whether propped on a leather Brooks bike saddle or swaddled in the leather bucket seat of a Bugatti, communication takes place through honks, swerves, fingers, waves, blinking lights, and physical impact. Which of these primitive actions you can access depends not on your wealth and education, but on the means by which you entered the intersection.

The same word comes to mind when I observe a cyclist dumped in the middle of an intersection fearing the approaching driver talking on his phone as when I think of a patient dreading being treated like a cadaver while under anesthesia: *powerless*.

COGNITIVE DISSONANCE

The power dynamic resulting from the separation and institutionalization of knowledge in these ways devalues the knowledge that people with cancer derive from undergoing treatment. Perhaps as a result, some survivors respond unfavorably to analyses of cancer by individuals who are presumed not to have experienced the disease themselves. I've learned this when giving talks and not coming out as someone who has gone through surgery, chemotherapy, and radiation for fear that my personal experience would discredit my views, make me seem less "objective." In this trade-off, some survivors then think that I'm an outsider.

Bristly survivors make a valid point. For how *could* you imagine the scene of the radiation room? The frail gown that had surely covered someone for whom this very treatment hadn't worked now inelegantly smothers your unease about the dose the machine is emitting and strains to catch the shiver that threatens to displace the crimson rays from the tumor. The soft-rock radio's ionizing thrum replaces the technicians who moments ago trussed you like a Christmas turkey before saying *that's probably good enough* and pressing the button to elevate your scarcely clad prone body higher into the frigid cement vault before bustling down the leaded hallway to cluster in the teddy bear–garnished booth as the machines start to tick and squeal.

I, for one, would not have been able to grasp being an object in other people's daily work lives—a slippery-veined wriggly mound from which to draw blood; a back-wrenching load on a difficult-to-steer bed needing conveyance from one department to another—had I not gone through the experience myself. I won't soon forget the doctor who meticulously peeled and then sucked on each in a pile of Hershey's kisses as he reeled off the statistical likelihood that radiation treatment would work, versus the likelihood that it would produce more and other kinds of cancer. Certainly his view of those statistics differed from mine. Maybe chocolate would have sweetened my end of the deal, but he didn't offer.

Experience differs again from an outside observer's social science account of cancer treatment. The humiliation of being told by a group of giggling nurses who can't put in a catheter that they wished you were still under general anesthetic would not be conveyed by a series of data on catheter implant success and failure rates. Not exactly predetermined, each of cancer's scenarios funnels possible experiences. From the radiation room to the support group, each new role offers new requirements of physical and emotional discipline, masochism, and passivity. For these reasons, a kind of recognition emerges among people who may identify as cancer "survivors," akin to the knowing winks that parents of adult children give to those quieting screaming toddlers.

In an ideal world, a cancer diagnosis would come with an explanation of cause and move on to successful treatment. All the small embarrassments could disappear with a bit of psychotherapy if the treatment offered a cure. Would that I could describe that idyllic situation in this book. In our parallel hackneyed universe, cancer's uncertainties define the structure in which millions of people live, in which decisions are both offered and made: whether to join a trial, have a screening, or take a dangerous and expensive drug.

This book unpacks the head-spinning ricochet that characterizes a cancer "journey." It revolves around the stamps put into my passport by the immigration officials at the gates of the kingdom of the ill: *Diagnosed with a late-stage cancer at age thirty-six, after three years of misdiagnoses by three different doctors.* Nearly three-quarters of the seventy thousand or so adults under the age of thirty-nine who are diagnosed with cancer each year have late-stage cancers because cancer is wrongly thought of as an old person's disease. Not uninteresting, but not so very special. *Underwent hormonal therapy to be an egg donor for former partner.* Hundreds of thousands of young women have been egg donors. On average, each IVF (in vitro fertilization) baby born in the United States has been the result of four rounds of brain- and body-altering hormonal treatments on a mother or an egg donor. Not much research exists on those culturally acceptable treatments. Again, not a particularly unique story. *An out queer.* Me and millions of others, though the meaning of and phobias around that word have changed dramatically during my adult life. Now, a queer person is considered different from many, but no longer so stomach-turningly odd as to require eviction from an apartment. *Two small children living with her, one born three months prematurely and still hooked up to an oxygen tank; resided with parents during treatment.* Many adults in their thirties find themselves in this odd bind of trying to be adults while relying on the very family that may threaten to turn them back into children. *An anthropologist with expertise in medical anthropology and injury law.* We number at least in the tens, perhaps even hundreds. *Canadian.* Something of an outsider, though like thousands of my fellow denizens, I've lived in the United States for years. In other words, there is nothing special about my quotidian experiences in the cancer world. The orthodox details of my life—the very ordinariness of it all—make the story worth telling.

Any good anthropologist respectfully asks the reader to follow him or her on a voyage, and then on to an interpretation of that trip. Anthropologists who work in the field not only observe the lilt of the language and the voguish headgear, an estuary's time-polished obsidian, and one's bug-bitten ankles. The ethnographer calls attention to these social and physical features in order to offer insights into the larger processes of human interaction. The discipline posits that having been there, having at once observed and participated, provides a perspective not available in other ways. Tracing a finger along the blue line that represents the American River on a map of California does not equate to paddling the baroque rapids of Satan's Cesspool; the ethnographer aims to show how experiencing the crash of the wave can trigger meaningful insights not conveyed by the colored ink.

Travel, like reading and writing, results in a sometimes uncomfortable intimacy. A companion's smelly shoe or overly long description of last night's dream can intrude on one's pleasant sojourn. As I write, a droning voice in my head tells me that my efforts to present a likable patient won't translate well through my attempts to portray a trusty narrator. I worry I'll say something that rubs my mates the wrong way. Maybe I'll make a bad joke I wish I could take back, or I'll seem too sensitive and expose too much. Maybe something I say will reveal a not-so-pleasant side of myself.

I'm not an angry person in general, but the feeling of betrayal that washed over me when I found out about my misdiagnoses sent my conflict-averse and easygoing nature skittering to the brink. The snubbing of my concerns, making me feel like an idiot for even raising them, came at such an absurdly high cost to me and naught for those dismissing me. It's tough not to take that very, very personally, even though it happens all the time. The same part of me that never called my doctors out to their faces does not want you, my reader, to see me as hostile, ungrateful, or less deserving of survivorship than much brighter and kinder people who have died. Part of me is terrified to admit my ugly thoughts, occasional death wishes, and the fact that I sometimes have to bench press my frustrations away. At least a couple of readers will locate my problems in the lack of a stiff upper lip.

Having been raised as a reticent Canadian, I'm already tempted to recant the nonfictional status of this book and ask you to read it as fiction. Long after my diagnosis, even still, I tell as few people as possible that I'm a so-called survivor. It would be easier to play the role of a detached guide.

But the world outside wedges open the door and makes it difficult to stay closeted. At a party I attended last June, the head of our organization for women diagnosed under the age of forty with cancer read the names of those in our community who had died in the last few years. The reading of the seventeen names felt more like a memorial after a bombing than the usual way of understanding death as an individual, personal tragedy. Yet we *did* undergo a sort of massacre as, every month, we read email after email about those who suddenly landed in the hospital as cancer returned and pinballed from one vital organ to another, and as we attended funeral after funeral. That contradiction—the exaltation of community and connection against the grief that emerges at so many cancer events—still feels like a good solid kick in the spleen.

For this reason, we need to delve into cancer discussions that we'd rather hide from. And so, after looking long and hard from the canoe for seven years, I've leapt into the white water. I invite my readers to explore with me the very things we (read, a slightly lonely "I") most want to shy away from.

The stains on my passport do not provide me with a global or objective view of the cancer machine. However, they do reveal the route I've taken through a titanic subject. Each chapter in this book began from a curl of feeling—like a lock of hair pinned to a voodoo doll. I worked my way backward from the discomfort to decipher the structures that organized it. Walking down the hall for chemotherapy at the hospital, I tried to pass as a doctor. Anyone could tell that the slumped-over sick people crowded in the waiting room were the real losers. I noticed people, pinioned between experts' uncertainty and the social pressure to be optimistic, resorting to small forms of resistance. Although I was still a citizen of the first world, I fell out of sync with how my generation moved through their lives.

A more pernicious companion than my own skepticism joined me: the constant thought that things could have been otherwise. Anyone with invasive cancer might have had a higher chance of survival had we been diagnosed sooner, or so claim the ubiquitous ads for early detection. Over the decades, early-detection awareness has seeped into the public's often half-shaped ideas of cancer as well. One of my retreat friends with terminal ovarian cancer learned to respond to the constant, distressed inquiry, "But didn't you have a Pap smear?" Her community wondered whether her imminent death wasn't her own fault, whether their own medical obedience could save them from her fate. Discussing how she took that question as a nearly physical attack, Alice fretted, "A Pap smear has nothing to do with ovarian cancer." The fact that a Pap smear would have done nothing for her doesn't quell the search for an alternative world in which she might had survived, just as Lerner insists that chemotherapy might have worked for Kushner.

Historians have a word for the surrogate world that would have resulted from a mere tweak in the course of events, such as an earlier diagnosis or no exposure to a carcinogen at all. The "counterfactual" offers a window into imagined, possible worlds. Counterfactual historians fill tomes with these alternative histories: Booth's pistol misfires and President Lincoln lives on, or Adolf Hitler dies at birth. This little nook of possibility for a different life can become a living, breathing escort in the cancer world. It takes up residence right at the base of your throat. For example: everyone knows that we are all exposed to a torrent of carcinogens every day, yet no one can tell you which, if any, caused a particular cancer. One "races for the cure" while knowing that the production of the race T-shirts required the use of carcinogens. There may be a cure someday, and you may live to see it, but only if you can work out the right course of action—a certain drug, trial, diet. Someone might be held accountable for a misdiagnosis or an exposure, and for that, you might yet win a compensatory award from a court of law. But in the grand scheme of things, cancer is no individual's fault.

Cognitive dissonance—or the mental pressure created by opposing truths held in tandem—happens precisely when one tries to hold together the factual and the *might-well-have-been-or-still-be-otherwise-if-only* counterfactual. One can't live in a world in which every detail could have been, or could yet be, otherwise. One can't actually vote while psychically living in a world in which Lincoln hadn't been shot and the Ku Klux Klan had not murdered generations of African Americans. One can't pick up the painkillers or apply for Social Security disability insurance when lost in a world in which one's lover hadn't been diagnosed.

Cognitive dissonance, a defining feature of cancer, can't be resolved, only spun out and examined. No one knows what causes any individual cancer, although we have suspicions and part-data, and certainly we could be doing much more to address the National Cancer Institute's claim that two-thirds of cancers are caused by environmental factors.[40] Accepting the contradictions of cognitive dissonance comes with a certain optimism—*you may survive!*—but it also carries the potential for unmooring. The loopy feeling brought on by a cancer diagnosis has many causes. Somewhere, nowhere, and everywhere, cancer hides in plain sight. We don't want to admit that it runs through so many of our institutions and holds together our ways of life. Who can blame us?

A friend and colleague of mine, Derek Simons, writes about intersections—real intersections with traffic lights and painted lines. At any moment in an intersection, steel and rubber traveling at high velocity can come into conflict with delicate flesh. Simons examines the ways in which physiological, technical, aesthetic, and political vectors coincide with the material conditions—the concrete, the asphalt, the speeding projectiles—that both necessitate and obviate these injurious collisions. He refers to the dissonance between the taken-for-granted quiddity of road violence and its savage consequences as an "elegiac politics."[41]

The dissonance between the total social fact of cancer and the ugliness of the suffering it causes offers an opportunity for an elegiac politics. The suffering ultimately needs to be okay not because it is fine, but because it happens and thus needs to be acknowledged. I want to usher cancer and its identities out of the closet and into a space not of comfort, or righteous anger, but of mourning, a space where the material humanity of suffering and death informs communicative and collective action.

ON STEROIDS

After my treatment, as I distracted myself with afternoon TV and wondered if my career lay in ruins, the absolute last thing I wanted to do was write a book about cancer. I wanted to *move on.* But the terms *indolent* and *relentless* that doctors use to describe cancer also depict the treatment hangover. Seven years later, I still can't eat curry or drink rooibos tea—let alone watch afternoon TV—without feeling that wave of nausea. I spend thousands of hours and dollars each year on cancer-related issues. And it could have been much, much worse. The scholar's antidote to confusion lies in research, and my study took on an insatiable quality.

First, I read every history I could find. I read about early cancer treatments. James S. Olson describes the women who had access to the latest, most aggressive breast cancer treatments of their age as "a sisterhood of guinea pigs."[42] Their treatments involved the removal of the adrenal and pituitary glands, the cracking open of the sternum to remove the internal mammary chain, cauterization with hot irons, and the removal of ribs, collarbones, and shoulders—in some cases following the discovery of tumors less than a centimeter in diameter. General anesthesia had barely been developed, with doctors and patients alike becoming addicted to the opiate painkillers. Cancer patients—part experimental subjects, since they were dying anyway, and part people desperate enough to try anything—were given massive doses of radiation and injections of radioactive elements to see what effect these might have.[43]

Progress, I found, isn't at all clear-cut. Cancer patients were sometimes caught up in larger professional turf wars, such as that leading to the development of massive radiation labs. While difficult to discern in the present, one can see from the history that far from a lucid teleology of discovery, science is a cultural project that takes place within political and ethical infrastructures.

When I couldn't fully locate cancer in historical study, I expanded my search. I attended oncology conferences all over the country. I also reviewed hundreds of trial reports to understand the current research, who funds it, how it fits within a history of oncology research, how it is interpreted and communicated, and, just as important, what is *not* being done. I also craved other kinds of first-person accounts.

My research took me to an archive in rural Maine where I pored over marine biologist Rachel Carson's tiny cursive. Written as she was dying of cancer, her letters to a close friend describe her fear that her disease would discredit her research on the environmental causes of cancer and that her work would be dismissed as advocacy rather than studied as scientific research. I drove out to Carson's oceanfront property and snuck down her driveway to see where she had written her bestsellers, *The Sea around Us* and *Silent Spring*. I also went to Harvard to forage through the letters and studies that Rose Kushner collected in the 1970s. I wanted to know how other people had done it—how they understood cancer, how they lived and died with it.[44]

I amassed memoirs and graphic novels; plays and art; patient pamphlets and public health websites; histories of cancer advocacy, the insurance industry, medicine, and allied professions. I scrutinized the story of how the radiation research carried out in Marie Curie's tiny lab and resulting in her death progressed into contemporary treatments. I studied the medical, legal, and sociological literature on medical errors, how physicians, hospitals, and insurers handle them and what recourse patients have had in such cases. I also examined other diseases, and sought to fit cancer within a broader context of how medical anthropologists understand disease. I was at a buffet in Vegas: ravenous, stuffed, and empty all at the same time, somehow still unsatisfied.

Several experiences, both during and after treatment, helped with that feeling somewhat—at least they helped me to accept the raggedyness of the cancer I was finding in these places. I attended six weeklong retreats, as well as several shorter ones, and support group meetings. I listened as people tried to pick up the shards and fit them back into life stories. I became an unwilling funeral junkie. I swam, ostensibly for "women with cancer," though I couldn't get up the nerve to ask anyone to sponsor me, so I just paid the fee and did my laps. I still have the bag: *I swam a mile for women with cancer,* as if all those "women with cancer" suddenly turned into charity cases who need a mile of splashy (and not in a good way) front crawl.

I wanted to believe I could cobble together an adequate treatment if I just looked hard enough. Short of that, my internal scholar has heavily pressured me to box up my findings and observations to provide, if not The Solution, at least An Explanation. But if the plot has a pudding, it molds to the disconnects, the cognitive dissonances, that make the disease, let alone a cure, so elusive. The chapters that follow examine how a culture that has relished such dazzling success in every conceivable arena has twisted one of its staunchest failures into an economic triumph. The intractable foil to American achievement, cancer hands us, on a silver platter and ready for dissection, our sacrifice to the American Dream.

CHAPTER 1

Living in Prognosis

The Firing Squad of Statistics

After receiving my pathology report and full diagnosis, I found a set of prognostic charts in my burgeoning cancer library. Each listed the survival chances for a variety of subtypes of cancer. The left column specified tumor size (<1 cm, 2–3 cm, 3–5 cm, >5 cm), and the horizontal lined up the number of positive lymph nodes. Each box in the chart contained a number, such that the reader could correlate the characteristics of his cancer to the likelihood that he would be around in five, ten, fifteen, and twenty years. Ironically, no matter how hard I stared at it, the table could only mask the very thing I obsessively wanted it to disclose: Would I be in that percentage of people who had a recurrence just two years after treatment or in the 20 percent who would survive for the next twenty?

At my next appointment, I asked Dr. Slideshow the somewhat naive, somewhat urgent question, "What does it mean?" The doctor responded in a way that was both helpful and not helpful, depending on the moment that I recall it: "Exactly what it says." Banal as a winter day or the color of the ceiling, survival statistics offer a smidgeon of information, but not much to cuddle with.

How could something be at once so transparent *(you will live or die)* and so pig-headedly confusing *(will you live or die)?* The prognostic skullduggery reminded me of a short story by Maurice Blanchot, a French philosopher whose life spanned nearly the entire twentieth century. World War II offers the backdrop for "The Instant of My Death," in which a group of Nazi soldiers remove the French protagonist from his chateau and place him before a firing squad. At just this moment, a distraction in the bushes demands the attention of the German lieutenant. The soldiers disband and scatter, while the main character lives on within an impossible ambivalence. Blanchot writes: "There remained . . . the feeling of lightness that I would not know how to translate. . . . I imagine that this unanalyzable feeling changed what there remained for him of his existence. As if the death outside of him could only henceforth collide with the death in him. 'I am alive. No, you are dead.'"[1] In the instant of his death, or "The Instant of My Death," two deaths implode, one inside, "I am alive," and one outside, "No, you are dead." In the meantime, the integration of the manifestly unnarratable event of one's own death (no linguistic philosopher would accept the claim "I am dead") preoccupies his (the soldier's? Blanchot's?) posthumous life.

The prognosis epitomizes the haunting character of death that transpired in this eponymous nonexecution.[2] An attorney friend of mine, Mary Dunlap, who died in 2003, wrote a book-length manuscript while living with cancer, "Eureka! Everything I Know about Cancer I Learned from My Dog." Ever the optimist, Mary found hope in her dismal prognosis for pancreatic cancer: a 5 percent survival chance wasn't nothing. In the last chapter of her book, she handwrites: "On Monday, Maureen [her partner] and I were confronted with the news—predictable to many, but surprising to us—that the cancer discovered in my pancreas has moved into my liver. Today I am an asymptomatic person with an almost invariably deadly cancer."[3]

When Mary found that her cancer *had* spread (had, indeed, been spreading), her health status retroactively shifted. *I am alive. No, you are. . . .* In one swift motion, the cancer prognosis detonates time, which scatters like so many glass shards.

Having harbored cancer in one's body all that time before diagnosis, when one thought one was quite well, thank you, mystifies both past and future. One young blogger, who identified herself only as "cancerbaby," wrote as she was dying of ovarian cancer: "The vernacular drones constantly. And for those who speak it, the talk is loose, as it should be. Rendered mute, you can only listen to the din. It swirls around you, looping endlessly in patterns and figures you can't quite recognize—a language you once studied, but cannot speak or master."[4] Many, many people I have spoken to who have gone through cancer diagnosis echo this sentiment.

Unable to specify with certainty the behavior of any one particular cancer, oncology relies instead on statistics. Cancer and prognosis form oncology's double helix. Patients might receive prognoses at a doctor's visit or look them up in books and charts. Others may not want to know how they line up before the firing squad of statistics. One rarely knows if treatment has ended for good or if a next round with the "palliative" rather than the "cure" box checked on the medical treatment forms will be needed. A prognosis seems like a fact, if only a scrap of flotsom frenziedly bobbing in the rapids of cancer treatment. But its stunning specificity ("34.7%") shields the bloodlessly vague platitude: in five years, you, yourself, will be either dead or alive. The prognosis purees the I-alive-you-dead person with the fundamental unknownness of cancer and gloops it into the general form of the aggregate. The individual cookie cut from the dough is both prognostic subject and cancer object.[5]

Living in prognosis severs the idea of a timeline and all the usual ways we orient ourselves in time: age, generation, and stage in the assumed lifespan. If you are going to die at forty, shouldn't you be able to get the senior discount at the movies when you're thirty-five? Does the senior's discount reward a long life, or proximity to death?

Sometimes comfort lies in data. Taking numbers at face value, prognosis offers mortality odds, odds that one can potentially beat. Other times, when data feel vacant, literature provides a different sort of clue about the mysteries of living outside of normal time. Data and narrative each have their place, though neither ever really assuages the stupefaction of living in prognosis.

VANQUISHED ODDS

At my first week-long cancer retreat, I gazed at the other seven participants. Lisa (all names changed), about my age, with a two-year-old daughter at home: breast cancer. Kai, from Montreal: leukemia. Sharon, from Ottawa, worked for Canada Health: breast cancer. Then there was Tina, a nurse: oral cancer. Alice, mother of a twelve-year-old, had ovarian cancer and was about to start her third course of treatment. Beth had received a high-dose bone marrow transplant a decade prior in Montreal and had been ill ever since. Kate, an English educator twenty-five years older than me, was diagnosed the same day as me but with metastatic disease.

I coped throughout the week by indulging in a compulsive, downright sick guessing game of "who'll die first?" Unlike my father, who at weddings delights in predicting out loud how long a marriage will last, I told no one of my hunch—which, as it turned out, was right. It seemed as though the bearing out of my wretched little assessment made these women's excruciating deaths more reasonable, if not fair. Rationalization offers one of the few explanatory tools we have to account for death.

Perhaps I can attribute, even justify, my own window of survival to the treatment, my vegetarian diet, my good constitution, the surgeon's skill, or possibly even my kindly nature and goodwill. Many explanations and secret theories belie objective measurement. Some breast cancer survivors credited the Halsted radical mastectomy long after most surgeons abandoned the procedure in favor of less invasive surgeries. Who knows? Just because it was overall less likely to work than other treatments doesn't mitigate the fact that it may have saved some who would have died with the alternative surgery.

We assume survival—until we don't. You don't really think about it until you are called into the position of survivorship (by age, illness, anxiety, prognosis), until you are asked in some way to inhabit the category, to live amid those who are not, in fact, surviving. I know the muted exhilaration of the survivor. Each morning that I wake up not dead or sick, I'm happy and miserable at the same time: Pleased to be waking up at all. Blissed out to have landed on the vitality side of that prognosis. Repentent about my good cheer as my mind wanders to the three people from my support group currently dying. It's not quite that one's own survivorship is contingent on others' deaths. But the contemporary cancer discourse of survival against the odds seems to veer too far in the other direction, neglecting those in the category whose deaths have built those very odds.

The medical community identified the term *cancer survivorship* in the 1980s as a way to distinguish the medical needs of people who had undergone cancer treatment.[6] Since then, the term has absorbed new social meanings. Cultural and personal investment in the Survivor runs deep, and on several occasions I have witnessed people in support groups discussing their dismay both at the term and at the implicit taboo against critique. As one person said, "It's as if being against the survivor rhetoric means being against living."

The dictionary reflects the uneasiness of these discussions. *Survivor* can mean, on the one hand, someone who has survived a dehumanizing and degrading experience of terror, or on the other, someone who outlives others. Whereas the first definition gestures toward survival of the kinds of histories that have led to various stripes of identity politics (based in race or gender, for example, in racist or misogynist cultures), the second overlapping definition reflects living beyond an event in which others die (the veteran of a war, the cancer survivor, the widowed survivor of her husband).

I initially resisted the moniker *cancer survivor* because I didn't want an identity built on the backs of those people who didn't survive.[7] I thought it all seemed pretty arbitrary—after my diagnosis, my mom would say that she wished it was her, instead of me. But then the next year it was her as well. Survivor-style math doesn't allow for substitution.

Once in the emergency room at Stanford Hospital the nurse said to me, "Oh, I'm a sister." I couldn't tell if she meant she was queer or if she had had cancer, but either way it was a powerful, not unwelcome, call to identify. Don't get me wrong—I'd rather survive (usually). And a touchstone for commonalities can be good. It's just that the form that contemporary survivorship takes in relation to statistics—*survival against the odds*—combined with enthusiasm for one's own potential agency in cancer's battles, hides the conditions of probabilistic language, and in so doing leads us away from an opportunity to think through other possibilities for identification. Maybe I'd prefer something like *cancer* survivor as opposed to cancer *survivor*. The distinction is perhaps ham-fisted, but I mean to indicate with the former category that people who have gone through certain of the hoops of cancer to some extent share an experience that has potentially identity transformative effects. The latter category transfers the emphasis away from the commonalities and toward the individual, particularly through a triumphant ideal of the human spirit. That part of the cancer survivor identity struck me the wrong way.

Physician Bernie Siegel bows to such restricted language in his *Love, Medicine, and Miracles: Lessons Learned about Self-Healing from a Surgeon's Experience with Exceptional Patients,* in which he suggests that there is a right attitude needed to survive cancer.[8] In portraying cancer survivorship as a moral calling, Siegel implies that dying results from a personal failure. Siegel-style literature offers another form of torture to people with cancer: *Did my mind declare war on my body? Am I a cold, repressed person?* (Okay, don't answer that.) The huge and punishing self-help industry preys on fear and adds guilt to the mix. As one woman with metastatic colon cancer said on a retreat I attended, "Maybe I haven't laughed enough." She added, "But then I look around the room and some of you laugh a lot more than I do and you're still here." She died a year later, though she laughed plenty at the retreat.

Another version of *attitude v. cancer* can be seen in the ubiquitous language of battle. Self-avowed cancer survivor Kristine Chip echoes a common refrain: "I had a quote 40% chance for survival for 5 years and 25% for 10 years. Now, did I live by those statistics? No. Did I let them influence the way I battled the disease? No." Chip instead turned inward: "With a positive attitude and hope, you can conquer anything."[9] Chip specifically does not battle other *people* who will die so that she may live. Rather, she configures her agency in relation to statistics about her disease.

The very possibility of surviving odds emerged relatively recently. Not coincidentally, the culture of the cancer survivor rose in tandem with the consolidation of cancer statistics and their disclosure to the patient through the last couple of decades.[10] The term *survivor* itself, however, has had a longer life.

In 1624, John Donne wrote about the survivor in his masterpiece, *Devotions upon Emergent Occasions*.[11] The chapter title of Meditation XVII (Roman numerals seem apt) slays me: "*Now, this bell tolling softly for another, says to me: Thou must die.*" He languidly, almost pleadingly, writes of the communal nature of survivorship:

> Who casts not up his eye to the sun when it rises? but who takes off his eye from a comet when that breaks out? Who bends not his ear to any bell which upon any occasion rings? but who can remove it from that bell which is passing a piece of himself out of this world? No man is an island, entire of itself; every man is a piece of the continent, a part of the main. If a clod be washed away by the sea, Europe is the less. . . . Any man's death diminishes me, because I am involved in mankind, and therefore never send to know for whom the bell tolls; it tolls for thee.[12]

After Donne, *survivor* loses its communal reference, coming to describe not the individual reminded of his mortality by the death of another, but rather the one distinguished by his longevity. The survivor exists as temporally dislocated from the collective.[13] The combination of Siegel-type notions of the exceptional patient and the ways in which prognoses have come to situate individual patients underpin and enable Chip's notion of survivorship.

The noted biologist Stephen Jay Gould wrote something of a *how to survive statistics guide* after his diagnosis with abdominal mesothelioma. In "The Median Isn't the Message," Gould shows us that hope can be found in the "right skew" of a curve that describes his own

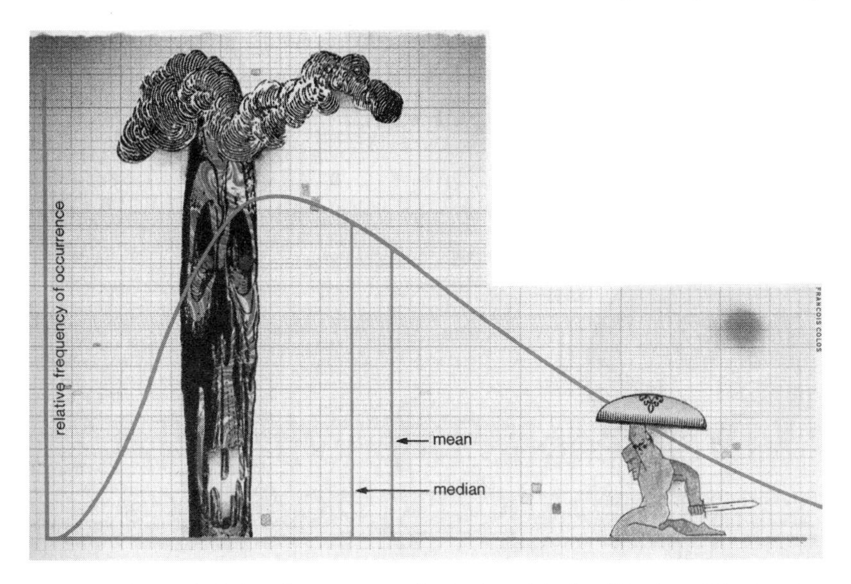

FIGURE 2. Francois Colos, diagram appearing in the original publication of Stephen J. Gould's article "The Median Isn't the Message" (*Discover*, June 1985, 61).

gloomy odds in which half of those diagnosed will die within only eight months (fig. 2). The gradually declining curve to the right, though, indicates that some of those who survive the first eight months will live for years and even decades. As he points out, "There isn't much room for the distribution's lower (or left) half—it must be scrunched up between zero and eight months."[14]

Everyone hopes to be represented by that right side of the graph, which floats gradually back down and eventually correlates with those few who live out a normal lifespan; that is, they die of something else. Gould did indeed remain in that latter side of the graph for twenty years. Early-twentieth-century novelist Hilaire Belloc wrote that statistics offer a "victory of sterility and death."[15] In my estimation, that victory can be experienced in the plummeting feeling of the search for oneself in the graph. Or the victory might be one step removed; after all, the graph encourages this self-centered search for oneself in a way that Donne's communalism would not brook.

This graphed representation could not differ more from another version of survivorship: the Holocaust memorial. Museums, web pages, documentaries, and Hollywood movies have all developed a unique material culture that aims to breathe historical life into those who underwent the brutalities and genocide. The familiar images of barbed wire; emaciated, bald bodies with loosely hanging striped uniforms; piles of corpses; bodies in mid-crumple after a shooting—these stand as markers of precisely what we must remember, the deaths and the specific vicious way in which those deaths occurred.

The last few Jewish survivors have been ascribed the role of bearing witness to the Nazi devastation. Their tattoos and their children—fleshy repositories of that history—haul the burden of ensuring that history "never again" repeats itself. At the Holocaust Museum in Washington, D.C., observers are ushered strictly through the displays and one can't shy away from much. You arrive on the second floor to a pile of the thin black and brown midcentury shoes taken from people before they entered the gas chambers. Hundreds? Thousands? At once universal—anyone could have worn them—and also specific, each bears the particular moldings of the foot upon which it was worn.

Each single, anonymous, stiffened shoe tossed into the haphazard pile recalls the body and life that inhabited it. One shoe, thin at the heel, must have rubbed a callus; another, irreparably worn through, would have let the frozen dirt cut directly into the sole of its owner. The sheer height of the pile, emphatically not a bell curve, raises a sense of sickening disbelief.

The dead bodies depicted as data in Gould's graph orient mortality, too, though shorn of fleshy references. But the stories of those who died before or after the eight-month median—those in some way described by the graph—dissipate into the universal, timeless curve. The stories lent to the prognosis will come to be inhabited by other people—others who will wear those stories in their own ways, leave their own imprints. The search for oneself in this chart will always end in disappointment, for numbers are not shoes. A number will not mold to your arches; it will not record the shape of your life.

The graph abstracts the lives it represents, painting Gould as a victor against the *odds* rather than as one who literally vanquished those who landed to his left. In reading the graph, we can all hope that we might find ourselves on the right side of the graph, even though we know this is logically impossible. Yet justifying one's own life in the numeric death of the collective makes a dangerous bedrock for hope. Fickle adulterers, numbers make love with the generations who move through them. These data have no allegiance.

Statistics render another sort of violence by abstraction. Gould's disease is virtually always caused by asbestos exposure; according to historians, the disease exists only because of a massive, decades-long cover-up by the asbestos industry. In different circumstances, mesothelioma might easily have never existed, which would have led to a different curve entirely (a flat one). The spread of the disease was enabled, arguably, by the impersonality of aggregates—it is as if a gun was shot into a crowd, and fifty years later someone from that crowd keeled over and died. Given this cloak of anonymity (who was it who had the gun all that time ago?), a would-be assassin might well be more likely to shoot.

Gould's graph offers a seemingly objective view of the natural course of a cancer, rather than a glimpse into the politics of diagnosis—a politics that could easily fill a museum in the nation's capital. Ovarian cancer, for example, is known as a particularly aggressive form of cancer because women often die relatively soon after diagnosis. But like most cancers, life chances have to do with how far the cancer has advanced at diagnosis, and so the label *aggressive* masks the fact that patients and doctors may have ignored subtle symptoms until the cancer advanced to a stage at which it was no longer treatable. In other words, skipping over the causes of cancer gives it an apolitical mystique. Statistical aggregations provide a logic through which bodies become interchangeable numbers for which nothing need be felt, neither guilt, nor pleasure, nor horror. They enable prediction.

Donne's bell can neither notice nor toll for a statistic. Donne can't rationalize survivorship. Gould aims to comfort us with the possibility that in the coin of life in prognosis, we *could* each flip tails, even if some of those in a group of one hundred will invariably stare at the nickeled eyes of Thomas Jefferson. The Holocaust shoe project refuses statistical logic altogether; it's not about the six million who died, but about each one of those people who died.

Built of the dead—people we've never met nor could meet—survival prognoses contain homogeneous units with only one variable: alive or dead. These Frankenstein numbers do more than scare each of us. They become something sinister: they feed on our friends', acquaintances', and enemies' deaths, and they will feed one day on each of our deaths, just as they feed now on our lives.[16] The statistics that offer the promise of beating the odds also evacuate the politics of prognoses.

STAND UP AND BE COUNTED

After my treatment, I went to the hospital to see if I carry a cancer gene. The genetic counselor congratulated me on my negative result; I had won the genetic roulette and could avoid a horrid conversation with my offspring about what I had done to them. But a strange chat still ensued. The genetic counselor told me she was pretty certain I am a carrier of *something,* they just don't know what. She then showed me a chart that detailed my two sisters' patterns of cancer risk, which increased a couple of percent each year until the chart ended when each turned seventy-nine. How weird to see my little sisters' lives as a bar chart on the desk of a genetic counselor who knows nothing, absolutely nothing, else about them. I tried to picture my younger sister at seventy-nine. Would she still live in Vancouver? Would I get to see her? Would she still be my little sister? If I died, would she still be my sister? Then I chided myself for my narcissism.

My other sister, younger still, has an even higher risk for cancer. I couldn't get my head around it until I realized that it is all about time: the older sister has lived cancer-free for eight extra years, and so has weighed in on one side of the calculated risk, while the younger sister has to live through those still risky years. Irony ensued when my oncologist told me that even at age 110 I will have a higher risk for cancer than the "general population." Even my most doddering imagined future carries a threat.

In projecting a misleading solidity, the numbers don't count only what's already out there. They become a basis of evidence for arguments about cancer by virtue of the preset categories for data collection.[17] Numbers can seem equivalent and then tradable. Before you know it, you can exchange lives for other things, especially money, forgetting that the numbers once represented real people, with real communities and real histories and complex genealogies. Taking an objective count can be as misleading as it is illuminating.

I don't particularly want to join the head-counting tribe, but since numbers so often define this disease, it's worth examining them.

As the numbers stand now, one in two American men, and one in three American women, will be diagnosed with an invasive form of cancer during their lifetimes. Each day, over 1,500 Americans die of cancer, and a quarter of all Americans will eventually die from this disease. While more men will ultimately develop cancer, under the age of 39, women are significantly more likley to develop invasive cancers.[18] Cancer has been the leading cause of death for Americans under 85 since 2001, and is the largest killer of women aged 34–70 and of men aged 60–79.[19] Of all diseases, leukemia is the biggest killer for men under 40; after 40 it's lung and bronchus cancers. Breast cancer is the main killer, period, of women aged 20–59.[20]

Currently, more than thirteen million cancer survivors live in the United States.[21] Overall, cancer death rates are slightly declining: between 2004 and 2008, death rates decreased 1.3 percent per year.[22] Some people consider the falling death rate the result of decreasing smoking rates, others attribute it to the success of early detection, and still others consider the decline meaningless given its minuscule size and the wide spread of sundry diseases it covers.

Different cancer registries use different categories to collect data, including the site at which the cancer first presents; stage at diagnosis; the patient's age, race, and education; and the geographic location of treatment. The American Cancer Society estimates absolute numbers of cancer deaths each year as follows: lung and bronchus: 160,340 (with a median age at death of 72); colon: 51,690 (median age, 74); breast: 39,510 (female), 410 (male); prostate: 28,170.[23] Cancer incidence rates, as opposed to death rates, offer quite a different lens. For example, the lung and bronchus cancer incidence rate, with 226,160 diagnoses annually, is about 41 percent higher than the death rate, while there are nearly three times the number of colon cancer diagnoses (143,460) than deaths each year. Breast cancer incidence is about six times the annual death rate for both men (with 2,190 diagnoses) and women (226,870); the prostate cancer incidence rate (241,740 diagnoses) is nearly ten times the annual death rate. About 360 men a year die of testicular cancer, with a median age of forty-four. Over two million Americans a year are diagnosed with nonmelanoma skin cancer, a disease with fewer than a thousand deaths annually; meanwhile, the 76,250 cases of melanoma each year correlate to about 9,180 deaths a year.[24]

Although the numbers vary from year to year, certain trends emerge. For example, testicular cancer incidence rates have increased by at least 75 percent since 1975 (although death rates have decreased to less than a third), and over the same timespan rates of brain cancers and central nervous system cancers have doubled for those aged 65 and over. Mortality rates for children under fourteen have declined by 66 percent over the past four decades, but incidence of cancers for those aged 1–19 increased by 19 percent between 1973 and 2002.[25] Similarly, rates of thyroid and rectal cancer are increasing. For prostate and colon cancer, incidence rates spiked with the introduction of screening, and then decreased. Between 1975 and 2003, incidence rates of prostate cancer nearly doubled while death rates decreased by about 15 percent (from 2.5/100,000 for men under 65 and 227.5/100,000 for men over

65 in 1975 to 1.9 and 196.9, respectively). Over half of pancreatic cancers are diagnosed at later stages, when the five-year survival is only 2 percent.[26] Some cancers have been clearly linked to hormonal use, asbestos, cigarettes, hair spray, and nuclear fallout, but stats in themselves remain obdurately unable to produce causal explanations.[27]

It might be tempting to stop, draw conclusions, and compare different types of cancers. But any such attempt would be immediately stymied. Cancers, for example, are often graded to determine how aggressive they are. Then again, doctors will often tell a patient with an aggressive tumor that he is lucky, since chemotherapy tends to work better on more quickly dividing cells. Although cancers are listed in the registries by the organ that hosts the initial cell division, these categories mislead, since even tumors that start in a particular organ can be a completely different type of cancer. Occasionally physicians can't tell where a widely metastasized cancer started. Such categories can have significance for detection, though, as witnessed by the recent introduction of the term "below the waist" cancers. This term calls attention to the way that curtains of discretion can affect the spread of the disease and the likelihood that one will seek advice for symptoms that most people don't want to hear about, let alone talk about.

Already, the statistics of incidence and mortality confuse. Add to this race, stage at diagnosis, time to recurrence, a three-to-four-year time lag in collating cancer data, and the fact that many states do not keep adequate registration records, and cancer becomes virtually impossible to track. And of course, although statistics mark diagnoses and deaths en masse, the actuality of "one here and one there" means that each case alters, for better or worse, the flourishing of whole communities.

To be sure, each cancer comes with its own unique way of torturing people. Some cancers present so rarely that virtually nothing is known about how, why, and when they spread. Others may begin in different organs but attack in similar ways, such as by causing loss of a vocal chord, making it difficult to walk, or changing physical appearance. Two people with random cancers might find solace by sharing similar prognoses rather than the etiology of a disease. Debate rages about whether very early "precancers" should fall under the category "cancer" at all (a question I take up in chapter 7). This debate carries dramatic implications for the statistics, not only in how the data are listed, but for policy decisions that affect screening and treatment protocols that are based on extrapolations from population data.

People with good prognoses die, and people with bad prognoses live, so churlishness about who gets to carry the "real" cancer card can only take one so far. Besides, people who survive benefit everyone facing discrimination and counter the cancer-diagnosis-equals-death-sentence perception. Nonetheless, the very word *cancer* is so fraught that the fact that the cancer may be tiny and curable can be lost on a patient. Type of cancer can be confusing in another way as well: both Susan Sontag and my friend Jane "officially" died of leukemia, though the leukemia was the result of treatment for other cancers.

In their 1981 book *The Causes of Cancer,* Richard Doll and Richard Peto list three types of cancer of "outstanding importance" that, as of 1978, accounted for half of all cancers: lung, large bowel, and breast.[28] These still remain the top killers, seemingly intractable medical and social issues despite the billions spent on antismoking campaigns, research, education, early detection, and treatment.[29]

Race offers another way to parse the statistics. Overall, African Americans have more cancers, as well as higher mortality rates.[30] Some researchers ascribe this difference to biology anchored in racial characteristics.[31] Other studies find that once African Americans have access to screening, their cancer incidence and survival rates become comparable to those of whites.[32] Such examples show that the categories used to collect data may be misleading if experts attribute disease patterns to race or age alone rather than considering access to healthcare or environmental factors.[33]

Risk does not deal fairly. Still, in some ways the risks of getting or dying from cancer can be measured against social status. Educational status matters more than race for absolute death rates. Less educated people are more likely to smoke (by a factor of three) and more likely to be obese. Whole groups of people, depending, say, on who might be eligible for spousal healthcare benefits or which jobs come with benefits, are excluded from healthcare coverage. One person I spoke with who was diagnosed with cancer at the age of thirty-three traces his symptoms back to when he was sixteen. However, as the son of a working-class single mother and then as a contract worker in the computer industry, he had no insurance until he got married at age thirty-three, three months before he collapsed in a subway station, which led, finally, to the diagnosis of his cancer. Minorities who have experienced, or interpreted, discrimination are less likely to visit doctors for checkups or to follow up on health concerns. One study found that nearly 80 percent of nurses did not want to touch their gay and lesbian patients.[34]

The Mautner Project, subtitled the National Lesbian Health Organization, finds that "lesbians are likely to receive substandard care, or remain silent about important health issues they fear may lead to stigmatization. . . . Lesbians may be one of the most medically underserved populations in the U.S."[35] Another study, one that used actors and scripts, found that given the exact same symptoms and age, women were less likely to be treated with the standard of care that men received, blacks less than whites, and black women were the least likely to receive medically indicated follow-up. This was true regardless of the race and gender of the doctor.[36] Systematic discrimination is also disguised by the fact that the cost of medical insurance is the same no matter how actual care received measures against the standard of care.

The statistics, vast enough to argue for the significance of a researcher's findings, or to claim a political agenda, also serve to shore up a notion of the disease—or the sum of the various diseases—that we implicitly agree to call cancer. The numbers create categories that might be inhabited and battled in terms of odds. Others have found more fluid ways to live with, and inside of, the new versions of time presented by the data. Often, this brings us to narrative.

IT MUST GO ON

Prognostic time demands that we adopt its viewpoint, one in which the conclusion haunts the story itself. Familiar dramatic narratives offer a pleasurable consummation. Knowing from the beginning how a Shakespeare play ends, we can anticipate that end throughout. By disclosing the eventual death of the protagonist in an opening scene of her play *W;t,* Margaret Edson offers the omniscient opportunity to witness Bearing's journey into that experience. In this way, the play mimics other artifacts of cancer culture in which endings and beginnings are entwined. The clinical trial report states survival statistics, while the medical malpractice archive documents injuries and deaths. In these archives, the punch line of the future is dissipated, dissolved into the past—we know the end of the story even as we read it from the beginning. The temporality echoes the double action of prognosis: causing and evacuating the terror of a potentially limited future.

Vivian Bearing, *W;t*'s terminally ill English professor, offers a grammar, rather than a chart, for approaching death. She speaks about Donne's Holy Sonnet VI: "Nothing but a breath—a comma—separates life from life everlasting. . . . Death is no longer something to act out on a stage, with exclamation points. It is a comma, a pause."[37] The pause indicates the blip between time lines—the one that leads toward an inevitable death, and the other in which there is no death. Amid all the ways to mark illness—the check boxes on forms, the numbers, the wigs, all the things that purport to carry meaning but can as easily occlude it—the comma, for Bearing, carries both significance and mystery equal to impending death. Punctuation provides comfort.

In Donne's poem, where death merely interrupts two forms of life, punctuation provides the structure of inevitability and the means of mourning. But in its own ambition toward timelessness, it also provides the structure for the narrative of life passing into death through the meter of time and recitation.

Using the time-arresting medium of photography, Hannah Wilke, who died of lymphoma in 1993, challenges the viewer to ask related questions about destiny, the future, possibility, and inevitability. Wilke began her project of self-portraiture in the early 1960s, as her mother was dying of cancer, donning Greek robes and photographing herself in sensuous poses, or sticking chewed gum on herself and photographing it, perhaps offering a 1970s New York art-scene version of a Dutch vanitas painting. If Wilke's early images reflect Western archetypal beauty, their meaning shifts dramatically in light of the two-decade series of images that ends with larger-than-life photographs of her middle-aged, positively not beautiful self in hospital gowns, receiving chemotherapy, and losing her hair.

The series of images comes full circle: Wilke foreshadowed the end at the beginning, when she juxtaposed her self-portrait with an image of her dying mother (fig. 3). The artist is young—youthful and white as a sixteenth-century Bronzino, her eyebrows plucked high and perfect; her stereotypical red-rose lips puckered with half a smile, triangulating the nipples of her breasts; her mass of dark hair tumbling around her head as if she were aroused. She looks directly at us. Audacious. Challenging. She reiterates a scene—an icon—a caricature.

Her mother, in contrast, looks down and across, as if toward Wilke's right breast. That gaze triangulates the young Wilke's right nipple and the mother's vertical mastectomy scar, rutted against her dark skin with the cluster of red welts, which must be skin metastases, edging into the taut skeleton of her shoulder. The vivid color in the photograph—black, unkempt wig (surely?), reddened lips—hints at an ersatz health.

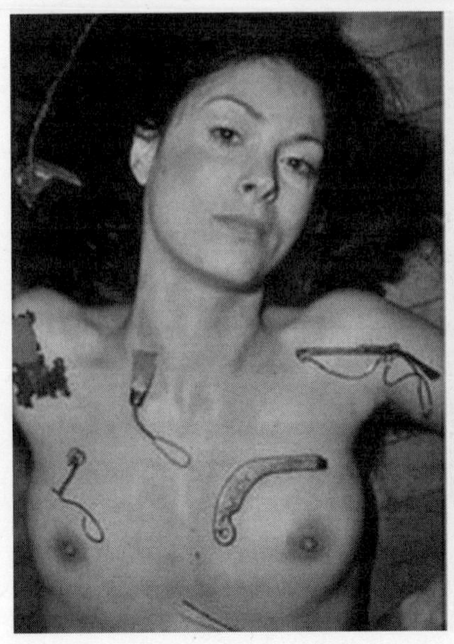

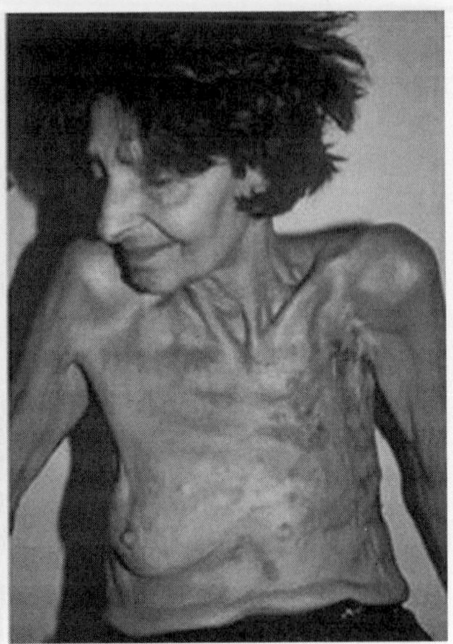

FIGURE 3. Hannah Wilke, *Portrait of the Artist with Her Mother, Selma Butter,* 1978–1981. Diptych, two cibachrome photographs, 40 × 30 inches each. Hannah Wilke Collection & Archive, Los Angeles © Marsie, Emanuelle, Damon and Andrew Scharlatt/ Licensed by VAGA, New York, NY. Reprinted with permission.

Thirty years later, Wilke's final, hyper-staged photos cite the Madonna theme again. In one she uses a pale blue hospital blanket as a shroud that covers both her bald, tilted head and her now sagging breasts (fig. 4). The depths of this image do not conceal a held child, however; the cancer legacy stops here. The photos together force the question: did Wilke foresee her cancer future?

From this vantage point, we can read the first photo only in light of the later one. We know what future they embodied: Wilke haunts us with a near-inevitability.[38] But if her ironically posed grace in the Madonna photo shows the certainty of disease and death, it also iterates the mocking of time afforded by the medium of photography. Photography, as Roland Barthes theorizes, gives each of us a prognosis. A short time before he was killed by a truck as he left his classroom at the Sorbonne, Barthes wrote:

> One day, leaving one of my classes, someone said to me with disdain, "You talk about Death very flatly."—As if the horror of Death were not precisely its platitude! The horror is this: nothing to say about the death of one whom I love most [his mother], nothing to say about her photographs, which I

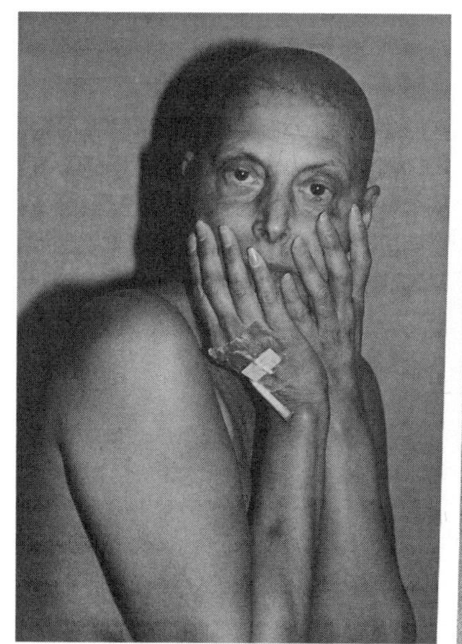
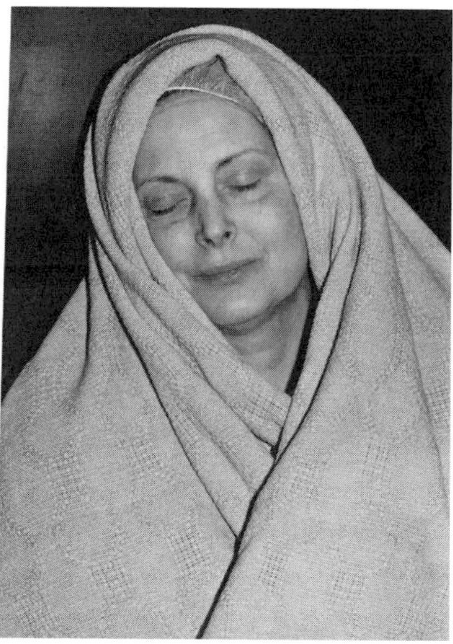

FIGURE 4. Hannah Wilke, *Intra-Venus Series #4*, 1992–1993. Performalist self-portrait with Donald Goddard, chromogenic supergloss print, 47½ × 71½ inches. Courtesy Donald and Helen Goddard and Ronald Feldman Fine Arts, New York.

> contemplate without ever being able to get to the heart of it, to transform it. The "thought" I can have is that at the end of this first death, my own death is inscribed; between the two, nothing more than waiting; I have no other resource than this *irony*.[39]

He can see it, but he can't get at it. He has nothing to say; he can't transform it. He can only wait. Here again, as with Bearing's comma, the seeming timelessness of the photograph counters the time of life's passage. Wilke's images suggest that prognosis affects every dimension of time, not just the future; the past becomes equally mysterious and unknowable.

Lucy Grealy makes this point explicitly in her memoir *Autobiography of a Face,* capturing the eeriness of the past under life in prognosis, the sense of how her life's truth and relevance might be "revealed" through diagnosis. Grealy was diagnosed with Ewing's sarcoma in her jaw as a child and underwent years of harrowing surgeries that attempted to reconstruct her face, disfigured by radiation treatments, until she died of a drug overdose at age thirty-nine. Here, Grealy recalls a precancer childhood memory that becomes epiphanic after diagnosis:

> As I sat there on the playground's sticky asphalt I experienced time in a new way. . . . A year before, my class had gone on a field trip to a museum where I became fascinated with a medieval chart showing how women contained minute individuals, all perfectly formed and lined up like so many sardines in a can, just below their navels. What's more, these individuals contained more minute versions of themselves, who in turn held even more. Our fates were already perfectly mapped out within us. . . . It's impossible for me not to revisit this twenty-year-old playground scene and wonder why I didn't go right when I should have gone left, or alternatively, see my movements as inexorable. If the cancer was already there, it would have been discovered eventually, though probably too late. . . . Sometimes it is as difficult to know what the past holds as it is to know the future, and just as an answer to a riddle seems so obvious once it is revealed, it seems curious to me now that I passed through all those early moments with no idea of their weight.[40]

Trying "to know what the past holds," what alternatives and what necessities it contained, can become a near obsession when a person with advanced cancer faces the flimsy pages of a medical report. When a patient learns, for example, that her cancer, though present, was undetected in earlier tests and thus unannounced in earlier reports, this realization turns the faulty reports into the material remnants of lost opportunities—of times when treatments might have been less invasive, more efficacious.

No matter how far one's cancer has spread, virtually everybody wishes they had been diagnosed sooner. At the retreats I attended, people talked about their alternative, possible pasts: the shame of not having done self-exams, of delaying tests because of being too busy, or of not wanting to ask more of already overworked people. Sharon said: "I wasn't politicized enough and aware enough to ask." Liz talked about the junctures when her doctors didn't believe her reports about her symptoms. Not believing them herself, she decided to collect evidence of her yet undiagnosed leukemia herself, storing blood in her refrigerator and photographing it. Despite the action she took on her own behalf, regret and shame filled her memories: "How could I have just let it all happen, with all these signs—how could I have, you know, gone for my course in Toronto when I had to get up five times because I was bleeding so much?" Alice asked, "How could they have missed two tumors 11 cm and 10 cm that were fused together? On my CT scan they thought my tumor was my uterus." Tina, a nurse, asked: "How could I have had so much trust—how could I have been so lackadaisical about my own health?" When she needed to book her surgery, her nurse-colleagues told her not to book it for the fall since they were short-staffed. So she delayed and later wondered, "I'm a nurse, for God's sake. Why couldn't I advocate for myself?" Here is Jennifer: "When doctors did not do exams, I did not want to ask them to touch my tits." And Christine: "She told me I was too young to have cancer, and so we just watched it metastasize." And Lynn: "I showed him the lump and he said since it is painful, it is not cancer." Beth: "I don't know why I didn't insist. I guess I just didn't know."[41]

The "how could" discussions expressed a yearning for an alternative narrative that offered better odds. The women's stories recalled moments, imagined crossroads—places at which a different action could have resulted in a different life. Despite the possibility of illness, *well* people, presumably, entered these life-altering junctures. Advocacy, diagnostic tests, trust—had my friends stayed well, they never would have given such things a second thought. Entering the nexus, not one of those women perceived herself as at risk for having cancer.

CONCLUSION

If I hadn't been the "1 in 207" women who at my age have my stage and type of cancer, the rifle's spray of statistics would have laid claim to someone else who didn't do self-exams, whose physicians were careless, who delayed her medical checkup, who had no symptoms until it was too late, or who had no medical insurance. The stats don't really care about that part. They at once describe and mask description. A single number implies both anyone (who could be the one with cancer) and everyone (in a culture and biology of cancer).

Survival odds and grammar offer various ways in which prognoses come to be made meaningful through the counting, recounting, and uncounting. As fragments, they also create partial knowledge and cast silhouettes that hide other tricks, as the subsequent chapters describe. The prognosis yokes the survivor to the past and future, but confusingly. The illness adage of "living in the moment" nearly entirely misses the point. Living-in-the-Moment may provide a small resistance to the march of time. But it also mystifies the ways in which daily newspapers, retirement savings plans, and pharmaceutical advertisements alike ask us—even require us—to live in prognosis out there in the wild world, walking before the firing squad. I am alive. No, you are dead.

CHAPTER 2

Poker Face

Gaming a Lifespan

When my partner's sister showed up at our house all bald after her chemotherapy, I demonstrated my unvarnished social aptitude with the ridiculous joke, "Hey, you could totally be a lesbian!" I had picked up the culture of stigma, and this prevented me from genuinely recognizing her, even a few years later as she sat in a wheelchair shortly before her death. When my cousin Elise was undergoing chemotherapy treatment while in her early thirties, I couldn't even mention cancer, couldn't (wouldn't, didn't) say I was sorry or ask her how she was doing—even though it was so obviously what was going on. I was thirty-five, for God's sake, a grown-up, yet cancer was so unthinkable that I couldn't even acknowledge her disease. Whatever rationalizing spin I try to give it, I sucked in all the ways I had to deal with later when others made similar dumbish comments.

I don't blame people for not knowing how to engage with a person with cancer. How would they? I obviously didn't. Despite the fact that each year 72,000 Americans between the ages of fifteen and forty are diagnosed with the disease—double the incidence of thirty years ago—many of my friends in their thirties had no personal experience with cancer.

Everyone who has "battled," "been touched by," "survived," "become a shadow of a former self," or otherwise inhabited cancer clichés has been asked to live as a caricature. As poets recognize, clichés shut down meaning. These turns of phrase allow us not to think about what we are describing or hearing about. If we know roses are red and violets are blue, why would we bother to take a close look? News articles, TV shows, detection campaigns, patient pamphlets, high-tech protocol-driven treatments, hospital organizations, and everyday social interactions force people with cancer to live in and through these clichés. These venues overlap to form a broader network of ways we think, and refuse to think, about a revolting way to die.

I'm not opposed to social grace. A quick "You look good" followed by "Oh, thanks" offers a mutually welcome segue to the next discussion topic and enables propriety to mask the confusion about how disease should be acknowledged. It saves us from getting snot on a work shirt or accidently oversharing an existential crisis with a mere acquaintance. Still, the awkwardness—no, the devastating denial—contained in these conversations offers a window into the larger social confusion about how illness fits in with the broader economic and political infrastructures that contour American ideas, even ideologies, of a lifespan.

It's no wonder shame is such a common response to diagnosis. As usual, the *Oxford English Dictionary* helps—shame: "the painful emotion arising from the consciousness of something dishonouring, ridiculous, or indecorous in one's own conduct or circumstances . . . or of being in a situation which offends one's sense of modesty or decency." We know cancer will happen, yet when it does, it seems dishonoring or indecorous. I don't refer to its side-effects here; the physical breakdown of the body virtually epitomizes "indecorousness." Judgments about proper decorum *(be a survivor, wear a wig, look good!)* can help illuminate the ugly downside of America's will to health.

My economic class, my age, and certainly my nationality buffered me from thinking about survival until I was suddenly the one who might *be* survived. Diagnosis beckoned me to attend retreats, camps, and support groups. Diagnosis made me share an infusion room—do all kinds of things, really—with many people who didn't live for much longer. Diagnosis accompanied me in reading their obituaries, attending their memorial services, going to the garage sales of their things, writing on their memorial websites.

To be sure, diagnosis (as opposed to death or just plain old life) comes with its benefits. I got a kayak, albeit with a leak, as well as two weeks of adventure camp where I learned how to use it, all for free thanks to a group that offers young adult cancer "fighters" an experience designed to empower them to "climb, paddle, and surf beyond their diagnoses, defy their cancer, reclaim their lives and connect with others doing the same thing."[1] Even so, things can go bad. During down moments, I think about how at least my life insurance could pay for some cool things for my kids, or that maybe I don't have to worry about saving for a down payment for a house, since in order for a home to be a good investment one should really plan to live in it for five years. I can look down from a superior place at all the people scurrying around on projects I have determined do not matter—and then go and do the laundry or shop for groceries just as everyone else does. Like Bette Davis's character dying of a brain tumor in the 1939 movie *Dark Victory,* one can consider oneself the lucky one, not having to survive the deaths of those one loves.

(Sometimes one can't help but devolve into a self-centered, unremitting fear. To ground myself in my ordinariness, I like to keep in mind what a driver once told me when I asked him what it was like to chauffeur celebrities such as Oprah Winfrey around New York. He fingered the St. Christopher amulet hanging from his rearview mirror and declared, "They like to think they are important. But after every funeral I've been to, people do the saaaaame thing. They eat.")

The child survives the parent, the doctor survives the patient, the healthy survive the sick. But how have we come to take this mode of lifespan and survivorship for granted, as something to which we are entitled? Even a century ago, some—heck, many—of us would have died youngish, in childbirth or of some illness. Devastating though it may have been, people weren't shocked. Even in the present, we don't exactly live in medical nirvana. The United States is not in the top ten for the longevity of its population. According to some studies, it's not even in the top forty.[2] Yet despite such statistics, the United States spends more on healthcare than any other nation. Part of Americans' dismal life expectancy results from the broad lack of access to healthcare as well as documented discrimination against the usual suspects: African Americans, women, younger people, and queers (not to mention those groups that remain not so well documented). Other factors affect even those with excellent access to excellent care: high levels of toxins in the environment, and in turn in human and animal bodies; cigarettes; guns; and little safety oversight of food, automobiles, and other products. Physician Peter Pronovost lists medical error after heart disease and cancer as the third largest killer in the United States.[3]

In short, despite the insistent rhetoric, American economies simply do not prioritize health. No particular logic demands that a population's general health *should* trump other national concerns. So what do we get when we notice that it doesn't?

The anxious dissonance between the bleak median state of health in America and the upper and middle classes' general sense of entitlement to health and longevity plays out in the different, even contradictory, modes of time in which we each must live. On the one hand, lives correlate to a greater and lesser extent with a standardized, assumed timeline: birth; marriage; children; working, saving, paying taxes; kids' college bills; retiring; dying. On the other hand, we have various links with immortal systems. The state, for example, underpins our expectations of a lifespan by helping some of us if we die early through various forms of financial aid to those it understands as legitimate dependents. In this sense, the immortal state (or an employer) can take the part of linking our "survivors" to the immortal timeline of capital. Still, enough people drop out of line with this standard story that a pervasive insecurity shores up a uniquely American security state.

Unpacking the dissonance offers insights into how notions of health are shored up and made to seem like an entitlement, when health is in fact the unspoken tenet of a lifespan, one that is often cast aside as an externality. No one feels this more baldly or sees it more starkly than those who have slipped off the bandwagon at the peak of the party onto the cold, hard cement.

CANCER BURDEN

If the organ that first harbors a cancer provides one way to chalk up numbers, age offers another vector through which to analyze the social dimensions of the disease. One of the most delightful characteristics of youth—that you are indestructible (until you're not)—is one of its greatest risk factors, as well. Cancer is the largest disease killer of adults under forty. One in forty-nine young American women and one in sixty-nine young men are diagnosed with invasive cancers.[4] The numbers are far from insignificant, especially given the social costs of the number of years of life (read, productivity) lost. Yet until about five years ago virtually no oncological attention was given to this demographic.

While cancer survival rates have steadily, if haphazardly, improved for children and older adults, they remain historically static for young adults. Adults under forty don't undergo regular screening, and as students or temporary employees, they often don't have access to regular healthcare. In cases where they do seek out care, younger adults have little experience advocating for a definitive diagnosis. Furthermore, doctors often work under the misguided assumption that cancer is a disease of older people, leading to an immorally high number of delayed diagnoses and, in turn, the large proportion of late-stage cancers. This misinterpretation of cancer carries enormous financial and personal costs, costs that are more often dismissed as individual misfortune—an act of God, perhaps—than as problems with the diagnostic process and access to healthcare.

Alison, age forty-one, spoke before she died of her months of being misdiagnosed by a pulmonologist at University of California, San Francisco, who claimed that she must have asthma rather than a metastasis to the lung of a cancer that she had been treated for three years prior. Afterward, she was confounded by her doctor's "lack of curiosity," but she said she didn't advocate too hard because she didn't want to hear that she had a metastasis.[5] Petra initially went to her ob-gyn to have a hard spot checked out when she was thirty-six. The doctor thought it was nothing but promised to keep tabs on it. The next year she went to the office again, though the original doctor was not available. The new doctor ordered a mammogram, ultrasound, and core biopsies; the ultrasound found nothing, and the day after a core biopsy located an eight-centimeter malignant tumor, the mammogram results came in: negative.[6]

Gene, twenty-eight, found out in 2004 that a brain tumor recurrence had been growing since 2000, yet no one had passed along the information. He has those original radiology reports, but the doctor left the practice. Jess's doctor pulled a silicone "practice" breast from the cupboard to show her the difference between a hard lump and a soft lump, diagnosed hers by feel as a benign cyst, and delayed diagnosis by over a year. A freshly minted thirty-three-year-old lawyer I spoke to had waited for six months until the insurance that came with a new job would cover her visit to a doctor. She was diagnosed with metastatic cancer and died six years later.[7]

Compounding these problems, younger people suffer from an intense "cancer burden." Often they have few savings on which to draw during long treatments; have young children to support; face job discrimination and job loss; and, if they survive, suffer from a chronic condition that may cost thousands of dollars a year even with insurance. Furthermore, the stereotypes about cancer lead to the profound alienation of young adults, who, often the youngest people in the chemotherapy room, need to cope with the inexperience and misinformation of their friends, family, communities, and at times, even physicians. Few clinical trials focus on young adults, and overall they have poorer outcomes than the older and younger groups with treatments standardized for those demographics.

As with the cancer category more generally, it barely makes sense to consider cancer in this demographic as one disease. Mean five-year survival rates for young adults (15–39) exceed 94 percent for Hodgkin lymphoma, thyroid carcinoma, and testicular tumors. Notable improvement has taken place in acute leukemias, while survival rates for numerous other cancers remain intractably low, particularly when controlling for stage at diagnosis. With metastasis, mean five-year survival in this age group slips to 89.7 percent for thyroid carcinomas, 86.7 percent for Hodgkin lymphoma, 73 percent for testicular cancer, 47.8 percent for ovarian, 31.6 percent for breast, 18.9 percent for colorectal, and 5.9 percent for lung.[8] (I examine various aspects of cancer and young adults in other parts of *Malignant.*)

The nearly complete lack of socioeconomic support that presses those with catastrophic illness entirely out of the system bears some examination, especially given the pivotal role young adults play economically. Having to watch the economy of accumulation from the outside—to decide whether to return to work or stay on Social Security disability, for example—might give new insight into the justifying logics of mortal lifespans in immortal systems.

Cancer itself parodies the capitalist ideal of accrual through time, and people with cancer inhabit its double consciousness. In the cancer complex, the relations among cell division, financial accumulation, and deferred gratification are anything but linear. For each postdiagnosis individual, the story will go one of two ways: You will have a recurrence, or you will not. You will die of cancer, or you will not. You will be ill for a long time, or you will not. If you defer your spending for too long, you won't get to enjoy it. But if you don't defer . . . well, what if you survive but have spent all your money on a new kayak and a trip down the Grand Canyon? What if you want to go back to work but can't because your employer found out you had cancer and fired you? What if you can't get insurance because of preexisting illness? What if your small business didn't survive the time you had to take off for treatments?

When I was in college, my dad offered me ten dollars to read a book called *The Wealthy Barber.*[9] In this book I learned the value of starting to save early in one's life. The book claimed that the barber or secretary who began working and saving at age twenty was far better off than the teacher or nurse who began working at thirty or the lawyer who spends all her money on Pebble Beach vacations. That extra ten years of working and saving, even with a low salary, adds up some forty years later to a princely sum on which to retire. The book aimed to show how people who live for seven or eight decades can hook into market systems that grow for a couple of centuries to their advantage. These systems value modest barbers who know how to play the system more than spendy lawyers who don't bother. The trick lies in time—specifically, in having a lot of it during which to watch one's savings grow inside the market.

The morass of young adult cancer, the confusion and dislocation, can be read as a collision in modes of time. In an aspirational, personal, and normative timeline, one supports one's kin. In losing one's relation to that, an immortal timeline ticks by as one misses the chance to put aside savings and get that promotion. These two temporal modes can compete and destroy each other with even the smallest trip-up in their assumed alliance.

The idea of lifespan justifies the pressure on young adults. After all, when else would one save for retirement or have young kids? The obviousness of this question indicates the centrality of the larger social fantasy that holds together the economic necessity of one's "productive years" in which one is assumed to be the most attractive, the most fit, the most able-bodied of one's life. Yet precisely when people have to drop out of those years because of the brute bad luck of illness, one finds, instead of the expected social supports, people holding their own fundraisers or websites auctioning massages and hula hoop lessons to pay for chemotherapy. As one twenty-nine-year-old who has been living in the cancer complex for fifteen years put it, "A fundraiser is where you invite people to a big fun event, serve great drinks, and do everything possible for them *not* to think about cancer."[10] You do want people to feel good and strong so that they will open their wallets, and who doesn't like good clean fun?[11]

GAME FACE

When it comes to interpretive rubber meeting the symbolic road, nothing beats an advertisement featuring cyclist Lance Armstrong (fig. 5). Armstrong inspired a generation of cancer survivors through his charisma, his cycling victories, and by pouring millions of dollars into his nonprofit, typographically loud, **LIVESTRONG** organization. To be sure, he cuts an ambivalent figure, both having played the cancer card *in extremis* to veer attention away from the numerous performance-enhancing exploits that led to his being stripped of seven Tour de France victories, and having funded needed cancer research. Armstong and

PUT YOUR LANCE FACE ON
What does it mean to put your Lance face on? It means taking responsibility for your future. It means developing a plan for the most important goals in your life. It means staying focused and determined in the face of challenges. When it comes to investing, it means the same thing. Lance makes every decision count. You can too. For more information, contact your financial advisor or visit www.lanceface.com.
American Century Investments
Past performance is not a guarantee of future results. Investment return and principal value will fluctuate, and it is possible to lose money by investing.
You should consider a fund's investment objectives, risks, and charges and expenses carefully before you invest. The fund's prospectus,
can be obtained by calling 1-877-442-6236, contains this and other
about the fund, and should be read carefully before investing.
American Century Investment Services, Inc., Distributor

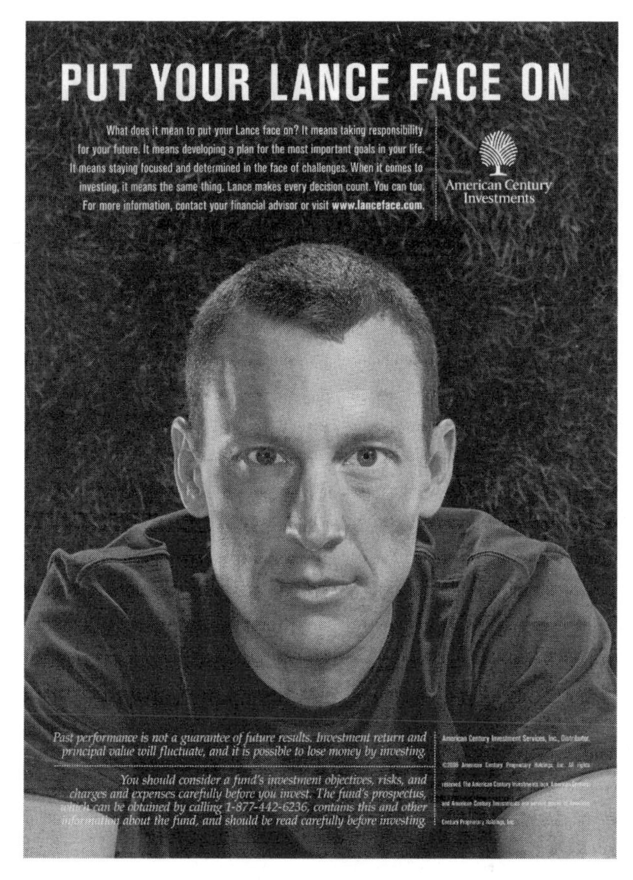

FIGURE 5. In 2006, American Century Investments partnered with Lance Armstrong to create a series of widely advertised Live Strong term funds. The company continues to maintain the Live Strong funds, despite Armstrong's ignominy over performance-enhancing drug use.

cancer cultivated a mutually beneficial relationship, partly demonstrated by the willingness of many cancer survivors to support him even in his fall.

In 2006, American Century Investments (ACI), a private firm managing more than $100 billion in assets, entered into a partnership with LIVESTRONG in which ACI donates to the charity part of the profits from a series of life-cycle mutual funds, "in which the type of investments vary according to the age of the investor."[12] As ACI boasts on its website, "LIVESTRONG Portfolios make investing for retirement . . . as easy as identifying the approximate date you plan to begin withdrawing your money."[13] The pun of "life-cycle" aside, the magazine ad highlights Armstrong's role as a translational figure for the nexus of industry, cancer, and humanitarianism.

Armstrong claims survivorship as a key identity, reiterating continually that his greatest success and pride lie in his having survived testicular cancer. In his autobiography, *It's Not about the Bike,* Armstrong describes his active search, when diagnosed in 1996, for the best care available to overcome his prognosis.[14] He settled on a doctor who offered a then-new regimen that revolutionized treatment for testicular cancer, turning it from a high-risk disease into a largely curable one, even in its metastatic iteration. The coincident timing of his diagnosis and this new treatment underpins what he portrays as his own agency in finding medical care—another inspirational aspect of his cancer survival story. Armstrong's story is misleading, however, in that it overemphasizes the role of patient agency in the success of cancer treatment, a view that correlates with the advertising messages of cancer centers and, well, banks. It also overestimates the curative potential of treatments for most cancers, though we'd all like to believe in these inflated claims. And it propagates the myth that everyone has the potential to be a survivor, deaf to the reality that "survivor" implies, in the final analysis, "dier."

The Armstrong story comes with real social costs for many people surviving with and dying of cancer. Like so many cancer narratives, Miriam Engelberg's graphic novel *Cancer Made Me a Shallower Person* ends abruptly with the recurrence of her disease and her subsequent death. In one frame she holds a placard stating, "Lance Armstrong had a different form of cancer!" (fig. 6).[15] Her friends' and colleagues' comparison of her situation with Armstrong's offered only a terrifying denial of her actual situation.

The ACI advertisement summons you to gaze into the close-up image of a determined-looking Armstrong, and after thinking to yourself, *What the fuck?* you read that "to put your Lance face on . . . means taking responsibility for your future. . . . It means staying focused and determined in the face of challenges." Control over one's future weaves cancer survival, Tour de France victories, and smart investing into a common thread. But all this unravels, much as his own cycling success has, in the tiny hedge at the bottom of the ad: "Past performance is not a guarantee of future results. . . . It is possible to lose money by investing." Even the Lance Face can't see the future.

This warning, necessary by law, echoes a skill essential for capitalism. In a study of financial risk, Caitlin Zaloom finds that a market

I CONSIDERED CARRYING AROUND A SIGN.
LANCE ARMSTRONG HAD A DIFFERENT FORM OF CANCER!

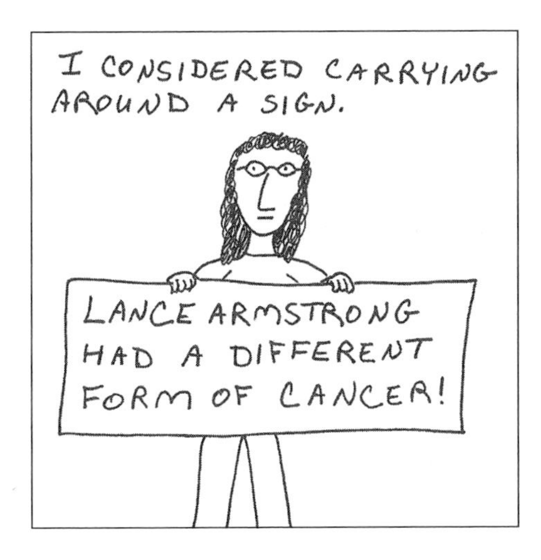

FIGURE 6. Cartoonist Miriam Engelberg captures the confusing, misleading, and sometimes undermining ideas about cancer and survivorship in light of Lance Armstrong's iconic status as a cancer survivor. (From *Cancer Made Me a Shallower Person* [New York: Harper, 2006], n.p.)

trader "must learn to manage both his own engagements with risk and the physical sensations and social stakes that accompany the highs and lows of winning and losing. . . . Aggressive risk-taking is established and sustained by routinization and bureaucracy; it is not an escape from it."[16] The ACI ad's conflation of Armstrong as athlete and cancer survivor proffers the ideal personification of market investing, since capitalism requires a valorization of focused determination and responsibility for one's future, even as one risks one's savings. By now a truism, liberal economic and political ideals require citizens to place themselves within a particular masochistic relationship toward time: we save money now for imagined pleasures and security in the future. Without this ethos of deferred gratification, banks couldn't remain solvent.

In Armstrong, age, class, gender, and a curable cancer along with his brilliantly choreographed cheating, masochistic training schedule, and dazzling marketing skill combined to form an icon of cancer survivorship. His status overshadows a simple fact: cancer can completely destroy your finances and your family's future. Sixty percent of personal bankruptcies in the United States result from the high cost of healthcare.[17] Cancer can be a long, expensive disease, paid for over generations. When your financial planner asks, semi-ironically, how long you plan to live, he calls up the paradox of survivorship. Middle- and upper-class Americans plan for an assumed longevity, and to be sure, a properly planned lifespan combined with a little luck comes with its rewards. But in times of trouble, the language of financial service starts to ring hollow, even for healthy youngish people. In a meeting with a Fidelity representative about my decreasing retirement account—and the decreasing value of virtually all of Fidelity's offerings—he kept saying, "As your retirement plan grows." When I pointed out that it had, in fact, shrunk by 45 percent, he stared at me blankly. When I asked him about people who don't make it to the age of sixty-five, he pleaded: "You really need to think about it as a retirement plan." In his training, the age of the investor offered the proxy for lifespan prognosis.

An implied lifespan grounds many economic benefits: you work now, we'll pay you later. Social Security benefits are based on how much you put into the system over years, and they last until you or your survivors are no longer eligible. Middle-class jobs often include not only salaries, but also "deferred payments" such as pensions, penalty-free retirement savings, and, for some academics, tuition breaks for children's college education.

If you croak early, some of these contributions may revert back to your estate, others are disbursed to qualifying survivors, and still others are recycled into plans that pay for the education of your colleagues' children. As with any insurance policy, the state or the employer calculates averages over the whole workforce and offers a salary package as a financial bet on your mortality. If you get paid a certain amount when you're old, it's because some died young. It's nothing personal; this is actuarial time.

Wait—I take that back. There is little more personal than your sex life, your orientation, and your marriage status, which greatly affect your survivorship. That is, if you say you are sleeping with one person and one person only, and if that person is of the opposite sex (as of this writing!), you are over a certain age, and you have sealed the deal with the court, your cancer card will play more lucratively. If you fill these criteria, you can pass on your benefits and enable your loved ones to pay off some of your medical debts or live out a more comfortable life in spite of your absence (and sometimes because of it).

Every American worker pays Social Security taxes in accordance with income rather than by the type of support they will be withdrawing from the system. Thus, the surplus skimmed from the nearly half of American adults who choose not to live with, sleep with, or bicker with someone over eighteen of the opposite sex—or at least to do so, by choice or exclusion, under the radar—underwrites the benefits that others receive. (Actuarially speaking.)

A Social Security check is one of the few dependable modes of retirement income now, in the insecure world of private investment for retirement (given that there are not many guaranteed pension programs left). The quarterly slip of paper that tells each working person how much money their spouse and dependents will receive each month if the worker dies or becomes disabled offers different measures of security. To some it will offer a sense of relief that her main "peeps" will be taken care of, and to others it generates an awareness of disenfranchisement, a reminder that his labor will not result in the same benefits for his social support systems and the folks who depend on him. With its two categories—married or unmarried—the quarterly chart offers the trappings of democracy: any adult can join the institution, and once you do, more cash is available to you. But in fact, those who join the system rely on the exclusion of benefits and the financial contributions of those who don't sign up.[18]

Several friends of mine have found a way around this status quo. One young man described the reasoning behind his recent gender change: he can now legally convert his girlfriend into a wife, legally bring her into the country, and offer her the protections of Social Security. For the same reasons, my lawyer advised me to marry a man, so that my husband could give the survivor-cash to my girlfriend. But the question is both more and less one of who can marry whom—regardless of who fits in the box, it's still an exclusive relationship with benefits, reliant on those buttressing it from the outside.

Health is not just physical, but social and institutional, and the currency of survivor street-cred varies. Capital and kinship legitimate and augment each other in ways that require a fair amount of massaging to seem logical. The economic rewards and costs that underpin these notions of survivorship remind me of an idea common a few generations ago, which is that cancer results from a degenerate lifestyle (fig. 7). Few people would still argue outright that remaining single or living in sin counts as degenerate, though certain demographics still cling to the idea that same-sex couples deserve to burn in hell. But the systematic privileging of marriage results in an increased vulnerability for others, no matter how it is justified. More important to my argument here, the benefit structure encourages us to expect a certain lifespan. You expect to live until the children grow up; you put money away that you will have access to when you turn fifty-nine and a half. Lifespan becomes a financial and moral calling, one that the state will partially subsidize in disability and death for all citizens who fulfill its principles of economic and sexual responsibility.

All this rests on a basic premise: time and accumulation go together. You need the former to get the latter; in theory, the older you get, the

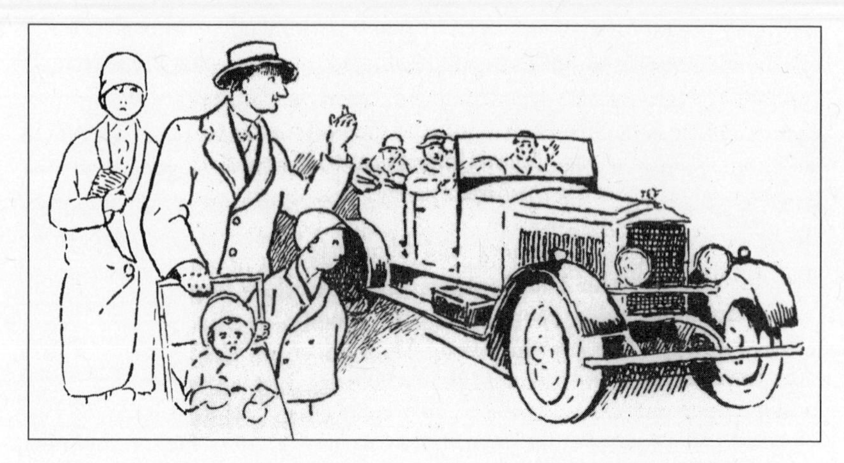

FIGURE 7. A 1930s car advertisement portrays the wise man as investing "his money in a handsome car . . . whereas his foolish neighbour invests his money in a wife and children." In reality, argues John Cope in his book *Cancer: Civilization: Degeneration—The Nature, Causes, and Prevention of Cancer, Especially in Its Relation to Civilization and Degeneration* (London: H.K. Lewis & Co., 1932), "The luxurious car brings with it the evils which arise out of inadequate exercise of the muscles. . . . In the end, the man who walks and marries is the gainer. He is healthier and in every way better for the exercise, and both he and his wife are less likely to become cancerous" (299.) These conservative notions of family continue to gain otherwise unjustifiable (in a free market economy) social support.

more stuff you have. No wonder people want to freeze themselves. Cryonics offers an obvious strategy to maximize capitalist accumulation. On my salary, I'll be able to pay for my kids' college tuition in one hundred and fifty years. If I could freeze my family and let my savings grow that whole time, I'd come back to life after all the work of accumulation is done, taking full advantage of both the deferral and the gratification. This may sound ludicrous, but it's the logical next step in the current situation. People already freeze their gametes in order to maintain their fertility until they've gained the financial security that education and accumulation (are supposed to) bring.

In its offensive use of disease to create business, the ACI ad bestows a comforting ideal of survivorship. As one woman wrote about giving Armstrong's autobiography to her dying mother, "I wanted her to be a courageous 'survivor' too. I think we find it less creepy or at least difficult when people assume the role of survivor, where they pretend they're going to live an easy and long life."[19] I get the appeal, I really do. The survivorship metaphor captures the ache of seeing someone sick and feeling completely unable to help. You want them to *fight;* you want to climb inside of them and join in when they can't anymore. But the throbbing desires that the term *survivor* captures do not leave room to recognize the structures of cultural and economic survival in which physical survival dwells. These underwrite a uniquely American insecurity and the fact that, every day, people lose medical insurance by losing a job or partner, and that many Americans can and will lose everything with a single diagnosis. And not because they didn't work hard enough.

STICKY FACE

In a series of experiments in the 1960s and '70s, Stanford psychology professor Walter Mischel and his colleagues undertook what would become known informally as the Stanford Marshmallow Experiments.[20] The research intended to figure out how attention could be strategically allocated, enabling a subject to delay gratification. Each experiment contained several control groups and differing situations, but for the sake of brevity, I'll explain the most general protocol. Experimenters gave each of several preschoolers a marshmallow (or pretzel or cookie) and asked the child to sit in a room that was either empty or contained various distractions. Once the adult left, the youngster could go ahead and enjoy the treat he had been given, and the adult would come back. Or he could wait, not eating the snack, until the adult returned and have both the initial treat *and* another treat. Behind a one-way mirror, Mischel's team sat back to watch the torment as each child sniffed his marshmallow, poked it, held it up to the light, sat on her hands, tapped his feet, chewed her lips, sang a song, or, glancing both ways, took a *teeeeny tiiiiny* lick. Many couldn't resist. Others waited an astonishing hour, shattering the myth that little ones can't wait. Years later, Mischel found that the children's ability to wait for their reward correlated to their life success.

Typical interpretations of this experiment maintain it demonstrates that deferral of gratification is a skill that can be learned, can be learned early on, and pays off. Arguably, though, in testing a practice that our political and economic system often rewards—deferring gratification—the experiment also naturalizes this political, psychosocial, and economic skill as unquestionably allied with success. Given that grade-school education does not specifically teach students how to strategically allocate attention, the fact that a child who has this skill can parlay it into success in a system that values it, while significant, is not particularly surprising.

For that very reason, the experiment gives insight into how we take for granted the bond between time and accumulation.

Obvious pitfalls prevent us from taking the connection of experiment and real-world success too literally. For example, anyone living in a major city would have been better off buying a small house in the 1980s or early '90s than tucking away their dimes in Citibank or ill-fated stock to save for a larger house. In other words, we can't really know until a decade or so later whether buying a home will equal eating or saving the marshmallow. Money saved has to go somewhere other than your mattress to keep up with inflation, and if it does, it goes directly into what the economist Susan Strange so aptly described as "casino capitalism."[21]

The marshmallow-equals-deferred-gratification-equals-success translation to real life can fail by several routes. You may have excellent deferred gratification skills that don't carry a big payoff. For example, the market may crash, leaving you to wish you'd bought that new car, so you'd at least have something. In this case, the means of deferral—the market—failed you. In the terms of the experiment, it would be as if the adult never came back with the extra reward. Skill at waiting matters here, but the practice of deferral also requires faith in both the process and the authority figures that do the distributing.

Or, the rendition from skill to success can fail this way: you did so well at school that you spent twelve years in grad school to become a research biologist, while your little brother, who barely slogged through high school, became much wealthier as an adman than you dare dream about. In other words, he found a better way to get marshmallows than allocating his attention into whistling a mournful tune waiting for the experimenter to come back. Or, the equation can fail because just as the experimenter returns, you topple over and die of excitement while using your marshmallow to sop up the mouth-watering juices pouring down your chin. In this case, you got to enjoy neither the marshmallow you already had nor the immortally deferred one.

The design of the experiment hinders its ability to do any more than gesture to these bigger issues. Its use of insubstantial snack foods, for example, nudges the interpreter to think about material gains rather than other kinds of satisfaction that could result from an ability to concentrate. (The experiment might have focused on an ability to learn math or fall asleep.) Its time limit of a few minutes and the lack of data on the home lives of the children render the possible failures detailed above not only into externalities, but as somewhat ridiculous. But they aren't. Too close an extrapolation from the experiment obscures the critical fact that what you do, when you do it, and how these things magically converge for some people all relate to a world beyond one's control—including the chance to have a home situation that enabled trust to begin with. When read in this light, the experiment reminds us that the stipulation to defer gratification, for a life-cycle retirement account, say, offers merely the opportunity to enter a routinized casino bureaucracy, not a means to show off an individual propensity toward managing the frustrative effects of delay.

Above all, let us never forget that without marshmallow eaters, the marshmallow business would go broke and we'd live in a dim, s'moreless world. The noneaters need the eaters, as much as vice versa, just as the married workers depend on the unmarried ones, and the heroic survivors depend on those not so lucky.

If wealth rots the soul, accreting tumors rot the host. Cancer just grows, sometimes as a tumor you should have noticed but didn't, sometimes as a tumor you can't help but notice but can't have removed. It may just live there; you may touch it each day. It may disappear, or it may wrap its way around your tongue. Its changing size may make it seem to be living or dying. Described by words such as *apoptotic* and *runaway,* cancer inhabits a competing version of time—not yours, not the one in which savings, Rice Krispie squares, and retirement exist.

Alas, the Lance Face can't look in the eye the cancer survivors whose bodies experience these fissures. Unlike many people who calculate their odds and cash out their retirement policies after diagnosis, unlike the friends of mine who told me that I was the inspiration for them to live in the moment and renovate their homes *(not dead yet!),* unlike those ads in *Cure* magazine that offer to buy the life insurance policies of people with cancer in exchange for a percentage, the Lance Face returns our focus to future thinking through sheer determination. The ACI ad applies this notion of cancer survivorship to banking products for its own ends, pulling the wool over all of our eyes.

BABY FACE

From cashing in the retirement savings to hours spent in the waiting room, from the prognosis to the too quickly dividing cells, cancer is always about time. But if cells reproduce, so do people, and if anything can provide a foil for cancer's temporality, it's the children—new ones who arrive as fast as the prior ones exit. Both the child and early detection campaigns work with embedded ideas of temporality that reflect

NOW
MEANS SPENDING $700 TO KEEP HIS MOTHER HEALTHY.
ER
MEANS SPENDING $200,000 TRYING TO KEEP HER ALIVE.
60% of cancer deaths can be prevented. Health care reform must include access to prevention and early detection. For all Americans.
ACTION NOW NOT LATER
Cancer Action Network
American Cancer Society
acscan.org

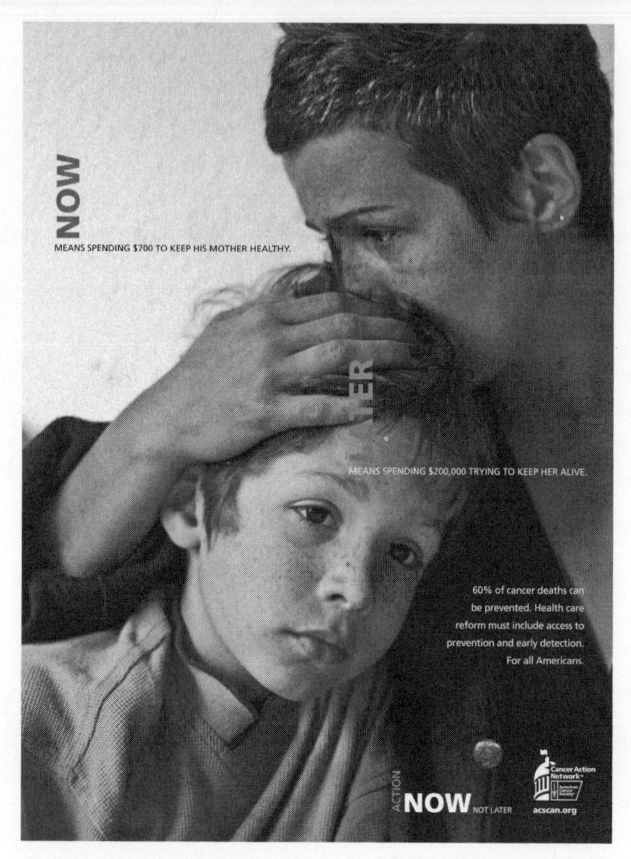

FIGURE 8. An American Cancer Society Cancer Action Network (ASC CAN) advertisement, circa 2009.

back on the bald insistence behind representations of lifespan. Recently, the American Cancer Society (ACS) played on the tropes of both in a widely distributed campaign intended to draw attention to the high number of Americans without health insurance (fig. 8).

The ad at once builds on a century of emphasis on early detection and implicitly critiques the logic of accumulation that I have been outlining. It presents a simple enough message: acting now by seeing a doctor means saving cash in the long run. Stuck between registers of accumulation, the ad cautions us to be careful what we defer.

Early-detection campaigns have always walked a knife-edge: they aim to provoke sufficient fear that people take symptoms seriously, but not so much that they bury their heads in the sand. An ad needs to inspire some confidence that medicine can work on the cancer (when diagnosed early), but not so much that a person thinks treatment will work if cancer is caught later on. Likewise, an ad needs to impart enough anxiety that the patient makes sure the doc does the test, but not so much that she doesn't go to the doc in the first place or that she pesters the doctor with benign symptoms.

Based on the current theory that cancer starts in one area of the body and may spread to distant organs, early detection encourages people to take advantage of the brief window of opportunity offered by even a small tumor. Early-detection narratives, suggesting future and past counterfactuals, seek to break the deeply held association between cancer and death with one simple directive: *You won't die if you just see your doctor!* The directive has a foreboding undertone: *It could have been different.* We can change the course of history—and if we can't now because we waited too long, we could have before.

The ACS ad highlights the key mechanisms of early-detection campaigns. A simple cost-benefit analysis maintains that it is cheaper to "keep his mother healthy" now, for $700, than it will be to "try to keep her alive" later, for $200,000. Early detection means saving money and saving lives: it's win-win.[22] The ad also relies on the myth that if you find and treat cancer later, you could probably have found it sooner, with the additional promise that cancer death rates and overall cancer expenditure could go down. The small print informs the reader that "60% of cancer deaths could be prevented" and urges "access to prevention and early detection. For all Americans."[23] The gap between "keeping" and "trying to keep" the mother healthy is unsettlingly similar to the hedge at the bottom of the American Century Investments ad: "Past performance is not a guarantee of future results." Like financial accumulation, cancer treatment offers only uncertainty.

To whom is the ACS message—*money and lives are being lost*—addressed? In other words, who cares? The difference between $700 and $200,000 might in fact invite incredulity. While there may be investments that increase twenty-five-fold over some unspecified amount of time, as a financial wager it's dubious, especially since it's unclear how the various pockets will lose and gain coin. Thus the ad must cite not only the Market, but also the other key referent of the future, the Child who stands to lose his mother.

English professor Lee Edelman has argued that the Child holds a critical rhetorical place in American politics.[24] The wide-eyed face of the Child has ideologically justified everything from marriage with its unequal distributions of wealth to the Patriot Act. Mothers used their children to curb drunk driving in the 1980s, and after the deaths of hundreds of gay men, only the presexual child Ryan White finally brought AIDS to national attention. From Megan's Law to denying gay marriage to expelling gay school teachers, political action has harnessed the power of the Child. The Child gains his potency in his abstract permanence and his winsome innocence, in his asexuality, in his disconnection from the market and his prepolitical sensibility.[25] This Child, not as a person but as fetishized ideal, plays a critical role in laying out expectations about life course.

Without portraying a child and referencing its archetype, the ad would uneasily tangle with the "who cares?" question, since the state doesn't generally care about any individual's health. Such is the premise of the private insurance system and the reason that some forty-five million Americans remain uninsured, with sixty million more underinsured. Even given recent legislation that may change this for the moment, to ask the state to care for any particular individual using a market logic can't work. Not only does the pre- and postcancer money come from different, incommensurate pockets, but with only a few exceptions, health insurance, we've decided, is not a benefit to be distributed by the state. The ad needs, then, to appeal to another logic: humanitarianism.

While his mother might be blamed for not getting insurance, this boy has done nothing to deserve losing her. The young woman on her own may generate resistance (why doesn't she have a [better] job?), yet children remain outside the market exigencies that underlie the moral economy of who has healthcare. The ad purveys the message that "we" owe *him,* if not his mother, at least the initial $700, while it also assures the self-interest of saving ourselves $200,000. The "who cares?" question is both artfully raised and clunkily avoided.

Such ads can easily be understood as rhetoric, mere attempts to lacquer political ideals onto a ruse of sentimental innocence. Had the ACS portrayed a person of color, a homeless person, or a childless queer person, the ad would certainly have been less palatable. If strategic reference to children's safety achieves a broader goal, then so be it. But the representational power of the Child is especially potent, for none of the other cast of uninsured characters would help us make the rhetorical and political leap toward a cancerless future.

In bringing our attention, justly, to the huge effect that insurance has on mortality rates and pointing the way to a future fantasy in which all Americans have insurance, the ad diverts attention from the way statist ideologies justify the market distribution of medical insurance. Indeed, in an internal contradiction it supports, rather than challenges, these same ideologies.[26] The ad, ultimately, recants the ways in which the ideology of the Child denies benefits to huge swaths of the population (as in the justifications for marriage benefits) and forecloses a more earthy discussion of who has insurance and who does not and why both insurance and healthcare are so expensive.

STRAIGHT FACE

The Young Adult, too, holds a critical rhetorical place in U.S. politics. Years ago at a funeral I attended for a grad school colleague who had died of leukemia at thirty-three, her cousin comforted herself in a speech with the idea that Chaney had been lucky, for she would not have to experience the horrific event of turning forty, as the cousin recently had. Chaney would not have to pass that invisible, ineluctable birthday that drew the speaker one step closer to disposability. Virtually any comment at a funeral gets a special pass, but this remark is telling for its unashamed embrace of the fetishization of Young Adulthood, of the person at the height of intellectual potency and reproductive fertility, with boot-strapping promise, still marching up the sunny incline of the hill.

Like the Child and the Cancer Survivor, the Young Adult cuts a high-stakes ideal that can be exploited, as Lance Armstrong's vast empire demonstrated. Still, the fetishization of Young Adulthood is all the more insistently enforced given the lack of, or finely parsed distribution of, social support. As heirs to these ideals of a lifespan, the best, and worst, young unmarried survivors can do is to fail our families by leaving parents to survive us (a crime against nature) or leaving our dependents without support. Regardless of who is listed as kin in the last line of an obituary (" . . . is survived by . . . "), those relationships are local. The broader economy, miraculously, has protected itself from being failed or survived by the illnesses of it citizens.

Legitimate, financially supported survivorship relies on kinship models. Specifically, marriage entitles one to benefits, some of which I have mentioned already: insurance, or increased odds of insurance, through a spouse's employer; survivors' benefits for the spouse, such as Social Security; and government and employer benefits for children. Quite distinct from individual success and hard work, these selective gifts result not from performance but from kinship. They also shore up the notion that some lives are more worth living than others and some lifespans more worthy of completion (if only by proxy). To put it coldly and without ascribing intent, not everyone deserves to survive or to be survived.

The early-detection trope routes the promise of a cancerless world through the fetishized child and the market *(pay now, save later)* and consolidates the notion that the problem of cancer can be solved through these ideals, rather than seeing them as part of the problem. The ACS ad shrugs off the same questions that all early-detection ads do: about missed cancers (especially in this mother's age group), about the expense of treatment, about the causes of the disease. It also describes cancer as white and straight, and early detection as a duty of individuals and in the interests of the state. Given the conservatism of the ACS (some of the country's top industrialists have served on its board of directors), one would not expect something so radical as a prevention statement that focused on the chemical, industrial, and medical causes of cancer. Still, the ad does more than not make waves; it erases the underlying politics of the disease.

The market relies on a notion of the future, which in turn drives ideas about expected lifespan. Retirement and children, the two carrots of futurity, are the key symbols of a life well lived. The productive reproductive young adult takes center stage in these ideals. Early-detection campaigns also play on some version of the defining market ideology of "pay a little now, save a lot later," coming close to promising that, despite everything, we can succeed against cancer, both as individuals and as a society. But the disease also enables a unique insight into the disparities in the distribution of goods underwritten by the fantasies of fairness that justify the market.

Despite cancer culture's nearly panicked generation of future thinking, the disease places futures radically in danger. In the United States, the redistribution that cancer entails—the massive expenses incurred and the mammoth profits made—puts the whole system at risk of failure. Lance's poker face shamefacedly disguises the cancer that threatens the underwriting ideologies and promises of the market (lifespan, futurity, deferral). A culture may not have cells that can divide, but cancer has it by the pocketbook.

CHAPTER 3

Cancer Butch

Trip Up the Fast Lane

I didn't set out to test-drive a sports car. Commuting one morning in my work-a-day Honda Civic, I noticed rows of BMWs and a huge banner inviting me to *Come and drive one! Raise money for breast cancer!* I screeched into a U-turn: I had always wanted to try out a BMW roadster. The showroom, decked out with pink roses, ribbons, helium balloons, and a huge array of finger foods donated by Whole Foods, reminded me of a movie star's funeral, only the centerpiece was a BMW 3 Series instead of a coffin. That car would spend the summer purring through air-conditioned dealerships across the the southern swath of the United States being signed—yes, written on—by test drivers. The gleaming hostess, a cancer version of Vanna White, exclaimed, "You can drive as many times as you want to," with the confided aside, "but you can only sign once." That I was in North Carolina only added to the novelty of the experience.

Near the door, another exhibit—"The BMW Pink Ribbon Collection"—featured the usual array of logo'ed stuff—towels, coffee mugs, sport bags, caps—all embossed with the words *The Ultimate Drive.* A fellow test driver said, with real feeling, "It's really beautiful, they did such a good job this year." I took a pamphlet inviting me to "Show you care with style."

Beckoned more by style than care, I turbo-charged down the highway minutes later, encapsulated within exquisite walnut and leather. (This was no CT scanner tube.) Five minutes after that, I accidentally diverged from the specified route, thus driving uninsured the same stretch of freeway on which my own car had been totaled by a semi the previous month. (For a minute, cancer seemed less dangerous than the current risk.) At least I was Earning-a-Dollar-a-Mile-for-Breast-Cancer. I turned pink at the thought.

It can be hard to untangle the motives of the breast cancer–corporate care nexus. I bought a Hansen's grapefruit soda the other day, which bade me to "Save lives, Send tabs": If I disengaged the pink opener from the can ("use extreme care!"), washed it, put it in an envelope, and sent it, they'd donate a dime to the cause. The right postage stamp would earn another two cents. Although it is difficult enough to find out how much money these campaigns collect, it is nearly impossible to figure out where that money goes. Nevertheless, BMW raised $9 million through its campaign, and I was able to drive the car I've long fetishized.[1]

Despite the thrill, something about the campaign struck me the wrong way. The advertising for the event made it seem as if a cure were just down the road, although survival rates have barely accelerated in the last century. Nor did the atmosphere of self-congratulation and celebration leave space to mention several known carcinogens that the auto industry has lobbied hard to allow in gasoline and in car manufacture (a paradox perhaps made easier to swallow after the collective loss of brain cells from decades of inhaling leaded gas fumes). And the whole event, with the pink, the products, the dealer's marketing strategy, doubled down on the same traditional femininity that seeps through the entire complex of women's cancer, such as the pamphlets that let women know how soon after mastectomy they can return to "washing walls."[2]

It reveals my own messed-up romanticism to admit my reaction at diagnosis: *Why can't I have a cool disease, like HIV/AIDS?* I wanted a queer disease, a young-guy disease. Susan Sontag wrote in the 1970s of the varying licenses bestowed by different diseases: "The tubercular could be an outlaw or a misfit; the cancer personality is regarded more simply, and with condescension, as one of life's losers."[3] Not only does a cancer diagnosis tend to relegate one to the world of loserdom, but breast cancer in particular drags one by the hair into the territory of gender. When diagnosed with breast cancer, the literary theorist Eve Kosofsky Sedgwick thought, "Shit, now I guess I really must be a woman."[4]

Moving between self-elegy and elegy of her friend Michael Lynch, a gay man living with HIV/AIDS, Sedgwick examines diagnosis and gender in her article "White Glasses." She details her cross-country search for a pair of spectacles. She wanted those very glasses that Michael wore as a flaming signifier, to augment her own self-identification as a gay man. But on finally finding them, she realized with dismay that on a woman "the pastel sinks . . . invisibly into the camouflage of femininity."[5] In the end, the glasses merely reinforced the very codes of femininity that Sedgwick aimed to shuck. In a similar way, breast cancer—not the breast itself—sinks her further into the obscurity of white womanhood.

You can spend your whole life creating an identity different from the one people smear onto you (girl, husband-seeker, spinster, mother, whatever), and then one charming little diagnosis threatens to suck you under, into the archetypal death doled out by the feminine body. Like a huge "we told you so," diagnosis provides the capstone to the argument that biology defines you. "They" (whoever they are), with hurtling finality, shamed me into accepting the truth of my sex.

Then again, gender signifiers provide an easier conversation topic than does mortality. "Shit, I am woman (fine, have it your way)" is more palatable than "I'm also *person*—animal, mortal, finite." What would it mean to acknowledge—*really acknowledge*—the sheer number of people who literally rot from the inside out each year, with no way to stop it, while so many known causes of cancer continue to be pumped into the environment? Just like Sedgwick's white glasses, which sank "banally and invisibly into the camouflage of femininity on a woman," cancer everywhereness drops into a sludge of nowhereness. The focus on pink and breasts and comfort conveniently displaces sheer terror, as do the ubiquitous warning signs. While the gay activist slogan *silence = death* decreed public outcry, for cancer, ubiquity = death. Now, *that's* terrifying.

BOMBSHELL

In *The Cancer Journals,* feminist Audre Lorde compiled journal entries, poetry, and analysis to explore her experience of breast cancer in the 1970s. The book brought cancer out of two closets: the personal closet of disguise and the political closet of cancer production. Lorde believed that the pressure toward prostheses and reconstructions tended, on the one hand, to prevent women from coming to terms with the multiple losses that accompany the disease and, on the other, to make women feel the lack of a breast as a stigma: a sign of shame, a token of lost sexuality, and therefore an indicator of cultural worthlessness.

In considering mastectomy as a gendered stigma, Lorde poses the counterexample of the Israeli defense minister Moshe Dayan, who wore an eye patch to cover an injury sustained in World War II. To Lorde, the patch was an insignia of Dayan's suffering and thus his strength and courage: "The world sees him as a warrior with an honorable wound, and a loss of a piece of himself which he has marked, and mourned, and moved beyond. And if you have trouble dealing with Moshe Dayan's empty eye socket, everyone recognizes that it is your problem to solve, not his. Well, women with breast cancer are warriors, also."[6]

For Lorde, the signifier of the scar presented opportunities for communicative and collective action. *The Cancer Journals*—a critical part of both the history of cancer and the history of feminism—offers an exhilarating read. Lorde called it as she saw it, unapologetically. When offered a prosthesis to stuff into her bra, she responds, "For me, my scars are an honorable reminder that I may be a casualty in the cosmic war against radiation, animal fat, air pollution, McDonald's hamburgers and Red Dye No. 2, but the fight is still going on, and I am still a part of it. I refuse to have my scars hidden or trivialized behind lambswool or silicone gel. I refuse to be reduced in my own eyes or in the eyes of others from warrior to mere victim."[7]

To Lorde's list one might add the many carcinogens that have been researched since her death in 1992, as well as an extensive list of unresearched substances (such as bisphenol A [BPA], found in 93 percent of American bodies), many of which were grandfathered into the National Toxicology Program (NTP).[8] Since 1980, the NTP has published, through the National Institutes of Health (NIH), the go-to biannual report on known or suspected carcinogenic chemicals. The document neither leads to nor advocates for any sort of regulation; instead, it simply lists dangerous products, such as the flame retardant hexabromocyclododecane (HBCD), often found in insulation and electrical equipment. (HBCD remains unregulated, and is commonly found in grocery store foods, though European companies have discontinued its use.) The latest Report of Carcinogens lists "known carcinogens" such as formaldehyde and "anticipated carcinogens" such as styrene. The peer-reviewed report, which draws from peer-reviewed literature, has come under vicious attack by Congressional Republicans, who aim to kill the NTP altogether.[9] Prostheses, Lorde notes, disguise these issues, asking even those who have taken the fall for these politics to graciously accept an illness that may well be a measured sacrifice to the ideology of economic progress.

Trained as a soldier, Moshe Dayan received his eye injury—and his eye patch—as a young man fighting against the profascist Vichy regime. Audre Lorde, a black lesbian, received her mastectomy as the result of a disease that was, at the time, barely utterable, let alone funded, researched, or understood.[10] Without dismissing the horror and humiliation that Dayan reports having felt after his injury, such that he could not be fitted for a glass eye, one can note that the eye patch signifies an event, a quick and clear cause and effect. The mastectomy scar, in contrast, verifies not a singular event, but an inchoate process. When I was in treatment, I longed for the solidity of a verifiable enemy.

In making cancer survivors into warriors, Lorde strategically transforms cancer into an event, taking it from the banal, everyday slow death into the language of crisis.[11] On the personal level, every diagnosed individual experiences this cataclysmic moment. Only at the level of the aggregate can cancer be chronic, endemic, or statistically representable—descriptors that leave out the human element altogether. A few years after Lorde's book appeared, the activist group ACT UP made the personal political, taking to the streets to ensure that precisely this representational catastrophe did not arise. ACT UP was not about to allow HIV/AIDS to become the new "cancer."

I think Audre Lorde would have reveled in the archive of images that proliferated since her book, and more so after her death, beginning with Deena Metzger's 1977 portrait "The Warrior," which depicts her mastectomy and the tree branch she had tattooed around the scar. This poster-postcard image reached virtual cult status during the 1980s (and Lorde certainly must have seen it). Metzger aimed to alleviate some of those awkward moments in public/private places: saunas, dressing rooms, places where women congregate and undress, places that merge the ultimate privacy of the body with the (potential, sidelong) gaze of peers. In these places where unveiling occurs, no matter how politely one approaches the space, hair growth is surveilled, sexual object choices assumed. Communication takes place through the furtive glance as well as through projected assumptions learned years ago from gossip about the high school gym locker room.

Corporate models have also displayed breast cancer's scars. Among the first was Matuschka, who posed with her mastectomy scar in a specially designed white gown on the cover of the August 15, 1993,

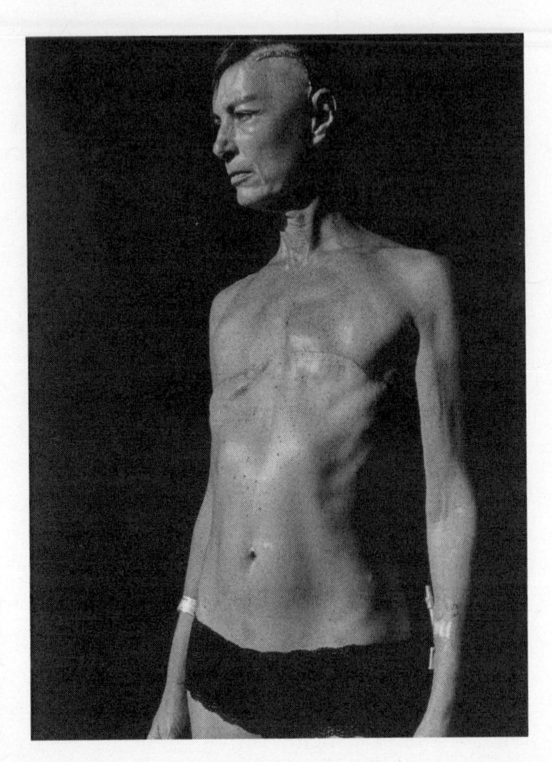

FIGURE 9. Lynn Kohlman, a model well known in the 1970s for her androgynous look, died in 2008 of brain cancer at age sixty-two. (Photo courtesy of Robin Saidman)

New York Times Magazine. Lynn Kohlman, a model in the 1960s and 1970s and then a photographer, upped the ante a decade later, posing with no top before her death of brain cancer (figs. 9–10). Her naked torso reveals thin mastectomy scars, and her shorn hair divulges a crescent moon of staples. No disguise here. She kept herself public in the journey from the front of the camera to the back and again to the front, and in so doing she moved along on another kind of expedition. She writes, "Cancer has been an unexpected gift that has brought with it dramatic change and transformation. . . . I never believed in my beauty as a model, but here I am, 57 years old, with a double mastectomy, hair fried from radiation, never feeling more beautiful! . . . I have gone inside out."[12] With this last statement, she presumably means that she has matured in the way she locates her own beauty. When I showed these images to a colleague alongside ones from her youthful modeling days, she said, "Kohlman is right. She is more beautiful when she is older."

The same weekend that I discovered the photos of Kohlman, an ad

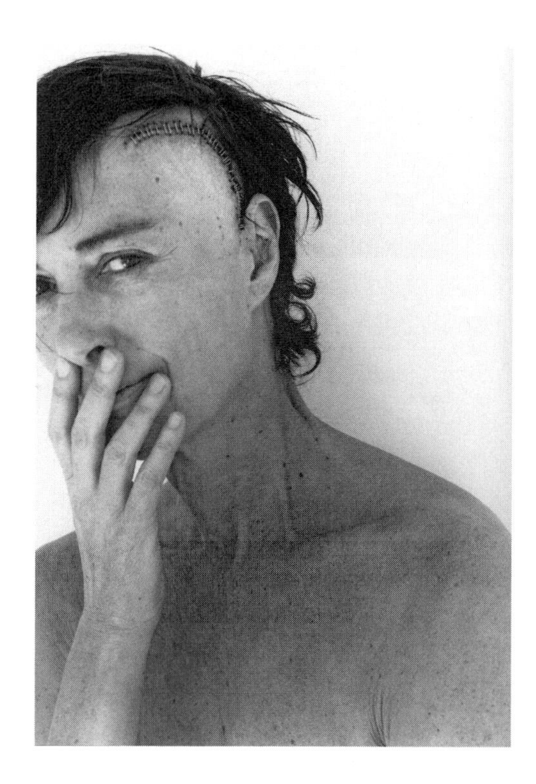

FIGURE 10. Kohlman's brain surgery required thirty-nine titanium staples. Her *New York Times* obituary reported that a body piercing fan complimented her on them in the streets of Manhattan, saying they were "'really nicely spaced and even.' She gave him the name of her doctor." (Photo courtesy of Mark Obenhaus)

for Mount Sinai Medical Center appeared on the back cover of the *New York Times Magazine* (fig. 11). I always notice such ads because I find the for-profit nature of hospitals so bizarre; they sell health as if it were a raffle ticket or cotton candy. This ad in particular caught my eye because the stitches on the iconic American baseball look nearly identical to the stitches I'd just seen on Kohlman's head, and indeed, the ad explicitly invites one to compare the embroidered ball to a sutured body. With its layered whites, its smooth texture, its aesthetic perfection, the incision seems much shorter than one expects on a baseball, yet so much longer than one expects on a head. In both images, the beauty lies in the purity of the visual effect and the startle of the upscale visual pun.

The U.S. government has appreciated the political impact of a publicly visual culture of injury at least since WWII, when it banned any images relating to posttraumatic stress disorder or other illness while still allowing patriotic images of amputated veterans to proliferate.[13] In a similar way, Kohlman's photo aestheticizes the bedlam of illness.

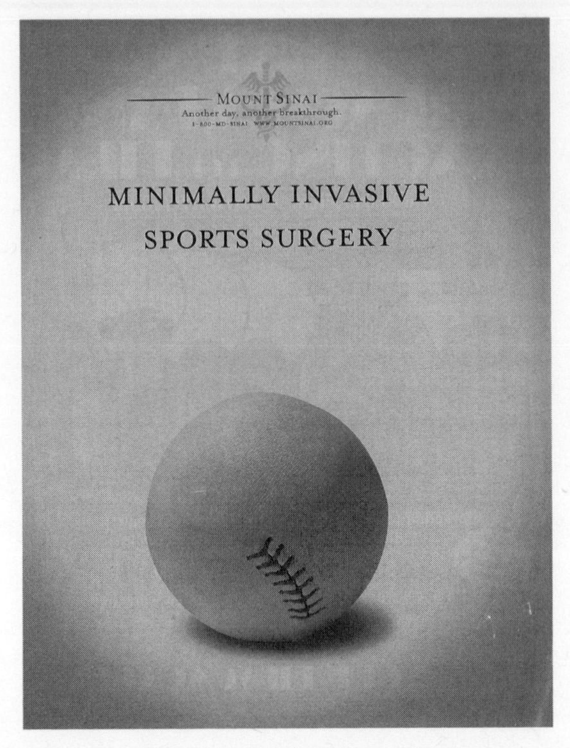

FIGURE 11. Mount Sinai Medical Center advertisement, circa 2009.

Going one step further, the baseball offers a purely theoretical injury, suggesting that Mount Sinai can just make it all go away.

For months after my first mastectomy but before the second, I repeatedly found myself in front of the mirror—appraising with clothes off, evaluating with clothes on. With a shirt on I wanted the second breast off; with the shirt off I wanted the breast left on. In public, I could not seem to find a way to negotiate the clear statement that having only one breast seemed to make. Not wearing a prosthesis seemed like an implicitly political statement, though the politics lay simply in the shape of the body rather than in any actual action. I did not want to feel permanently warriorlike. But when I wore the tacky puff of nylon stuffing I had been given, it wandered around my chest like a puppy searching for a teat. Besides, I did not want to have to wear a prosthesis just to seem as though I were *not* making a statement.

I liked the remaining breast: as my squash buddy said in the changing room one day, "Why would you get rid of a pleasure point?" and

I agreed. Then again, breasts had forced me to live in a sort of social drag. Rather than being a welcome harbinger of womanhood twenty-five years before, breasts stole my tomboy youth.[14] Not only did they require a cumbersome bra and add weight and heft that had to be dragged around the soccer field; they also came with a set of expectations about my behavior. Though certain of the perquisites of the phallus seem attractive (making more money, being taken more seriously), I do not want to actually *be* a guy. Nevertheless, if the second breast were to go, my body would approximate, albeit inexactly, my body image, absent the moral baggage of an unnecessary surgery.

Though unsure how to negotiate these politics and implied politics, I knew I didn't want either the reconstruction surgeries *or* the Amazon look. I especially didn't want anything that belonged in a litter searching for nourishment—so I did opt to have the other one removed.[15] As I lay in the hospital bed, shaking with pain, head clasped between two ice packs, the awesomely attentive nurse confided, "Vomit is my least favorite bodily fluid." (I had to agree, though sperm comes a close second.) The surgery was minor compared to the first mastectomy, yet illness carries its own license and I used it shamelessly to call my friends and ask them about things I had never had the courage to ask before. I suddenly needed to know the story of a friend whose girlfriend had died of cancer. It wasn't that I didn't want to know before, but I had no go-to etiquette for such questions. Like many people, for fear of seeming nosey or saying the wrong thing, I just never asked. The stories I now sought were about dying: about how people experienced dying in their lives; about how I could get close to those tales, snuggle up, and make them a part of me too.

Although having no breasts seems illicit, neither pleasure nor shame covers the range of emotion. My body can now fold into positions that it could not have before. Months after surgery, I was still surprised when I could do a tight yoga twist or hold the kids really close, and I suddenly realized that it was because my breasts were not in the way. But just as having breasts did not make me feel particularly girly, *not* having them doesn't make me feel more manly (or perhaps I should say boyish, given my lack of whiskers—*yay!*—and biceps—*bummer!*). Still, my femme colleagues take pains to assure me that this gender disjuncture is a good thing.

So, about a week after my second surgery, and after about two seconds of thought, I took my shirt off in a yoga class full of strangers. Of course, the possibility of performing that act was part of why I opted for the surgery: it would have been unthinkable with one breast. But once I did it, I could not stop squeezing the incident for meaning, imagining it as a communicative action.

On the one hand, it was a bow to Audre Lorde, and to the activism since her death, which has brought out in public once-shameful acts such as gay kissing. On the other hand, the act implicitly held a dare, and a question: Can women not show their chests in public because they are women, or because they have breasts?

I remember my horror at seeing, just after my diagnosis, the diagrams of mastectomies in the pamphlet they gave me: straight scars stretching across a narrow, pectorally challenged, smooth chest: not butch, and intensely not hot.[16] It took me two days to gather the courage to look down after my first mastectomy. If shock value spurred the disrobing in yoga class, what actual value that shock carried was uncertain at best, as I was in a roomful of strangers in the small Canadian town I was visiting. Perhaps I wanted the honor that Lorde claimed, the warrior pride. Or do the scars address the great denials of our culture: illness and death? Are they some medal of hardship that I now get to bear, like Jesus's scarred palms on a female martyr? Do the scars render visible the cultural sacrifice of cancer, showing that, because I bore the disease, six other women will escape it? (And can I please choose who they will be?)[17]

I know, that's a lot to read into a sweaty shucked T-shirt. Besides, I did not feel very honorable. Unlike the transgender queer who chose mastectomies, and unlike the prizefighter Rocky's demand to "cut me!!" to drain his swollen-shut eyelid so he could continue the fight, I remained just an unremarkable person who had that very morning searched her bag for a bra before remembering that she didn't wear one anymore.

As part of a militant strategy to bring AIDS out of the closet in the late 1980s by injecting gayness into popular culture, ACT UP staged events called kiss-ins, in which bystanders were invited to read the lips of kissing queers. ACT UP sought to normalize definitively queer behavior by increasing straight people's exposure to the prosaic, if pleasant, act of smooching. Such actions eventually tweaked the homogeneous, heterosexual public sphere, subtly changing what was considered acceptable public behavior. Read within this history of gay bodies in public, my taking-off-the-shirt moment may, at least for the sake of reflection, signify something other than debased narcissism.[18] Perhaps it could be read as a tiny, hard resistance to the layering on of social shame to the experiences of gender, possibility, and cancer.

Just as swathing the act in vanity misses the point, so does dismissing it solely as a reaction to shame. Perhaps my display was a call not for, but *to,* attention: a call to consider cancer as a communal event. It put into the public domain what every dimension of the cancer complex had told me should be kept private. And not public as in a magazine image— a staged photo that can be cropped, moved around, published, stared at, censored, discussed, and debated, an object that takes on its own life—but as a person in a room with other people. The act could be read as an attempt to mess with the cultural distinctions of public and private and what's at stake. I wanted a groupthink outlet. Because when I took the shirt off, the breast question faded behind the marks of cancer—scars left from radiation and the drains and the Port-a-Cath. I may have wanted to feel tough for bearing all of that (go, cancer butch!), but it was nothing like the suffering of women who had surgeries before anesthesia or chemotherapy before antiemetics.

Lorde bristled at the way her lambswool prosthesis was intended to make her appear whole again, but the absence of the breasts introduces a new set of interpretive problems for this odd mix of gender and illness. Had I not undergone a second mastectomy precisely to make myself feel and look whole again after the first mastectomy? Hadn't I now regained some of the sense of freedom I'd felt during my last shirtless summer at the age of six, when I learned to read the raised eyebrows of conservative Canadians?

Perhaps with this little social experiment I requested (desired? challenged?) a response from this tiny public culture of a yoga class in a small mountain town. As my shirtless girls used to say, "Look at me!" (Of course, they were five and three and so could be excused for such unabashed behavior.) But I could also have been saying something like: "Look or don't: I used to have another body that you couldn't look at, but now I have this body that you can, because its breasts have been taken off and in that place remains a flat space that is sort of coded male but really is very different, and when I take off my shirt you can see that, and anyway, why should males get to hoard masculinity and shirtlessness to themselves?" (I guess I can't blame the yogis if they didn't catch all that.) Or maybe I just wanted my body to be witnessed as a material bearer of carcinogenic culture, that artifactual statistic distributed with a spin of the wheel of fortune. I guess I both did and did not want something to happen: maybe I wanted to be kicked out, or be asked on a date. Something; anything.

SAFE-KEEPING

The San Francisco activist group Breast Cancer Action (BCA) decries the BMW campaign that gifted me with my coveted ride because it takes on the breast cancer cause while selling a product that pumps known carcinogens into the environment. In driving the BMW, I found myself in the middle of a cycle: a company sells a product that causes cancer, and then, to help find a cure for the disease that it is helping to cause, the same company raises awareness for the disease by selling more products that cause it, all while seeming to care about the cancer they are causing. You can nearly see one of those flowcharts with arrows pointing from one thing to the next and before you know it you are back where you started. And not in a good way.

So driving cars causes cancer. What does driving a car emblazoned with a cheesy pink ribbon do? For one thing, it increases the hypervisibility of breast cancer. It bears noting that the pink ribbon derives from a grassroots movement in which Charlotte Haley, inspired by the HIV/AIDS movement, sewed and distributed peach-colored ribbons to raise awareness about cancer and raise funds for prevention, like a pastel version of Betsy Ross. When Haley, not wanting to go commercial, refused to work with cosmetics icon Estée Lauder, Lauder had her lawyers design a new ribbon based on focus group research: hail the birth of the pink ribbon as we know it. In her history of the ribbon, Sandy Fernandez cites Margaret Welch, director of the Color Association of the United States, as saying: "Pink is the quintessential female color. The profile on pink is playful, life-affirming. We have studies as to its calming effect, its quieting effect, its lessening of stress. [Pastel pink] is a shade known to be health-giving; that's why we have expressions like 'in the pink.' You can't say a bad thing about it."[19] That said, not one country has found it health-giving enough to use in a national flag.

Though pink was considered a version of red and thus a boy's color in the early twentieth century, by the 1950s Americans definitely understood pink as a girl's color.[20] By this period, corporations widely adopted pink as a signifier for heterosexual womanhood through their introduction of special "women's" products. In the 1950s, Carte Blanche marketed a bright pink credit card to husbands as "a special HERS card to give your wife all the credit she deserves."[21] Nevertheless, like all credit cards at the time, it always bore the husband's name: he determined how much credit she deserved, while divorced women could rarely get credit at all. Because of the color's iconic use in signifying, and even constituting, heterosexual femininity, and perhaps also because of the use of the pink triangle to stigmatize gay men in the Nazi Holocaust, the gay pride movement, and particularly gay men, have actively resurrected and resignified it. But these oppositional uses of pink operate only in the context of the color's overwhelming coding of hetero-normative girl- and womanhood.

Despite Estée Lauder and other cosmetic companies' use of breast cancer to garner publicity, and their sponsorship of classes to teach women (and now men) to use makeup to make themselves presentable through cancer treatment, the cosmetics industry lobbied vociferously against the 2005 California Safe Cosmetics Act (S.B. 484), which requires that companies reveal potentially hazardous ingredients of their products to the state government. When industries use breast cancer pink to build goodwill, move product, and cover up their production of carcinogens, it's called pink-washing. Jingle writers have made over breast cancer and then handed it back as something palatable, obscuring the links among the production, suffering, and obfuscation of disease. Breast cancer poses as an innocent disease; as one marketer said, being "free from sin," it offers a promising way to transfer its affect to a "feeling about your business."[22] Barbara Brenner, a former executive director of Breast Cancer Action, argued that breast cancer presents an undercover opportunity to sell sex, but I think it offers an opportunity to sell girlhood—femininity precisely *without* the sex.[23] This version of benign girlhood requires sexual offenders to post their addresses on a website, but it doesn't teach girls to take off their shirts while playing street hockey.

The toothsome BMW campaign sprawling among the booths in the parking lot and the large trailer sporting huge posters from each year's campaign traffic in cure lingo. Not one mention of illness or suffering or death sullies the experience. By emphasizing the vague promise of a cure rather than the disease itself, corporate pink-washing diminishes the experience of breast cancer, diffusing other kinds of emotion, thus rendering them illegitimate or, worse, illegible. Unpink fear can barely be heard over the din of survival rhetoric and pink kitsch. But why are we so eager to buy this story about cancer, even as the prevalence of the disease means that everyone must know someone who has suffered or died of it? How has breast cancer become a disease that harbors such innocence—for everybody involved? What are the costs of this innocence?

In the twenty-first century, the coinciding rhetorics of pink-washing, sentimentality, the war on cancer, and the survivor figure scatter the politics of the disease as much as the pink-washing campaigns hide the distribution of cancer profits such that personal risk and responsibility become the primary discourses for discussing the disease.[24] Women can undergo patented genetic testing that costs upward of $5,000, while analyzing breast tissue for chemical carcinogens is virtually unheard of and is certainly not paid for by insurance companies, despite studies that have shown that breast tissue around tumors often has a higher level of carcinogenic material, to which siblings and other community members may also have been exposed.

In these models of corporate care, everyone has a scripted role. The Caring Corporation invites the Consumer to walk the line between denial and inevitability, neither of which are useful, but both of which prompt purchases. The Game-Faced Survivor toughs it all out, making the best of odds, and the Good-Girl Survivor revels in narratives of the "gift" of cancer and the "freedom to choose" from among a range of treatments and hospitals.[25] Sentimental empathy offers a passive, feminized ideal, which pink-washes the Corporation into the Caring Maternal Figure. Of course people want comforting images of cancer, and of course people want to help. And of course, people always want to buy stuff.

The almost viciously feminizing effect of sentimentality impacts the provision of healthcare. Although we want to imagine the rituals of detection as being cloaked in the professional touch of a gynecologist, sexuality pervades the doctor's office. Several women, both queer and straight, have told me that they wanted to say something when a doctor neglected to do a breast exam, but did not speak up for fear that the doctor might feel awkward touching their breasts.

A study of the media discourse around testicular, breast, and prostate cancers found that men who survive testicular cancer consider themselves as having "cheated death."[26] Lance Armstrong, as we saw in chapter 2, played up his survivorship as a measure of his personal potency, though somewhat by chance chemotherapeutic agents proved to be very effective for even metastasized testicular cancer. More men, in fact, die of breast cancer than of testicular cancer (the five-year survival rates for metastatic testicular cancer are over 70 percent, compared to about 5 percent for metastatic breast cancer). As Armstrong

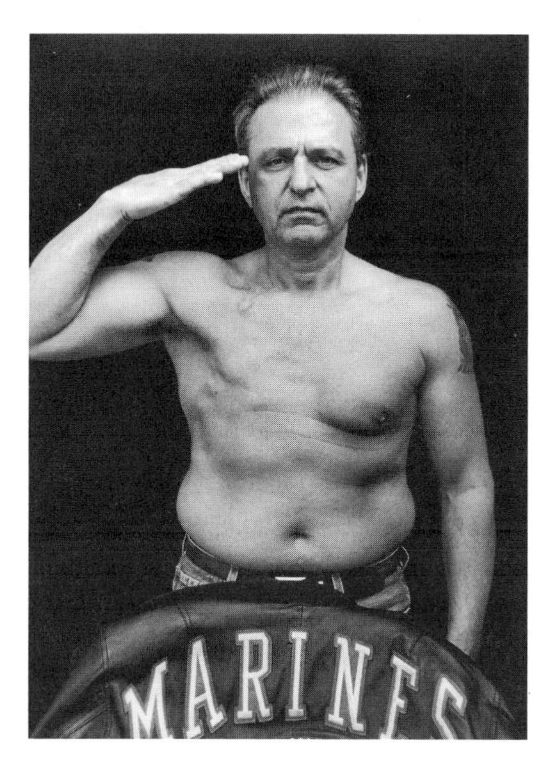

FIGURE 12. Jim Fontella, who as a marine worked at Camp Lejeune, a military installation where residents were knowingly poisoned through the water supply. Lejeune is at the center of the largest male breast cancer cluster in the United States (to date, over eighty men associated with that site have been diagnosed). (Photo courtesy of Patricia Izzo, www.izzophotography.com)

demonstrates, the myth of agency, in concert with the different biologies and cultures of disease, provides a critical space for men to be tough when it comes to cancer. But women's cancers (those of the reproductive organs) are less easily found and less easily treated than men's cancers, and death rates are nearly four times as high.[27] Although a guy could tough it out while his testicular cancer spreads and still have a very high chance of a cure, a woman toughing out her cancer will, after a certain point, have virtually no chance of survival.

To my knowledge, Armstrong prefers releasing images of his face to images of his cancer scars. Within the context of this history of gendered roles of protector, protected, and injury, Jim Fontella offers an ironic image of his mastectomy scar (fig. 12). Fontella lived at the Marine Corps Base Camp Lejeune in Jacksonville, North Carolina, believed to be the site of one of the largest water contaminations in U.S. history. (The U.S. Department of Defense is likely the nation's largest polluter, although it must vie for that honor with domestic oil and gas fracturing.)[28] Between 1957 and 1987, an estimated 750,000 to 1 million people living on the military base drank and bathed in tap water containing toxic chemicals in concentrations hundreds of times those permitted by current laws.[29] Camp Lejeune correlates with the largest cluster of breast cancer among men in the country.

Military men spearheaded a movement to gain reparations for the toxic exposures. Rather than focusing on their internal beauty, these middle-aged men are fed up with the betrayal of institutionalized friendly fire. Patricia Izzo's photograph of Fontella seems to say, "I protected America, and all I got was this lousy disease."

Despite Lorde's argument, mastectomy scars cannot offer a regendered version of Dayan's eye patch or Fontella's display, for the analogy skips over the heterosexual underpinning of toughness. Following the various definitions in the *Oxford English Dictionary* for *tough* and *butch,* we find that tough women are lesbians (note the reversal). Military scars signify if not the success of, then at least the obligation to masculine duties of protection, duties that are virtually definitive of manhood within the context of nation and heterosexuality. Women's mastectomy scars cite the amputation of gender, at once undermining nurturance and sexuality. Kohlman tames the threat through a coy look and a perfect body; Metzger tames it through a tree tattoo. These warriors take on a masculine sentimentality that is routed through recognizable femininity.

The endurance of *The Cancer Journals* and its continued resonance for so many people surely lies in the fact that it offers a way to inhabit cancer not as a victim, but as an agent. Lorde outlines a route through anger toward productive action. Yet I finished reading her book wanting still more. For one thing, cancer can be shut away behind prostheses, but it doesn't disappear. Cancer haunts us; terror underpins the spin of that cancer wheel, both for those postdiagnosis *(damn!)* and for those yet to find out *(could it be me?)*. For another thing, if we are warriors, whom are we fighting? What is our mode of resistance? Whom are we protecting? How might breast cancer culture be understood beyond the singular normative ideals of femininity, but in a way that does not take on a militarized masculinity?

BLINDSIDED

Lynn Kohlman's mastectomy images fall outside the pink charity mode, even if her language remains fixed on redemption. In one sense, these images bring cancer out of the closet by inviting scars out of the realm of private natural death and into the sphere of public, violent, and technological death. In a way, the images depsychologize scars by rendering them public, tough, and masculine. These scars display the trace of illness as a memorial of death. But the beauty of these images lies not in the way they mark mortality but, rather, in their hyper-designed quality: they draw attention to the markings that technology leaves on the body.

Also beautifully designed and engineered, BMW's ultimate driving machine features bulletproof glass, side-curtain air bags, and quick braking and acceleration to speed away from danger. It is a good thing, too. Even with safety features, nearly as many people are killed in car crashes in the United States as are killed by breast cancer each year: 32,885 in car crashes, and close to 39,970 of breast cancer.[30] Car crashes are the leading cause of death for people ages eight to thirty-four, after which cancers take the lead until the age of sixty-four. In terms of years of life lost, cancer is the main driver, car crashes take the back seat, and heart disease rides shotgun.[31] Canny, then, that a company with the reputation for producing some of the most aggressive members of the automotive fleet would have chosen breast cancer as its cause célèbre.[32] The physical and metaphoric versions of the ultimate drive juxtapose a masculinized car crash aesthetic against the pink-kitsch sentimentality of breast cancer.

By the 1950s, middle-class Americans experienced a vastly increased risk of public death (car crash fatalities reached the century's peak), as well as increased exposure to more realistic representations of violence through spy stories, westerns, and media images. At the same time, deaths due to illness became less and less visible—almost, as one social anthropologist described, "smothered in prudery"—as dying was moved from the living room to the hospital.[33]

Throughout the twentieth century, the automobile served as a critical cultural and material node for allying masculine characteristics with mechanical agency, and it has powerfully constituted gender in relation to heterosexuality, both socially and physically, in cultural domains as varied as auto racing and the rise of suburbia. Twentieth-century artists, from the Futurist Filippo Tommaso Marinetti to director David Cronenberg, portrayed car crash deaths in the service of masculinized fantasies of speed, power, agency, and the limits of human performance. No shame adhered to the car crash deaths of James Dean or Jackson Pollock, which in fact enlarged their statures while disguising the more widespread issue of automobile danger.[34] Fantasies of masculine prestige, liberation, and heroism invest car crash deaths with significance. Jackson Pollock provides one of many examples. Although he died rather ingloriously by hitting an oak tree with his head, the crash that ejected him became a key element in the interpretation of both his life and art. The fact that he killed his female passenger was virtually never mentioned in the significant media coverage of the event.[35]

Car deaths and cancer deaths meet in elaborate structures that give them layered meanings invested with fantasies about ideal gender types. Kohlman references a masculine aesthetic in this tradition, bringing attention to the scars and staples as technological enhancements and offering an intervention to the strict gender norms operating in the representation of breast cancer. Opposing reconstructive surgeries, and different from Matuschka's white-robed aesthetic, Kohlman's images bring the mastectomy into an aesthetic of the beautiful death. Far from engaging in the war against industrial pollution that Lorde envisioned, Kohlman instead cites the technobeauty dreamed of by Marinetti or documented by street photographer Weegee, and the mass violence of repetition iterated by Warhol: she offers an unveiling that usually is done in private or with trusted friends, family, and physicians. She takes her scars outside the realm of sadness and sentimentality and makes them matter as spectacle. Coming out of the domestic space, Kohlman shows and tells, adding to a personal and cultural archive of possible people. Her scars pose not as ugly to be covered, nor as ugly to be embraced, but as beautiful—both in themselves and on this classically beautiful androgynous woman.

Kohlman's chest is far from masculine, and she plays with the camera. Kohlman redeems her impending death by means of feminized norms, reclaiming her inner beauty as a response to and representation of the threat to her life. Beauty—in its varied guises—stands as a central narrative in the rhetoric of breast cancer culture, with regard to the valuation and evaluation of death. For example, when actress and singer Dana Reeve (most famous for her marriage to *Superman* actor Christopher Reeve) died of lung cancer in 2006, the shocked commentary revolved around her beauty and lack of culpability.[36] The reportage noted that Reeve, as a nonsmoker, did not deserve lung cancer. She was young, rich, and most of all beautiful—and so beautiful so recently, and still so dead of cancer. No one put it better than Edgar Allan Poe: "the death of a beautiful woman is, unquestionably, the most poetical topic in the world."[37]

Much of breast cancer culture parades as the pornography of death, with its constant representation of young women in sexualized poses on everything from the medical posters pinned in the doctor's office, to the covers of cancer magazines such as *Mamm* and *Cure*, to the ubiquitous cards showing how to do a breast self-exam. A recent ad by the Breast Cancer Fund of Canada featured a young, purposely slimy teenage boy named "Cam" who offers the free service of doing breast exams ("1-866-Ring-Cam"). Playing on the long-standing joke of the groping peach-fuzzed adolescent, the ad collaborates—even in its purported irony—in the same model of gender that has belittled the disease.[38] Is any other medical procedure sexualized in this way?

The very politics that leads to corporate use of breast cancer renders certain kinds of death innocent and tragic. This construction of innocence can be politically savvy, as when prioritizing children's issues such as car seats or safety regulations on school buses. But cancer is still perceived against all evidence as a natural illness, and the sentimentalization of tragic personal stories (rendered only more poignant in the case of the very beautiful) focuses on the suffering of individuals rather than on the culture that produces cancer, often through the very trappings that constitute beauty—the cosmetics, the cars.

As long as cancer remains an individual rather than a communal disease, as long as it is buffered by cultural fear of suffering and death, stigma can be the only response. And stigma gives rise to stigma. As Erving Goffman wrote, the stigmatized bears the burden of acting "so as to imply neither that his burden is heavy nor that bearing it has made him different from us; at the same time he must keep himself at that remove from us which ensures our painlessly being able to confirm this belief about him."[39] The stigma, the sentimental individuation, and the warrior offer triplet figurations. Slippery military metaphors insist that individuals, rather than the culture, suffer from cancer and that cancer can be fought—battled—and represented as outside of the very culture that produces it. Within that nexus, the Caring Corporations maintain the illusion of their own innocence.

CONCLUSION

Upon diagnosis, Sedgwick recognized the way in which the mammary ineluctably brought her under the umbrella of a gendered disease—and the violence of that gendering. *Shit, I am a woman:* I am the person whose wheel of fortune pointed to the illness not only of cancer but of femininity. Mastectomy offers a recuperation (of sorts) to that pregendered preadolescent space. This space ended with the coming of breasts, when girls' performance in math and sciences and sports tends to drop off and a heterosexual interest in boys is encouraged.

What if, instead of drowning breast cancer in a sea of pink and fundraising, those interested in mourning the toll of the disease took examples from other movements? Probike activists in many cities have revivified, for a short time, cyclists killed by cars by chaining a white bicycle to the spot where they met their death.[40] This move, like the HIV/AIDS quilt or the photos on the back pages of the *New York Times* of those killed in the World Trade Center, foregrounds a living presence, a material body, in the face of sterile statistics of accumulated deaths, a reminder of the embedded, invisible violence of the streetscape and of the structures that produce these deaths on a mass scale. If the Caring Corporation lionizes the individual to keep us from detecting the patterns, these communities honor the individuals who suffer from the patterns and in so doing draw attention to both.

Unlike Dayan's eye patch, which marked the end result of injury, the cancer scar can never really be the insignia of a survived event. The scar can only be temporary. The scar marks unpredictability. As the scar on the chest fades, are little cancer stem cells gathering force, reduplicating? One has no idea until later, just as no one knows now who harbors incipient cancers. The loss, ultimately, has less to do with a body part; cancer takes one's imagined immortality. Cancer is about the way U.S. culture shrouds terror under a scarf of rosy hopefulness.

Vito Russo, an HIV/AIDS activist, talked at an ACT UP demonstration about living with a disease that is cast as shameful from the beginning: "It's like living through a war which is happening only for those people who happen to be in the trenches. Every time a shell explodes, you look around and you discover that you've lost more of your friends, but nobody else notices. It isn't happening to them. They're walking the streets as though we weren't living through some sort of nightmare. And only you can hear the screams of the people who are dying and their cries for help. No one else seems to be noticing."[41] I have no idea what it would be like to lie, night after night, in the cold bog of a WWI trench not knowing when an enemy might approach. Still, I can see why those metaphors have such descriptive power. When you're ill, you feel under siege.

ACT UP did not focus on how beautiful they all were. Instead, ACT UP acted out about all of the issues that affect people living with HIV/

AIDS: the cost of drugs, housing, and medical insurance; the discrimination. They rioted, they educated, they stormed the National Institutes of Health, they unleashed power. They were arrested and they made news. The slogans from that era sound ballsy even decades later: "Bring the dead to your door—we won't take it anymore"; "George Bush, you can't hide, we charge you with genocide"; "This is an angry funeral, not a sad one"; "We are dying of government neglect equivalent to genocide." At one ACT UP demonstration, the artist and activist David Wojnarowicz wrote on his jacket: "When I die of AIDS, throw my body on the steps of the FDA." At the height of the HIV/AIDS crisis, deaths from the disease spurred countrywide riots, and people were pouring ashes on the lawn of the White House. The disease was public and angry, but most of all, it was a collective enterprise, bringing together people who then exercised their social power.[42] ACT UP's war—nevermind the limits of the metaphor—spurred a successful social movement.

In a pre–ACT UP era, Lorde asked: "What would happen if an army of one-breasted women descended upon Congress and demanded that the use of carcinogenic, fat-stored hormones in beef-feed be outlawed?"[43] Lorde leaves this as an open question, but I suspect that such women would have been ridiculed and dismissed as radical bra-burning dykes, just as the antinuclear activists were a generation ago by those who presumed themselves immune to cancer.

Ubiquitous breast cancer marches offer a strange space for reflection, one that is not quite mourning and not quite triumph, not a wake but not a celebration. But what if queers had sat around sipping Hansen's soda for a cure to HIV? Would the HIV/AIDS death rate in the United States now be a third of what it was two decades ago? Yet cancer continues, and we are just marching (and marching), throwing our pink around. Was HIV/AIDS any more of a genocide than cancer?

To raise money for cancer, I'd like to drive a scratched-up and dented car with photographs of tumors and of careers in ruins because of time spent in hospitals, trailing vomit and sperm out the exhaust pipe. Even in pacifist Canada, cigarette warnings sport graphic details of blackened lungs. Whom are we protecting here in the United States? But if I found such a car and, channeling my very toughest inner butch, had the guts to drive it, my display would be dismissed as a political statement. Meanwhile, the BMW pink car-lot celebration passes as care. And so, if I die of cancer? Forget burial—just drop my carcass on the steps of BMW HQ.

CHAPTER 4

Lost Chance

Medical Mistakes

Mike sat at the bar telling me about the blow job he insisted on every two days from his partner, a Hollywood agent about whom he was also writing a book. Reading numerous textbooks on personal injury law for the book I'd written on the subject still left me ill-prepared for my experience that afternoon: my lawyer going into increasingly drunken detail about his life in bed and in elevators. Some people love sex stories, but by then I had already heard far too much. The timing was just off. Still, it didn't feel right to prudishly cut off the conversation; in my role as Good Plaintiff, I attempted a lame smile because I had to depend on Mike to figure out the next step of my medical malpractice case. Abruptly, he turned to me and said that we would be suing for wrongful death.

When a patient walks into the oncologist's office with a diagnosis, the oncologist tends not to be interested in how things could have been otherwise, at what earlier point the cancer might have been found. Doctors rarely consider counterfactual pasts. The physician looks forward, treating the patient and the disease as they appear in front of her. It's safer that way.

The past tends to be a preoccupation of patients and of lawyers who wonder how and when things could have gone differently; law has the power to rewrite a story of the past, to take back a mistake by offering compensation to the person who suffered from the error. A compensatory award pays for the expenses that result from an accidental or negligent mistake. It symbolically recognizes and atones for the added hardships.

The law takes on a key practical and statistical quandary: how should the costs of the predictable human errors inherent in the practice of medicine be distributed? Quite simply, doctors can maim and kill people with the slightest slip-up, the tiniest moment of inattention.[1] Some doctors make more mistakes than others, with more or less grace, and with more or less associated attention to detail. Even the best and most motivated physicians make errors in diagnosis and treatment that could, in retrospect, have been avoided. A nonspecialist patient can't really know the quality of her physician; good manners or a caring demeanor do not solely lead to good medicine—nor does a patient's affection for her physician imply the doctor's competence. Because no one collects systematic data on physician skill and efficacy, it's virtually impossible to know how well one's own doc did in medical school or how many mistakes he has already made.[2]

Medical malpractice law arose specifically to acknowledge that physicians should not be held criminally responsible for errors *and* that the patients should not go untreated or personally pay for those mistakes. Accepting the truism that *accidents will happen because doctors are people too,* this area of law offers a way, albeit expensive and time consuming, to ensure that the costs of these errors will not be borne solely by the patient. The law lays out a system in which each consumer will pay a bit more for a service, and when the inevitable accident happens, the court redistributes the money to the person who suffered that inevitable mistake. Unlike a no-fault insurance system, which allocates resources regardless of a specific site of fault, medical malpractice law (or med-mal) requires the plaintiff to show that the care he or she received fell below the usual standard.

In theory, the threat of litigation inspires individual doctors to do their best work and it provokes systematic improvements in medical service delivery. Ideally, insurance premiums would be priced a little above the costs of payouts, and those companies wouldn't make undue financial profit or find themselves overcome by greed. Good in theory, but as with most systems that predicate their success on the good behavior of humans, it hasn't really turned out.

Doctors generally work in complicated systems, and fault for error can be distributed in many ways. Consider a recent case in which a wrongly administered chemotherapy drug (in place of another drug) into a patient's epidural shunt killed a young man.[3] Does fault lie with the system designer who neglected to use color coding or geometry to avoid confusion between types of infusions? Or perhaps the nurse didn't check the drug name properly, the technician misread the prescription, or someone misstocked the shelves? Should the doctor be blamed for her illegible handwriting, or were the names of the different drugs too similar? Does fault lie with the insurance company that would pay for only a few minutes for a nurse to administer the drug, rather than whatever time was needed to ensure adequate attention?

Malpractice claims against an individual can miss the structural nature of medicine and the many different junctures to which cause could be traced. That said, the doctor lends a human face to a medical bureaucracy. One might suggest that the generally high compensation that physicians enjoy makes up for the complex negotiations between patient and industry interests. The ability to cure in certain cases accompanies the possibility of being singled out as a causal force of injury.

The legal relationship between patient and doctor is not one of mutual agreement about the possible costs and benefits of a treatment (a misunderstanding that can result from an informed consent form that lists possible side-effects to a medical procedure). Rather, it pertains to a patient's right not to be injured. In order to assert that right, the court requires the physician and patient to take an oppositional stance, one in which each side argues their case as strongly as possible in an effort to win. Thus, doctors and patients who were initially assumed to work together toward the higher goal of patient health must inhabit divergent roles that may be highly uncomfortable for both. Many doctors feel unfairly blamed, even when they know they have made mistakes, whether due to a slip-up or because of structural constraints.

While many people stand by the notion, popularized especially by insurance companies, that Americans abuse the legal system and scurry around with frivolous claims, the heyday of plaintiffs' law is well behind us. The question remains: Who should pay for the inevitable mistakes, whether perpetrated honestly or carelessly? Current debates about the medical malpractice system focus on the difference between medical and legal understandings of error, and each seems to misunderstand the other. On the one hand, if physicians shouldn't be blamed for accidents, should patients just absorb the costs, including the cost of extra treatment, follow-up appointments, co-pays for specialist visits and drugs, and seemingly endless, often uncovered-by-insurance necessities such as physical therapy and durable machinery? On the other hand, an injured person must depend on medical expertise to make the case that their treatment was subpar, and to do so they need to hire expensive expert witnesses from those in the very field they are implicitly critiquing. This requirement makes it very difficult to bring a case. Who, then, will be responsible for improving medical delivery in this radically nonmarket economy?

Cancer offers a unique challenge to medical malpractice law. The fundamental unknownness of the disease requires both doctors and lawyers to rely on prognostic population data. But these numbers, seemingly the same, carry different meanings in these fields: for medicine, a prognosis characterizes an aggregated chance, but law seeks to specify an individual's situation. The cases that address missed diagnosis through a legal doctrine called "lost chance" show how numbers take on different lives in different arenas, at the expense of further mystifying life in prognosis.

GIMLET EYE

As I sipped my first-ever gin gimlet at a party in downtown San Francisco in June 2011, I spotted a doctor across the room. I immediately recognized her Farrah Fawcett hair and Nordic looks, relatively unscathed by the decade since I'd seen her. When I last saw Dr. Nordic (my primary care doc had sent me to her for a follow-up of a peculiar lump she'd found), I walked out of her office feeling humiliated and confused. I passed the coffee stand by the front desk of the office feeling as if my symptoms had been completely blown off. I remember thinking, at thirty-three but with the maturity of a twelve-year-old, "Well, if I do have cancer, that'll show *her*."

Still, I trusted her, or at least her position as a doctor at a world-renowned research university. Her own world-renownedness aside, Dr. Nordic did not tell me what to keep an eye out for; she gave me no list of red flags. Despite my snarky thoughts borne of our interaction, I never truly considered cancer as a possibility, but three years later I found out that it had indeed been more a likelihood than a possibility, since the largest tumor was in the exact same location. I never interacted with Dr. Nordic again, but because of the late stage at which the cancer was finally caught, the severity of the treatments ensured that she never strayed far from my mind.

That June night, six years after my eventual diagnosis, we both attended the soirée-fundraiser for an organization made up of people like me, people who had been diagnosed with cancer as young adults.

Two young women had founded the group some ten years before, specifically because this demographic tended to be ignored both medically and socially. A glimpse cast through my wide-rimmed, half-full glass refracted several memories: The bewilderment I felt in the first waking hour after my initial cancer surgery. The sound of her voice refusing me a biopsy (the only definitive way to have diagnosed that cancer), telling me they are painful and can spread cancer if it's present. The disbelief of hearing her, a preeminent cancer researcher, opining on National Public Radio on how she doesn't believe in screening. Most of all, the shock of what I experienced as dismissal, when high stakes for one person were made light of by another.

When Dr. Nordic point-blank refused to order the biopsy I requested at that original visit, my mother, also a physician, insisted on making an appointment for a second opinion. She spent hours on the phone with her doctor colleagues discussing the standard of care in a case like this one and lobbying the insurance company to cover a visit with another oncologist. She said at the time, "I want to be shown that I have nothing to worry about. Nothing would make me happier." Then Dr. Nordic relented and I canceled the appointment at the Stanford Cancer Center.

But instead of doing a core biopsy, she had two medical students do a fine needle aspiration (FNA)—a procedure known to take a great deal of skill and practice to do accurately and that isn't done at all in several countries because of the high rate of false negatives. I later found out, too, that there was no way of really knowing if they even got the right tissue, since they just pinched the area and inserted the needle. In instructing the students before she left them to carry out the procedure, she didn't suggest that this would be a baseline test or that we would keep an eye on it and check back in a few months. Instead, Dr. Nordic off-handedly commented, "I'm only doing this to please her mother." With the gesture of the FNA she may have evaded a lawsuit, but she didn't please my mom (who didn't realize until years later that a biopsy had not, in fact, been done, since I didn't know the difference).

From what I could gather through my furtive peeks at the party, Dr. Nordic had gained some weight. What had gone on for her during these last ten years? Did she see me there, in my best party T-shirt nursing my drink? If she did, would she even recognize me? After all, she has had hundreds of patients since seeing me, many of whom no doubt thank her for saving their lives. Maybe she had that vague feeling, "Hmmm, I recognize her from somewhere, but I don't know where." Then again, I had tried to sue her, so maybe that registered. Maybe she thought, "Well, you're still alive, so what's your problem?" At any rate, if she did notice me, she ignored me, and she left, with a noticeable limp, soon after I spotted her.

For a long time after diagnosis, I obsessed over why she hadn't taken me seriously. Wasn't I friendly enough? Did she think of me as a whiny patient who should just go away? Or maybe I wasn't insistent enough. Was the dismissal because of my dark complexion (race) or my sexuality? Did she just think I was too young to get cancer? It's true, as she reported in the note to my family doctor, that at the time there had never been cancer in my family. Then again, my family history was still emerging, with under-sixty-year-old parents and two younger siblings. Besides, genetics account for very few cancers.

As with financial planning and choosing a partner, one doesn't learn how to speak to a physician in school. Still, that interaction, in less than a few minutes, can change the course of your life. One study found, as an example, that when a patient mentions a specific drug, a doctor is more likely to prescribe it—both for good and for ill.[4] It doesn't help that on the doctor side, little medical training focuses on how to handle the fraught social exchange of an office visit. If determining when and where cancer exists takes skill and time in a system pressed for time, being a good, communicative patient also takes practice, though the literature on cancer diagnosis rarely touches on how this relationship, usually between strangers, bears on diagnostic procedures.

I had no idea how to talk to a doctor. So maybe in this case the misdiagnosis was my own fault. But I *had* gone in with a specific request, a biopsy, based on a concrete symptom. In fact, several years after that interaction I met another woman who'd had nearly exactly the same situation. She also had a fine needle aspiration that came out negative. However, her doctor had a six-month follow-up policy, and so an accurate diagnosis shortly followed.

The few oncologists who in the last couple of years have taken up the issue of cancer in young adults note that lack of patient education is a major problem affecting young adult survival. These doctor-patient interactions, even when resulting ultimately in a negative diagnosis, surely provide an opportunity for this sort of education.

As I began to meet other young adults who had gone through cancer treatment, I found that an absurdly high percentage of them had been misdiagnosed. At a day-long retreat, I watched a forty-year-old woman who had a diagnosis delayed for three years practice telling her family that she was dying. Her mother and two-year-old son hadn't believed her the first time. *No, really: I'm dying.* My cousin Elise stopped going to her young survivor group meetings because she couldn't stand to hear about the rampant misdiagnoses anymore.

I spoke to one thirty-five-year-old who had lung metastases surgically removed during Christmas break so that no one at work would find out that he had skin cancer. He described to me how easy it was to hide his cancer: "No one expects a young person to have cancer; you think of it as an older person's disease. I could never let on just how dire my situation was." His diagnosis had been delayed for two years because his doctor told him not to worry about the mole on his arm—so he didn't worry. After learning that the mole was actually a late-stage melanoma, he thought about bringing a medical malpractice suit. However, he discovered that the doctor had not kept records, so it would be the patient's word against the doctor's. Furthermore, his doctor—like others—carried only one million dollars' worth of insurance ("drivers carry more than that!"), which would not cover—by a long stretch—his losses as an executive with young children. His lawyers told him that juries tend to believe doctors. "Just as I did," he said.[5]

My patient self meets my anthropologist self here, drifting downstream with the alligators. I've collected stories of young adults' delayed diagnoses for a purpose beyond just some weird form of self-consolation. Although in my own case the misdiagnosis may well be explainable by a specific doctor-patient interaction, a faulty diagnostic test, a sloppy technician, a cocky and defensive doctor, or a jejune medical resident, in the context of the experiences of others, something bigger is going on.

MEDICAL ERROR

Medical errors vary vastly in scope, severity, and likelihood of being detected. Certain injuries must be reported to regulatory boards and investigated, such as when a surgeon removes the wrong limb. (Oops.) Most others require no such reporting, which is why studies on error drastically vary.[6] A 1999 study of accidental death in the medical system estimated preventable medical-error deaths to be in the range of 98,000 and suggested that this number is the "price we pay for not having organized systems of care with clear lines of accountability."[7] More recent work indicates that this figure vastly underrepresents the issue, which may in fact account for over 250,000 U.S. deaths each year.[8]

Two doctors found in 2009 that misdiagnosis alone, a small fraction of fatal errors, accounts for an estimated 40,000 to 80,000 hospital deaths per year.[9] Focusing on misdiagnosis of all diseases, a Johns Hopkins team in 2012 found rates "alarmingly high." Studying autopsies, the researchers extrapolated that 40,500 U.S. hospital patients die with an undiagnosed medical condition that caused or contributed to their deaths. Although two-thirds of all the misdiagnoses the study discovered did not directly contribute to those patients' deaths, the researchers note that nonfatal diagnostic mistakes cause lengthened hospital stays, unnecessary surgical procedures, and reduced quality of life.[10]

Few systematic studies have examined medical misdiagnoses specifically. One rare study in which physicians reviewed closed malpractice cases found that a cancer diagnosis was involved in 59 percent of diagnosis errors, of which 30 percent resulted in death. The overrepresentation of cancer misdiagnosis may well have been because these cases most clearly indicate an error to a patient, who consequently bears a costly burden. Breakdowns in the diagnostic process included "failure to order an appropriate diagnostic test, failure to create a proper follow-up plan, failure to obtain an adequate history or perform an adequate physical examination, and incorrect interpretation of diagnostic tests."[11]

Studying surgical errors, researcher Thomas Krizek found that "the probable incidence of error involves a staggering half of all patients admitted to surgical intensive care units."[12] Krizek reports that the 45.8 percent incidence of error, with a 21.2 percent incidence of serious error, is many times larger than the reported 10 percent error (3.7 percent serious) published elsewhere.[13] Krizek hypothesizes five issues that inhibit improvement in the quality of surgical care, including "inadequate data about adverse events, inadequate practice guidelines and outcome analysis, a culture of blame, a need to compensate injured patients, and difficulty in truth-telling on the part of surgeons." Each of these issues warrants closer analysis, but for my purposes, his most critical point is this: "The fact that the tort system is not very efficient (*of 480 patients in our study, only 3 with adverse events received compensation*) does not take away the awesome fear of litigation."[14]

LEGAL MECHANISM

Since newspapers report endlessly about doctors being sued over frivolous cases that upend the medical system, I had thought I'd have a pretty good shot at a settlement with a legitimate claim of misdiagnosis. Certainly Americans tend to use the tort system more than citizens of other Western nations because of the prohibitive cost of healthcare and the lack of a safety net. Some medical insurance plans, including Medicare and Medicaid (which cover 27 percent of Americans), provide for care, but 15 percent of Americans have no medical insurance whatsoever, while a further 10–15 percent have coverage that does not cover—by many thousands of dollars—standard cancer treatment.[15] Recent federal changes to the accessibility of healthcare may change this. But tort law offers a chance to recoup the crushing costs when one might not otherwise have been inclined to sue.

Despite this critical public health role, the system is unbelievably complex in practice. Courts make broad, politically influential decisions in a piecemeal way, drawing on the precedent of prior cases that have similar enough facts and concepts to apply to the situation in question. The legal record, an unruly record of history, policy, and personal stories, slowly defines which behaviors and product designs will be sufficient to balance humans' fragility against the material world's destructive potential.

Though they may seem like dry offerings, legal cases embody stories and regrets and attempts to change not just history but the ineluctability of time. Amazing nuggets of literature, judges' written opinions outline the dramas of people who feel that they have been wrongfully harmed, opine on the proper role of the law, and distribute wealth in an effort to restore justice.

People with wonderful names like Percy Pybus appear in the fat tomes of court reports, which record how courts made a tenuous sense of their stories by harnessing centuries of convoluted jurisprudence. In 1905, the nineteen-year-old Percy, while out on a joy-ride in his friend's dad's car, hit and killed nine-year-old Branch Lewis as he crossed a neighborhood street in Atlanta. When Branch's mother sued for damages, Percy was suddenly caught up in a larger conceptual issue being argued in courts at the time, namely, who should be responsible for the dangers of these new-fangled machines: the driver; the owner of the car; or even the owners of the garage where the car had been stored, who had handed over the keys.

With this case as precedent, the automobile came to be legally understood as an inherently safe machine that becomes treacherous only when driven recklessly, rather than as an innately dangerous machine over which an owner should maintain constant vigilance, as Branch's mother argued. From that point on, the driver, not the car's design or its owner, was considered the cause of injuries—until sixty years later, when Ralph Nader reopened the issue with his indictment of the automotive industry's resulting focus on whimsical tailfins rather than the slaughter on the freeways, in *Unsafe at Any Speed.*[16]

Similarly, in medical malpractice suits, plaintiffs harness previous legal decisions to make their claims. As an area of common law, medical malpractice dates back to the early fourteenth century, although it didn't become widespread until the rise of widely advertised medical promises and quack cures in the mid-1800s.[17] Physicians were protected from criminal claims in the normal course of practicing medicine after the mid–nineteenth century, when the law determined that anyone calling himself a physician would be legally shielded from criminal charges such as murder.

In 1853, long before the standardization of medical education and protocol, a certain Dr. Smith described the presumption of liability. He wrote that the physician hanging a shingle serves the community. When called on, therefore, if the "physicians and surgeons refuse to act, or they act unskillfully, the party employing them has a right to demand damages at a tribunal of justice."[18] Since that time, patients have had a legal right if not to the best care, at least to a standard of care. As a judge charged a jury in 1857, "The law did not require of the defendants eminent or extraordinary skill," averring "that this kind of skill is possessed by few."[19] In other words, because every physician cannot, by definition, give superior care, to require it would mean that many people would get no medical attention at all; hence, average care legally suffices.

Smith recognized a problem that has yet to be solved sixteen decades later, to wit, that gathering proof about the practices of experts requires the cooperation of those in their field, and doctors may well find testifying against a colleague, particularly someone prominent or senior, unwise for their own professional development. As Smith put it, "If in these cases of alleged mal-practice, it could be proved . . . that a patient died who might have been saved by his physician, . . . then an action might be sustained. Such supposable circumstances, however, are not likely to occur, for who, as a witness, would dare say, absolutely and without qualification, that death might have been prevented?"[20]

This early editorial points to two issues that continue to undercut the success of plaintiffs: first, a plaintiff needs medical professionals willing to testify against one another; and second, it is often difficult to definitively claim that fault for a death lies with the doctor (or the system he works within) and not with an underlying health issue.[21] In this need for expert witnesses, plaintiffs come up against a powerful professional culture around the admission of mistakes. One study found that only 30 percent of surgeons would testify against a physician who had removed the wrong kidney from a patient—demonstrating a stronger allegiance to protecting the interests of the profession, fear of professional censure, or concern for the physician who made the error than to ensuring patient well-being.[22] In my legal case, at least two physicians who concluded that a preventable misdiagnosis had occurred hesitated to testify against a prominent doctor (though I found two more who were willing to testify).

The language used by physicians to describe moments that might have gone better reflects this reluctance to attribute cause. A 2005 study, for example, found that surgeons discussing verifiable medical errors with patients used the word *error* or *mistake* in only 57 percent of conversations and offered a verbal apology only 47 percent of the time.[23] Physicians often prefer a passive voice ("a vein was cut" substitutes for "I accidentally cut a vein" and "retained surgical item" describes the forceps the doctor left in the abdomen; fig. 13). A language of side-effects and risk can serve the same ends. Insurance carriers and professional codes encourage these descriptions.

Dr. David Hilfiker, one of the first doctors to write on the subject of medical mistakes from a doctor's perspective, describes how hard it was to get his work in this area published and how it would be over ten years until other doctors spoke about their errors.[24] In a 1984 article describing some of the understandable yet devastating missteps he had made in his practice, he wrote: "We are not prepared for our mistakes, and we don't know how to cope with them when they occur. . . . This [medical] perfection is a grand illusion, of course, a game of mirrors that everyone plays. Doctors hide their mistakes from patients, from other doctors, even from themselves. Open discussion of mistakes is banished from the consultation room, from the operating room, from physicians' meetings. Mistakes become gossip, and are spoken of openly only in court."[25]

Liability insurance, which initially became available to doctors in the 1890s, offers one way to circumvent the personal blame game, at least in theory.[26] Insurance in one sense undermines the deterrent effect of personal injury law, since a defendant will not have to pay out of her

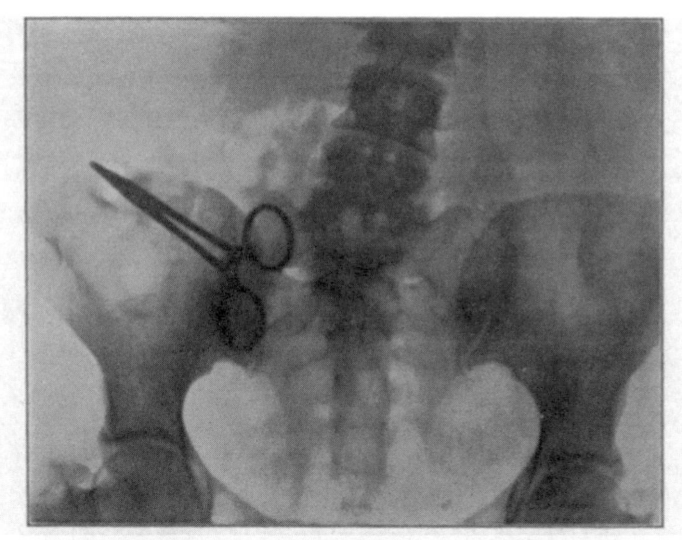

Fig. 100.—The x-ray film showing the forceps (hemostat) in the abdomen four years after abdominal operation. The patient was supposed to have a tumor till x-ray examination revealed the forceps. (Anonymous.)

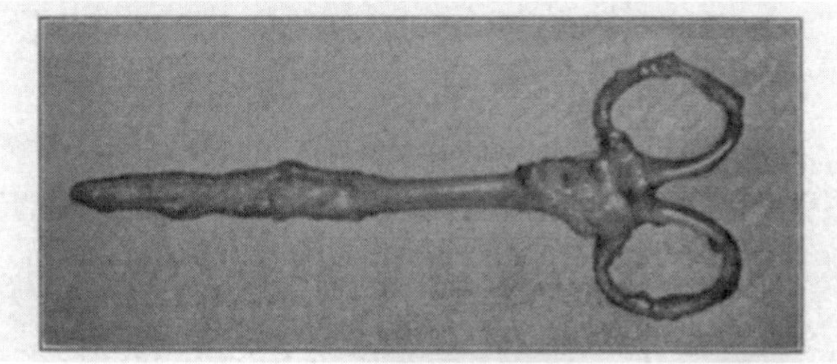

Fig. 101.—Rusty forceps removed from abdomen at a remote period. (From Keen. Bartlett—*After-Treatment of Surgical Patients.* The C. V. Mosby Company.)

FIGURE 13. In 1940, a doctor and a lawyer collaboratively offered a compendium of images of surgical objects left in body cavities after surgeries, including forceps, tweezers, scissors, drainage tubing, needles, and sponges. The book also includes case reports dating from the 1890s, including how an object was left and, if found, whether, and how, it was extracted. The authors make recommendations for avoiding such errors. (*Source:* Harry Sturgeon Crossen and David Frederic Crossen, *Foreign Bodies Left in the Abdomen—The Surgical Problems: Cases, Treatment, Prevention; The Legal Problems: Cases, Decisions, Responsibilities* [St. Louis: C.V. Mosby, 1940])

own pocket for a doctor's lapse. However, if a physician were able to admit that he had made a mistake and the patient could be paid out of that physician's insurance, the costs of a genuine accident might be equitably spread. One doctor admitted to me that it might be "naive and idealistic" but "I have always considered my [insurance] as the provision of justice to patients I may injure unwittingly, when I cannot pay enough to compensate for a mistake I make. They may be small incidents—taking only a moment's distraction—that cost the patient their health or life."[27]

My mother pursued a settlement after her doctor misread a mammogram and delayed a diagnosis by a year. Despite clear evidence of the cancer in previous mammogram images, the radiologist's admission that she overlooked the test results, and the personal consequences in terms of the severity of the treatment, lost income, and lower survival chances, the doctor and her lawyers fought the case, dragging it out and ultimately claiming that the fact that my mother was recurrence-free five years later proved that the oversight was irrelevant. To my mother, though, the months spent sick, sitting in the chemotherapy chair, and losing income from her own medical practice for a year of treatment were terribly relevant.

Insurance adds another powerful industry to the equation, and the med-mal phenomenon must be read in the context of insurance companies' efforts to bring about tort reform. One such reform, California's Medical Injury Compensation Reform Act (MICRA), passed in 1975, limits compensatory awards. The maximum one can receive for medical error that sends you home blind, without a leg, or having had a stroke is $250,000 (the amount hasn't changed since 1975), unless you can prove ill intent or that you have significant lost income, in which case you can claim those losses separately.[28] In addition, insurance companies have launched a media blitz ridiculing "frivolous claims" and set up in-house legal departments enabling them to battle claims and settle only at the last minute before a court case, deliberately driving up costs and scaring plaintiffs' lawyers away from taking cases. In my malpractice case, as the court date approached, my lawyer, Mike, became terrified that the defendants would, if they won, ask the court to make the plaintiff pay all the costs of the case. I couldn't find much precedent for this, and I couldn't tell if the risk was real or if Mike just wanted to get back to writing his book. Given the high fees of defense lawyers and doctor experts, though, these costs would have been exorbitant—easily well beyond a million dollars.

Movies often portray plaintiffs' lawyers as scrappy, all the more so when compared with the well-paid, well-secretaried attorneys of corporate defense firms. This representation results from a unique fee structure, which enables people access to the law who might not otherwise be able to hire an attorney. Namely, plaintiffs' lawyers front all the costs of the case, including court fees, expert witnesses (just one medical expert can cost about $20,000), and office and administrative costs. If they win the case, they earn between 30 and 40 percent of the award, but if they lose, they walk away with nothing. Physician defendants rely on attorneys hired by their insurance companies (or in-house legal departments); these salaried lawyers typically bill by the hour and are paid regardless of the outcome of the case.

In the states with damage caps, no sane plaintiff's attorney would take a case unless she could also claim some sort of reckless intent or she can make a large lost income claim, either of which would enable a settlement over and above the cap for the injury itself. As many commentators have noticed, this legal framework disadvantages people without a provable lost income—those who take time off to raise children or train for the Olympics, say, or those who have low incomes for other reasons.[29] Given the caps on damage awards, and the fact that most doctors carry only $1 million worth of insurance, it is virtually impossible to settle a case out of court for more than that sum. It is truly ironic that, while basing large fees on the inherent value of life, the medical industry with its doctors, lawyers, and administrators has been able at the same time to lobby for caps on damage awards in most states, stunting that same valuation.

Partly as a result of the structure of the system, but also for many other reasons, most injured people don't sue. For one thing, it is extremely difficult to know if one has been subject to an avoidable gaffe. (Even if you strongly suspect so, it's easy to second-guess yourself. Maybe I just wasn't communicative enough with Dr. Nordic? Maybe I, not she, should have considered a follow-up?) One in five Americans report that they or a relative have experienced medical error, and only about 2 percent of patients who have been seriously injured by medical error sue, and of those only between 25 and 35 percent win.[30] Based both on the study results of medical error cited above and comparisons of medical malpractice outcomes to other kinds of personal injury cases in which plaintiff and defendant wins divide more equally, legal scholars and lawyers alike understand that juries disproportionately favor physicians. It is virtually impossible to argue after the fact that a test, had it been done, would have shown something specific. And of course, the doctors write and control all of the reports. And who really wants to believe that doctors make mistakes, or work within systems that make mistakes all but inevitable? I certainly don't.

At any rate, from doctors' and patients' perspectives alike, as well as those who end up as both, the medical malpractice system dismally fails. But just because it doesn't work very often doesn't mean it can't provoke other insights. In fact, these cases provide a unique perspective from which to understand how statistics translate between the legal and medical fields, leaving those living in prognosis clambering through a numerical imbroglio.

LOST CHANCE

The slim archive of medical malpractice law devoted to missed diagnoses focuses on a concept called "lost chance."[31] In these cases, the alleged injury is the lost chance at survival, or the difference in the prognosis had a cancer been found sooner, compared to the prognosis for the later-stage cancer. Courts in different jurisdictions vary dramatically in how they interpret lost-chance claims. Some courts require the patient to have died, while others accept that the loss of a chance in and of itself can be injurious. In one lost-chance case, the judge unbelievably decided that the patient's extended peace of mind in *not* knowing about the cancer was a benefit outweighing the injury of late diagnosis.[32]

Lost-chance litigation illustrates the structural constraints on translating medical uncertainty into clear lines of fault, and the resulting legal, medical, and personal quagmire. While the law must locate the *fact* of causation in any given case, oncology only presents future *possibilities,* delivered through prognoses and statistics as they appear in (imagined) populations of individuals whose medical histories have various degrees of similarity to the plaintiff's. Physicians have developed means to roughly correlate individuals and population statistics. Courts, in contrast, must figure out how to convert the concepts of chance generated by oncology into terms that can justify an adjudication about fault. The medical question takes a vague future form: *Given the survival statistics of other people with this cancer, what treatment might work?* The legal question takes a precise historical form: *In this particular case, did the doctor err?* Courts typically make this translation from the population to the individual by running the medical data through their own legal tests, such as the "more likely than not" test. But regardless of the legal test applied, a population-based statistic (other than 0 percent or 100 percent) can never reliably predict any particular individual's life or death.

The territory of litigation only partly relates to "what happened." Because events must be fit into legal categories, they necessarily become distorted, much like a cancer fitting into the boxes and forms uses to describe it on the path report. When a friend of mine requested a colonoscopy after her mother died of colon cancer, her insurance refused to pay for it because she was too young. She went ahead anyway, using her own money, and when the colonoscopy turned up a lesion, her insurance offered her a partial refund of her out-of-pocket expense. The precancer colon—known only through the language of numbers and therefore denied surveillance—was later deemed, after the confirmation of cancer, to have been worthy of surveillance.

Courts in states that accept the lost-chance doctrine have established frameworks for adjudicating how numbers about probability matter. In these courts, the plaintiff (that is, the patient) must have suffered a greater than 50 percent loss of chance of survival, which also drops the patient's overall chance of survival to less than 50 percent.

Lost-chance plaintiffs encounter several temporal problems. First, cancer spreads over time, but no one knows precisely at what point time matters and for whom. Did the cancer become incurable in July? Or not until October? Second, doctors use a loose cluster of indices to tell how far a cancer has spread, what a prognosis will be, and how to treat the disease. However, the instant a tumor grows from 4.9 centimeters to 5.0 centimeters, for example, the survival chance of its host does not necessarily diminish by the 25 percent indicated by a staging chart. As less than perfect spheres, tumors cannot be measured with complete precision; staging and the prognoses that result offer mere estimates at every vector. Thus, doctors have little to go on in making a judgment about how long a delay will have mattered in an outcome. A six-month delay in diagnosis may not make a difference—too short to matter. On the other hand, a delay of several years makes it harder to prove that initial symptoms were related to the disease that later emerged—too long to matter. Cancer exists in nonsensical time, and living in prognosis challenges individuals and institutions alike to conform to its hourglass. When one's time is potentially limited, it takes on extra significance.

The law requires that each side take a position with regard to the recent history. The doctor's role in court is to defend the course of time as it actually unfurled—to argue in various ways that things could not have been different: the right procedures were followed, the patient would have died even if the cancer were treated sooner. The doctor defends the justness of the reality as it plays out.

As in all civil cases, the burden of proof falls on the plaintiff, since the plaintiff is the one claiming that things should have been otherwise. This can be tough given that the lack of diagnosis is precisely the problem. If a doctor had, for example, biopsied a mole, there would be evidence about the malignancy, or not, of the mole. Without that biopsy, no evidence exists—indeed, a doctor may not have even written about the complaint in his notes. The plaintiff yearns for validation of her reality by the court in the form of awarded damages, even knowing that such a validation will not make the counterfactual narrative any less a fantasy. A damage award won't literally give back a lost chance.

The plaintiff must rest a claim of lowered survival chances on her concrete prognosis. Such numbers can never prove that an error will have caused a death, in part because experimental knowledge depends on reproducibility. In medical trials, results can be reproduced in a population study, but an individual person's outcome does not bear one way or the other on the legitimacy of a particular trial result. The population is produced by gathering a series of preset standards, such as age, stage, and spread of cancer. But the dividing cells, unique in each person's body, stand as the antithesis of such standardization (which indeed is why we need the population studies in order to understand a cancer's potential behaviors). Such communal data may guide an oncologist, but they don't much help the person standing in court.

One decisive 1991 California case makes this conflict clear. In *Elaine Dumas v. David Cooney,* the plaintiff's husband had died of lung cancer. Had his tumor been discovered at the moment of misdiagnosis, his survival chances would have been 67 percent. On the tumor's eventual discovery, his chances were 33 percent, and he died. The court didn't deny the reduced chance of life, but worried that legal acceptance of the lost-chance doctrine would destroy the very integrity of the tort system, which "attempts to ascertain facts to arrive at the truth." The court held that "if the acts of the defendants *did not actually cause* plaintiff's injury, then there is no rational justification for requiring defendants to bear the cost of plaintiff's damages."[33] Because medical statistics cannot provide this level of specification, certainties of causation were impossible to determine (he might have died even with the higher survival chance); the judge therefore dismissed the case.

From one perspective, the court's decision does not serve the cause of "truth" any more than an opposite decision would have; it merely claims that prognoses don't, and can't, satisfy burdens of proof.[34] An example from the futures market can help to illustrate this situation.

Historian Theodore Porter explains in his book *Trust in Numbers* how the development of commodities trading required uniform categories—a drastic switch from the previous notion of barter. In the stock market, you no longer gave a trusted neighbor a dollar for a chicken that you could see was healthy and plump. Rather, one gave a few dollars for a few anonymous, unknown, even future chickens. All chickens were considered equivalent, simply by virtue of an abstract notion of chickenness. In tracing this displacement of concrete things by conceptual numbers, Porter writes: "In the end, bureaucrats and traders managed to create what had never existed on farms, much less in nature: uniform categories of produce. Thereafter, wheat could be bought and sold on the Chicago Exchange by traders who had never seen it and never would, who couldn't distinguish wheat from oats."[35] Plucking a patient from a prognostic category parallels the selection of a grain of wheat from a silo, in that the attributions of each single granule will vary widely from the average. Past experience with the neighbor's farm produce has no bearing on the future success, or quality, of one's stock holdings, nor on the quality of the commodity being traded.

Similarly, courts must try to figure out—with little to go on—how the one particular patient on the stand may compare to others in the category, and the only way to do that is by laying out necessarily arbitrary standards of proof. Examining each case individually, as the court must, carries the implicit drawback of not being able to trace patterns or to make decisions about fair or just medical standards of care and how the medical system should be responsible for upholding these standards. In the end, the court can't pin down, blame, or hold cancer to account, any more than other experts can. Thus, medical malpractice law serves to strengthen the aura of cancer as a quasi-mystical, ungraspable cultural and biological phenomenon.

STATISTICAL MYSTERY

One example of the way in which the misunderstanding of medical malpractice law as a system of blame has worked in the derailment of the whole system can be drawn from Atul Gawande's acclaimed book *Complications: A Surgeon's Notes on an Imperfect Science*. This book provides a compelling account of his training to become a surgeon, and the reader gets an inside perspective on surgery's particular mode of physical labor, which requires cutting into other humans; the enormous risks of such endeavors; and the great faith we place in surgery's efficacy, as against the huge costs and side-effects, which nearly seem to require the "great man" philosophy on which the profession has modeled itself. While some debates in the profession have drawn an outside audience, by and large medical professional debates have remained internal.

His story brings together all the elements of a wonderful adventure—life, death, close calls, quick decisions, emergencies, and attempts to save lives in a system that seems often to work against him. In one instance, Gawande recounts his inability to perform an emergency tracheotomy on a patient. He readily admits his own shortcomings in the event: he does not call for help soon enough out of hubris, he doesn't have enough light or suction, and he is so inexperienced that he makes his cut horizontally rather than vertically. The patient survives only thanks to a last-minute stroke of luck, when another physician takes over and inserts a pediatric breathing tube.[36]

This example, coming early in the book, does critical work on several levels. First, it factually records a horrifying instance of an improperly trained doctor with ego pressures and insufficient institutional support involved in a potentially fatal procedure. Second, the reader understands this instance to represent a commonplace event in hospitals. Meanwhile, Gawande labors to convince us that the training of surgeons requires just such risk and cost to real flesh. Third, the incident provides an opportunity for Gawande to explain the procedure for the disciplinary review of such events (the weekly Morbidity and Mortality Conference, or M&M). And fourth, the story, together with others in the book, invites the reader to share in Gawande's experience as a surgeon, through its use of key literary strategies that subsume the power differentials between doctor and patient. (For example, he comments that once his patient is able to breathe, Gawande is as well, as if the held breath of a stressed professional were equivalent to a patient actually suffocating on the operating table.)

Through this conversational tone, *Complications* makes a hard-hitting political argument: a doctor is a flawed but, perhaps more for that, valiant creature. The reader cannot help but empathize with this narrative, in which the intrepid surgeon slogs away in a system that could be better. He rightly focuses on potential improvements to the medical system, but in so doing backgrounds the way in which power differentials infuse the meanings of illness in America.

The disciplining that Gawande received after this failed procedure consisted of a reprimand by a senior colleague. Gawande's feelings and the private interactions among the surgeons take precedence in the retelling. There was no informing (or even discussion of informing) the patient or the family about the long period of oxygen deprivation and extraneous cuts and stitches, no apology to the patient, no discussion of compensation, and no consideration of systematic changes that could have led to the situation being avoided in the first place. Rather, in thinking through surgical discipline and responsibility, Gawande turns to a posture about medical malpractice law: "There are all sorts of reasons that it would be wrong to take my licenses away or to take me to court. These reasons do not absolve me. Whatever the limits of the M&M, its fierce ethic of personal responsibility for errors is a formidable virtue. No matter what measures are taken, doctors will sometimes falter, and it isn't reasonable to ask that we achieve perfection. What is reasonable is to ask that we never cease to aim for it."[37] The reader, however, learns little about what this "personal responsibility" actually means.

Gawande sidesteps the two most controversial questions raised by his book. First, what should happen to those patients who provide the meat on which surgeons practice their highly remunerated craft? While readers may agree that practice on real patients is a necessary evil, they may also want some recognition of the human costs of on-the-job training. In discussing how people unwittingly donate their bodies to the cause of training surgeons, Gawande readily admits that he would never allow a student to cut into him or a member of his family. A discerning reader will see class and education differentials affecting the receipt of medical care. Second, had the botched tracheotomy ended in a death, how would it have been explained? As an unpreventable accident? As an acceptable outcome of an emergency situation? As a compensable medical error? Even in the best-case scenarios, analyses and judgments are made behind closed doors, during the surgical M&M meetings. Surgeons will make mistakes, and when they do, they should not be taken to court.

Medical malpractice law operates on a parallel but opposite basis. In the law's alternative view, the court should be called on to adjudicate reasonable amends *precisely* when a doctor injures a patient.

In their understanding of the law, medical practitioners often confuse several issues. Gawande mistakes the individual surgeon who has to learn and who will make mistakes throughout his career for someone who should be responsible for those mistakes only to the profession (and not to the patient). He further confuses the compensatory function of law for a moral system of blame—a pervasive confusion in medical professional culture. While he admits to feeling shame (feelings in a man are good to see, although how would such sentimentality have gone over had the author been one of the 3 percent of surgeons who are women?), he ignores the questions of patient knowledge of error or whether patients being practiced on should pay reduced rates for care—a medical scratch and dent sale, so to speak.[38] Aiming for perfection is certainly an admirable goal, but structural challenges render it impossible.

Increasingly, the nostalgic view of a doctor's job does not match the realities of medical labor in a time-squeezing, for-profit system.[39] For example, two vastly different drugs, magnesium sulphate and morphine sulphate, can be written the same in prescription shorthand, MS (though they now appear on a "do not abbreviate" list). Or different drugs are stored in similar packaging and placed near each other in storage areas. The way that American health insurance works also means that patients change doctors often, making it virtually impossible for physicians and patients to build relationships or even for complete patient records to be maintained. Physicians, then, may not have the personal patient history necessary to make accurate diagnoses.

In the 1970s, a method for understanding medical error focusing on the root-cause was introduced. In early 1978, the engineer Jeff Cooper published a paper documenting his study of human error in anesthesia, which at that time led to the deaths of 3,500 Americans a year, even with a doctor dedicated solely to administering the drug and watching the patient during surgery. Taking system design into account, Cooper found that although oxygen monitors had been available for years, no one used them. Moreover, the machines were not standardized: on some, one turned the knob to the left for more oxygen, and on others one turned the knob to the right.[40] Cooper concluded that improved and standardized machine design could significantly reduce errors.

While widely discussed at the time of its publication, the study did not lead to systematic changes. Finally, Ellison Pierce, the president of the Society of Anesthesiologists, mobilized the society to focus on the problem after a friend's daughter died during a routine procedure. Like so many things, the issue had to become personalized for a powerful person to provoke action.

Here again, medical malpractice law has failed to step up to the plate. In many areas of injury law, a jury can find that an industry has "unduly lagged"; that is, an industry that fails to adopt new and safer technology can be found negligent. But, according to the late law professor Gary T. Schwartz, "in malpractice cases—and these alone—the jury is typically deprived of this power."[41] Therefore, the medical profession retains the power to define what will count as a negligent practice.

In one notable exception, in 1956 a judge examining a case in which a surgical clamp had been left in the body of a patient determined that it "requires no expertise to count" clamps, even though at that time it was not the usual practice.[42] Even as of this writing, 99 percent of hospitals still rely on those highly faulty counting procedures of the 1950s rather than using tracking devices that could detect left objects for less than $10 and a few seconds per surgery. One doctor has put it this way: "We've anesthetized them, we take away their ability to think, to breathe, and we cut them open and operate on them. There's no patient advocate standing over them saying, 'Don't forget that sponge in them.' I consider it a great affront that we still manage to leave our tools inside of people."[43] For better or worse, physicians serve as the gatekeepers to the standards of their profession and law seems impotent to assert protective changes.

Medical malpractice law can be used at least in theory to counter systemic discrimination in healthcare. When plaintiff Merle Evers presented her doctor with a breast lump in 1977, she was told to "go home and relax." Six months later she had a mastectomy, and five years after that metastasis appeared in her lung.[44] Myra Kennedy had a similar experience in 1983, when she was also told "not to worry," advice that was repeated a year later. By 1985 the cancer had metastasized.[45] In these instances, lawsuits could be seen as attempting to ensure that doctors do not dismiss women's concerns as simple misgivings but rather follow up reports of symptoms to ensure accurate diagnoses. Proponents of medical malpractice laws consider their activist nature a critical function, bringing attention to otherwise invisible injuries.

Gawande's book and Cooper's study negotiate a central mystery of medical practice: the fact that a doctor simply will not perform flawlessly every time. This is truly a bind—the very one that tort law was designed to acknowledge. Each patient has a right to an average, professionally acceptable standard of care, every time, in which mistakes, albeit inevitable, will be compensated for. The humanist quandary and tortured feelings of the physician (we want to do right, but we can't always; since we are doing our best, we should not be sued), shored up by the interests of the insurance industry, have somehow overridden the interests of the patient who has no recourse.

CONCLUSION: THE EVENT AND ITS TERRORS

Unlike the audiotapes that as kids some of us used to record and then rerecord music from the radio, the law's promise to rewrite history can offer only a palimpsestic attempt to tack a more satisfying conclusion onto the aftermath of a mistake. Even Madonna or Mozart can't completely erase Kenny Rogers or Shaun Cassidy.[46]

At the center of all personal injury law lies a plaintiff's counterfactual desire: *my heartbreak could have been otherwise.* By offering the potential to change the past through the offer of a more materially comfortable future, med-mal mirrors the promise of one of two outcomes of the five-year survival prognosis. In individual cases, the law's conjuring trick resides in rewriting history through the transfer of money.[47] Of course, the damages paid represent only the physical injury, and as such don't assuage grief or touch the betrayal, dismay, or terror felt on suffering medical error.

What I wanted from the tort system changed in relation to the course of the long history of my case. At first I wanted a way to make sense of what had happened—the structures that had made the missed diagnosis not only possible, but likely. Sometimes I wanted just an admission—no skin off Dr. Nordic's nose, I thought. I at least wanted her to know what had happened and to brainstorm on various routes to a counterfactual past and more efficacious future practices. Then I wanted to see how the legal aspects would all work out, how the events as I had experienced them would fit into the views of different medical and legal experts and ultimately into the system of law. Eventually, I wanted Mike to stop telling me about his sex life and I wanted to be free from these different systems of prediction and explanation—none of which seemed to be working all that well. All the administration and paper pushing that the suit required took reams of time and energy. "Moving on," as they say, provided its own counternarrative, albeit one about as satisfying as water-flavored ice cream.

In its most idealized form, medical malpractice law offers a place where standards of medical practice can be set and upheld through the close examination of those standards' failures. One thing is clear: as states continue to erode medical malpractice laws by placing caps on damages and shortening statutes of limitations, while continuing to leave responsibility for improving systems to hospitals themselves, we have fewer and fewer ways to make such often unknown medical mistakes visible as larger political issues. With no other way to collect data on cancer misdiagnosis, we also miss one of the few opportunities to study the major political and economic impact of diagnostic procedures. In the meantime, doctors remain stuck within a system that sets them loose with "little or no formal training on how to prevent medical errors and reduce preventable complications,"[48] in legal and medical systems that continue to enforce the notion that errors are exceptions to be disavowed or felt badly about rather than the norm in need of discussion, analysis, and emendation.

CHAPTER 5

The Mortality Effect

The Future in Cancer Trials

What happens if I get a placebo in the trial but later the medication is shown to work? This question appeared in a pamphlet designed to recruit people suffering from late-stage kidney cancer to participate in a trial. It echoes a key anxiety in the decision to join a trial: What if I don't get the better treatment? The answer: "If the study shows TroVax® prolongs survival and you received the placebo, you will be given the opportunity to be treated with TroVax®, following regulatory approval."[1]

The pamphlet doesn't mention that regulatory approval may take years, even decades. A person with metastatic renal cancer, for which the five-year survival rate is under 5 percent, has virtually no hope of surviving long enough for this drug to come to market. In the end, as with the vast majority of such trials, Trovax was found to be ineffective; the trial was canceled after nearly a third of the patients died.[2]

The gold standard of evidentiary medicine, the randomized controlled trial (RCT) refers to an experimental method in which researchers give groups of people different treatments and, after some time, compare the efficacy of the treatments. In a drug trial, for example, one group will get the new drug and a second group will get either the proverbial sugar-pill placebo or the usual standard treatment. Third and fourth study groups may also be added to the comparison. At the end of the trial, the researchers tally the survivors, measure the side-effects, and make a decision about whether to move the drug to the next stage of testing, a process that will require the recruitment of more hopeful cancer patients willing to try anything for a slim chance at survival.

That pamphlet offers one piece of cancer debris. In the world beyond ephemera, people fly with oxygen tanks to Texas or Argentina in their final months or weeks for experimental treatments or to join trials. Patients with carefully researched stacks of trial reports or with trial numbers diligently inscribed on a folded sheet of paper walk into the doctor's office only to hear her say, "Oh, no one followed that up," or "That's just not what we do here," or "There were not enough people in the trial to draw any conclusions," or "Yes, but those results are controversial, so we don't give that treatment," or "Yes, but the population was too varied to be of use in your case," or "Yes, but your insurance will not pay for that treatment." These collected stories epitomize the confusion and heartbreak posed by the constant promise of trials. In the long history of the rise and fall of various "miracle" cures, hundreds of thousands of patients have tried everything from radium pills to letrozole, interferon to Gc-MAF, often at great physical and financial cost. The stories demonstrate the excruciating position of patients attempting to navigate the grueling, expensive world of randomized controlled trials.

Used to test chemotherapy, pharmaceuticals, surgical techniques, and radiation, the RCT virtually defines oncology as a professional field.[3] The recent rise in stature of oncology coincided less with big leaps in survivorship than with more treatment offerings and more trials. People now stay in treatment longer and undergo more rounds of chemotherapy as the number and size of trials continue to increase. The "booming industry in clinical trials," as one doctor writes, "supports increasing interest in the development and use of various prognostic staging systems and clinical markers."[4] The constant reporting of trial results in the news media hints at their central role in shaping Americans' understandings of risk, suggesting that the things that caused cancer might have been avoided. As a result, many cancer patients carry excruciating self-blame and crushingly talk about their guilt, as if the cancer were their own fault, the result of drinking too much milk, say, or being overstressed at work. One twenty-seven-year-old three-time cancer survivor said to me, "I hate it when people talk like that; it makes me feel bad, and it's too late for me."

A lecture given at the annual San Antonio Breast Cancer Symposium (SABCS) in 2007 strikingly captured the paradox of late-stage cancer drug trials. Introducing his research with a roundabout acknowledgment, verging on thanks, of the people who partake in research trials, Mitchell Dowsett declared that "1,050 people would have to relapse before we had data."[5] Neither Dowsett's translation of lives into data, nor his use of the future conditional "would have to" fully accounts for the startling effect of this remark, which both predicts and underscores the necessity of the deaths. He foregrounds a fact usually left unsaid: the trials need—indeed, await—the cancer recurrences of their participants. One might draw an analogy to the organ transplant candidate wait-listed for a liver—literally waiting for someone else's fatal car accident or brain aneurysm. In each case, one awaits another's death, which spurs a new round of productive events.[6]

Researchers try to soften this paradox by noting that the recurrences would have happened anyway. Many scientists claim that the method requires this objectification—even, I suggest, instrumentalization—of the patient. This unfortunate by-product serves a greater good.[7] Physicians note that some RCTs have led to improved patient care: survival rates for several types of cancer have skyrocketed thanks not only to new treatments but also to the RCTs' ability to establish their efficacy.

Other theorists take issue with this justification. Historians, for example, argue that the RCT method will always produce a result. A nineteenth-century study provides an elegant demonstration of this point. The study, organized as a proto-randomized trial, examined the efficacy of bloodletting in reducing the severity of pneumonia. It found that the duration of the disease was an average of three days shorter for those who had been bled early as opposed to those who were bled later.[8] This finding did not in itself progress make, since later still, doctors found that bloodletting does nothing for fevers at any stage.

Furthermore, interests that can be difficult to pinpoint often corrupt the trial process. In histories of RCTs for many cancers, one finds promising Phase I and Phase II trials for inexpensive drugs that were then summarily abandoned, or conversely, multimillion-dollar Phase III trials that promised only incremental survival benefits. Anthropologists, meanwhile, trace the outsourcing of trials in the search for treatment-naive populations—that is, populations that do not take the many kinds of drugs that Americans do. Even if these turn up trustworthy data for a treatment-naive population, they don't accurately reflect the populations of the market for the drugs. Broader observations about the use and abuse of trials can be endlessly debated, but my point remains: a deeply embedded paradox structures the RCT.[9]

Two things I noticed while reading trial reports hint at the paradox I examine here. First, for decades cancer trials have mostly reported only fractional survival rates. The number of true breakthroughs can be counted on one's fingers and toes. Similarly, most "futures" that the trials lay out have been impossibly grim. In this sense, the trial offers not just a search for a better treatment, but a kind of shorthand for hope in times of desperation. The comment "I need a trial" substitutes for "I need a cure"; this common usage reveals the centrality of an ideology of the future, despite the trials' limited success. The vast numbers involved in the trials, the toxicity of the treatments for patients, the profits of drugs under patent for providers, and the incremental survival benefits consolidate cancer as a disease with a specific set of insights in relation to RCTs.

Something else came to my attention while I searched for information on my treatment course. I read a trial report written by one of the doctors, a pooh-bah in the oncology world, who had misdiagnosed me. An erupting chasm seemed to physically tear the papers from my hand as I realized that once in the category "diagnosed," I was useful. I don't mean that I became an interesting case in any way. On the contrary, I was a statistic. But as a statistic, I bolstered the gravitas and significance of her work. That recognition of the gap between the counter and the counted caused the rupture. No matter how much I wanted the trials to yield objective information useful to patients and doctors, our relationship to the data skewed at different tangents. She collects and publishes data—and even the kind of mistake she had made on me worked in her favor. I'm left to scrutinize her data to try to find what the future holds. Suddenly implicated in the stack of papers I had been working my way through, I realized that my use, dead or alive, was *as* data—just like those who populated (maybe peopled is a better word) the trial reports I was reading.[10]

Dowsett's comment creates a disconnect: one knows only after the data are in that 1,050 recurrences were suffered. Yet his phrasing acknowledges that he knows that there *will be* 1,050 recurrences, indeed, that there *must be,* and that these recurrences will occur in both the treatment and nontreatment groups. A subject in the trial may hope to be in the no-recurrence group, but only after the time has gone by will the subject know which group he or she actually was in. The researcher arranges these lives to figure out which treatments will be more promising, which pharmaceuticals more profitable. The final statistic will be hygienically inscribed by an omniscient observer who weighs out the benefits and the costs of a new treatment. Future cancer patients will be invited to stare at these statistics and attempt to slot themselves into one side or the other: survival or death. The RCT invites both patients and oncologists to live in a space in which both hope and progress are ubiquitous, virtually inescapable tropes.[11] However, the patient also lives in the real world, feeling better or worse, looking at the stats and making concrete decisions about treatments based on geography, timing, and money.

STRUCTURED COMPETITION

Belief in randomized controlled trials reflects a medical philosophy and a culture of health quite different from those of the nineteenth century, when physicians considered an individual's physical and emotional constitution more than particular disease characteristics in predicting the course of disease. A nineteenth- or even mid-twentieth-century physician might not have understood the logic of the RCT, let alone taken it for granted as the primary—practically exclusive—means of collecting medical evidence. Trust in numbers over clinical experience had to be cultivated, as did the techniques of collection.

The present-day appeal of the RCT surely lies in its elegant simplicity. Its commonsensical grounding remains so beyond reproach that even as physicians hotly contest the relevance of results and specific trials, the method offers medical practitioners a tightly shut black box; the method itself barely requires comment in the scientific literature. While some accounts locate the first RCTs in efforts to eradicate scurvy by comparing lime versus meat consumption, the historian Harry M. Marks traces the origins of the contemporary medical RCT to agriculture, where the method was developed by geneticist and statistician Sir Ronald Aylmer Fisher in the early twentieth century.[12] In trying to quantify improvements in agricultural methods, Fisher divided land into strips and alternated a specific treatment—for example, fertilizer—in one area with no treatment in an adjoining one. Through multiple replications, this comparative approach averaged out—thus canceling—random factors such as moisture or sun exposure, which might affect one patch of land more than the other if two large patches of land were simply compared over time. In this manner, the efficacy of the fertilizer—the likelihood that it would work on any individual sunny or windy patch of land—could be recast as a population probability in which sun and wind were factored out of the equation. Researchers celebrate the method precisely for its ability to eliminate any variable other than the one being tested.

This method of trials grew explosively after World War II.[13] RCTs are now used to study many things, from the potential benefits of physical exercise and eating greens to proper dosing of medications. Ideally, a series of controls such as age, gender, or stage of disease narrows the random factors, so that drugs can be more specifically tested for efficacy in accordance with these variables. Often, though, the quest for enough subjects requires broadening the group characteristics to enable more people to join. As trials move from Phase I to Phase III they require progressively larger groups of study participants. This affects the clinical value of trial results. In other words, if a drug is tested on a group including children, young adults, and older adults, clinicians will not know if it will work better on one of these groups than the others.

In the move from agricultural applications to medical ones, a windy or sunny patch of land translates into an old or male person, a disease becomes as measurable as an agricultural pest or the natural course of the growth of peas. The treatment of mobile, complicated individuals becomes as unproblematic as fertilizer spread on land. Remarkably, the RCT literature takes this shift from field to flesh mostly without comment. Still, the slippery markers make trials virtually impossible to compare, as oncologists readily admit. Often whole categories of terms—like what counts as "relapse-free survival"—vary from study to study, or even within studies, and among medical centers. Sometimes people in the treatment group are not treated: they fall into the category of "intent to treat," rather than "actually treated."

RCT logic is such a structuring principle of our time that its key requirement barely registers: two groups compete, one wins. Albeit evacuated of intent or skill, the trial reflects the logic of war (each side aims to outkill and outinjure the other) or the principle of sport, in which sides compete for goals, points, or marks.

In the RCT, patients compete in a contest that exceeds their ability to compete; they do not even know which treatment they get. The success or failure of the treatment will be attributed solely to the treatment itself. Stamina and fortitude of the patient, or weakness of the treatment, will be "randomized" out of the equation. Like its close kin statistical analysis, the RCT crushes life-or-death dramas in its drive for a result. The RCT erases the very human subjects that enabled its possibility, legitimating its dead through the promise of a future cure.

The simple yet unspoken premise embedded in late-stage cancer RCT logic holds that nearly all of the subjects in treatment trials will die. Even a trial for the most efficacious drug in the world will require the deaths of those in the untreated group in order to prove its worth. Thus the RCT asks its subjects to partake in the higher calling of what the philosopher Michel Foucault might have called "collective living on"—the sacrifice of oneself for the possibility of a social group. Each individual in a society, he writes, lives with the demand, "Go get slaughtered and we promise you a long and pleasant life."[14] This overlay between one's own mortality and the longevity of the society lies at the crux of the trade-offs in cancer research and treatment.

I witnessed exactly this pressure point at a lunch for cancer activists sponsored by Genentech in 2006. The representatives and scientists attempted to recruit subjects by claiming that the success of leukemia drugs in bringing about high survival rates in the 1960s and '70s was because of the large number of patients enrolled in trials—over 70 percent of known leukemia sufferers, as opposed to only 3 percent of adult cancer patients who now participate in trials (a tired statistic trotted out at many such events). In fact, chemotherapy does remain much more potent for liquid tumors, such as leukemia, than for many that take shape in solid form. But Genentech's representatives cajoled members of the audience not to let their diseases go uncounted, not to miss an opportunity to donate to the higher cause.

The RCT works in the service—or, depending on your level of cynicism, lip service—of collective living on, but who and what do we miss by rushing to that endpoint? Bodies lent to the cause of science suffer, and in many cases greatly, from cancer treatments, both standard and experimental. By promising a future it cannot know and asking patients to hurry to a sacrificial conclusion, the RCT ignores its own forms of violence and permission to harm. Its varied uses for science, capital, and professional advancement do not in themselves correspond with cures or better treatments.

To illustrate my point, let us return to Margaret Edson's play *W;t,* in which the English professor Vivian Bearing dies after a brutal course of chemotherapy for ovarian cancer. Certainly one could argue that Bearing's physicians should have cared for her more empathetically over the course of her treatment and death.[15] But the play also explores the fact that even if the medical community *had* treated Bearing more compassionately, the system still operates on the notion that the immortal logic of science trumps individual mortality. Bearing's doctors simply did not *need* to know anything about her except whether or not she would survive the experimental chemotherapy. She could have been anyone with ovarian cancer—it did not matter that she was Vivian Bearing, or that her cancer was diagnosed so late, or whether she was among the one in seven Americans who lives near a Superfund site.

In exchange for their deaths, the researcher renders individual subjects significant: he counts them. In counting them, he conjures a future—on the one hand, absorbing the individual into a potential yearned-for advantage, and on the other, further institutionalizing that fantasy of hope for the next generation of subjects. At the same time, the researcher will need to justify a new round of grant funding and consolidate his professional reputation. And in the final write-up of the data, those who read the numbers not only will not remember Bearing's name and profession; they also will not know her blood type, whether she smoked, whether the treatment was administered correctly, or even the critical details of her illness. Though some of this not-known information may be essential for future study, everything about her, short of a checked box on her cancer type and another on her treatment, will be gone. Despite the researcher's promise to bestow significance, at the end of the day Vivian Bearing as Vivian Bearing simply disappears. The deaths in the trial swing both ways, of course. Dowsett's 1,050 relapses were tallied from both groups: members of both the treatment and the placebo groups died.[16] It's nothing personal.

Elaine Scarry offers a telling insight into the political stakes involved in separating death from bone-and-blood bodies. As she notes, bodies on both the winning and the losing side of the Civil War have been explained as "the price of freedom"; in that sense, carcasses gain a mobility—and nobility—of attribution. The impersonal character of the dead body, she writes, "gives it a frightening freedom of referential activity, one whose direction is no longer limited and controlled by the original contexts of personhood and motive."[17] Once someone dies, they can be used in support of other interests.[18]

The cliché uttered at presidential inaugurations that "our ancestors died for this historic day" offers an obvious example of how potentially ignoble or unnecessary death is used to prop up a nationalistic history. The request for subjects to participate in RCTs mirrors this standard truism in American politics. The RCT brings almost a military, redemptive glory to an "unfair, unfashionable, unforgivable" death.[19] This point sheds light on the ramifications of impersonalized deaths in RCTs, a sterility of personhood that comes up over and over again in the way statistics are rerun and debated and in how the results are used for protocol, redone, or ignored. One doctor at the 2007 SABCS referred to the notorious difficulties in comparing RCTs with the comment, "It's a good time to be a statistician"[20]—meaning that disembodied results can be easily manipulated and endlessly debated because of the variety of statistical methods.

Grief about the mortality effect saturates patient-generated literature. As he was dying of prostate cancer, the writer and critic Anatole Broyard wrote: "While he inevitably feels superior to me because he is the doctor and I am the patient, . . . I feel superior to him too, that he is my patient also and I have my diagnosis of him."[21] Broyard, making himself visible—vital—in this dynamic, reclaims some of the power that the system leaches from him. Perhaps the physician reminds Broyard of a priest who decries sin in the face of the Black Death before falling victim to it himself.

In big cancer trials, the length of the trial will exceed the lifespan of nearly everyone involved, and by necessity the survivors cannot be predicted in advance. Even in one of the most successful cancer treatments ever, the use of Herceptin for a subset of breast cancers, many physicians expected another failure and expressed shock at the relatively high survival rates.[22]

Thus doctors stand in the awkward and horrible position of needing their subjects' deaths, sometimes withholding treatment, even when the treatment in question clearly extended lives. Nobel laureate Elias Canetti might be describing the principal investigator of a large cancer trial when he writes, "He is, as it were, an innocent hero, for none of the corpses are of his killing. But he is in the midst of the putrefaction and must endure it. It does not strike him down; on the contrary, one could say it is this which keeps him upright."[23]

Doctors do not necessarily enjoy this position, nor do they necessarily profit from it. But cancer deaths do support both the research and the researcher; they support whole industries and economies, however one measures success. Indeed, the bigger a problem cancer becomes, the more trials we need. Suffering and death undergird a system that works differently for different participants, constructing some members as experts and others as dependents. Stating the paradox of the mortality effect this baldly enables us to see how the RCT creates a temporal hierarchy in which the mortality of some props up, or allows, the immortality of the others. This mortality effect, however necessary, intensifies the hierarchies of medicine.

NERVE GAS

Medicine justifies this mortality effect with a logic: the costs to those in the trial will be made up for by broader social and medical benefits. Both the trial and the commonsense rationalization appear to be as objective as they are necessary. Then again, any logic has ways of discounting factors that don't fully merge with its worldview. Even cases that initially appear beneficial crash and burn in ways that should be more public. Edson and Broyard, cited above, offer one way to understand the patient's excision. The trials themselves offer another place to turn. Specifically, chemotherapy trials, with their high stakes, initial promise, high-tech medical and statistical infrastructures, yet overall failure, offer a unique place to see the excision of treatment injuries.

Where survival (or death) offers the endpoint of the trial, The questions of quality of life and quality of death often disappear. The radiation oncologist and historian Gerald Kutcher writes that complications are "presented as a stepchild of survival and characterized with qualitative terms like minimal and acceptable."[24] When a person counts only insofar as he or she lives or dies, the medical descriptions of suffering shift nearly invisibly. The consequences of this seemingly small elision are huge.

As a result, injuries gain a frightening invisibility and thus are easily misrecognized in the name of future progress. Current suffering and the questions it raises are illegible: Is the suffering due to the initial (natural?) cancer or the treatment? Are people dying of the cancer or the chemotherapy? To what extent is suffering acceptable, and who should decide? How are people living with, and dying of, cancer? Unlike survival rates, treatment injuries and complications have no complex statistical methods to measure them. This structure redoubles the assumption that suffering is by nature contextual, unquantifiable, and personal.

During my treatment, I took a chemotherapy drug called epirubicin every three weeks. Although doctors sometimes call it the "red death" (red for its color, death for its ferocious side-effects), I accepted this chunk of technology as the most aggressive treatment available. I met it in a dull hospital room that still nauseates me even to think about, a nurse's hands at one end of a plastic tube and a needle at the other. My insurance paid for it. A piece of the curative regime, epirubicin promised that something, *something,* was being done. I was glad to be partaking in this regimen, its promise.

Epirubicin became part of my self-image of toughing it out, toughing out the hardest possible chemotherapy because if I were tough enough, cancer would be scared away. I could handle the red death. About three years later, researchers determined that the red death only changed the survival stats for those with a small subset of cancers—a fact I knew through my reading, not because any of the treating docs mentioned it. The initial testing categories had been far too broad, which led to many hundreds of thousands of needless injuries before more precise data were gathered. The later results both do and don't mean that I shouldn't have undergone that treatment. I did want the most aggressive treatment available, and that was it. At the same time, it did no good.

Support group discussions, memoirs, graphic novels, and cancer stories reiterate the high physical and social costs pervasive to rituals of chemotherapy.[25] The treatment still involves severe side-effects for many people, even with vast improvements in antinausea drugs. Patients receive the drugs at the upper limit of tolerable toxicity, often measured in relation to body weight, in order to have the best chance of killing cancers. Many chemotherapy drugs come with maximum lifetime doses.

Chemotherapy treatment aims to kill cells as they divide. Despite the term *targeted chemotherapy,* the treatment takes aim at all quickly dividing cells, thus affecting not only cancer cells (one hopes), but also bone marrow, blood cell production, digestion, and hair growth—collateral damage, so to speak. Unlike surgery, chemotherapy offers systemic treatment, correlating with the theory that cancer spreads throughout the body in undetectable micro-metastases. Typical immediate side-effects include intense nausea, bleeding mouth sores, inability to fight infections, and exhaustion. Longer-term side-effects can include fatigue, cognitive impairment, heart injury, and leukemia. The remarkable success of chemotherapy after World War II transformed once-deadly diseases such as some types of lymphoma, leukemia, and testicular cancer into largely curable diseases, in the process turning these cancers (and those who have survived them) into oncology poster children who propagate the promise that with enough funding and enough people signing up for trials, all cancers will one day be curable. Chemotherapies for cancers of the lung, pancreas, brain, breast, and colon have been less successful.

Even so, refusing chemotherapy has a moral cast to it, as if one were inviting death by cancer; indeed, if a doctor does not offer chemo for Stage II, III, and IV cancers, no matter what the kind, it would constitute medical malpractice. At the same time, technical developments such as implantable ports for easier administration of drugs and better antinausea medication enable physicians to prescribe back-to-back rounds of different drugs, thus altering the toxicity trade-offs.[26] Chemotherapy offers another example of how the benevolent cast to RCTs render invisible the injuries and suffering from treatment.

Some examples from breast cancer history best demonstrate the tribulations of trials, because of the range in success. Following a 1976 trial in Italy, American oncologists largely, though not without controversy, adopted chemotherapy as a standard treatment. With a fourteen-month follow-up of 386 patients, the trial demonstrated a small increase in survival and was hailed by the media as "spectacular" and "monumental."[27] But as journalist and activist Rose Kushner documented at the time (discussed in the introduction of *Malignant*), and others have traced out since, oncologists disagreed over the trial's validity given the small number of patients involved and the inclusion of both pre- and postmenopausal subjects.[28] Nevertheless, the lack of other treatments, together with a general craving in the field to demonstrate medical progress after Nixon's 1971 declaration of the War on Cancer, led the profession to adopt as protocol CMF (combining three anticancer agents: cyclophosphamide, methotrexate, and 5-fluorouracil [5-FU]).

Since the 1970s the main change in the CMF regime has been the addition of a class of drugs called anthracyclines (among them my so-called red death). Despite a decades-long hesitation in testing anthracyclines because of their extreme side-effects, a 1998 study showed a 4 percent survival increase when they were added to the CMF treatment. This led to approval by the Food and Drug Administration (FDA) in 1999 and to widespread use of the drug soon after. For about ten years, anthracycline treatment was the standard of care for breast cancer patients at Stages II, III, and sometimes I, in hopes that each patient might be one of those 4 percent who received some benefit.

This changed again in 2007, when a team led by Dennis Slamon, an oncologist at the University of California, Los Angeles, announced that it had identified which people were likely to benefit from the more toxic anthracycline-based chemotherapy. In a presentation at the SABCS that year, Slamon claimed that "the use of anthracyclines in . . . treatment of all breast cancer is not supported by the existing data. Given the known long-term . . . toxicities of anthracyclines . . . other approaches to the . . . treatment of breast cancer should now be adopted."[29] This was indeed a breakthrough, as my interviews with oncologists during the meeting attest—although it is perhaps better thought of as a negative breakthrough, since it nullified one of the few "improvements" in chemotherapy of the past thirty years. It also made clear that between 1998 and 2007 nearly a million people were administered a toxic drug that has not helped them, a fact that went unmentioned at the conference. In fact, the scope and breadth of the resulting injury from the wide use of anthracyclines has barely been mentioned in the oncology literature more generally. How did these injuries get explained away? What could we learn by taking them seriously?

RCT methodology relies on a critical principle: that the cancers affecting all patients in a trial are similar enough that the patients can be said to have the same disease. Medical historian Charles Rosenberg has examined the historical contingency of such diagnostic categorization and concludes that diagnosis "labels, defines, and predicts and, in doing so, helps constitute and legitimate the reality that it discerns."[30] In other words, in the process of identifying disease categories, trials also construct them. The categories, reiterated and fortified, reverberate through treatment protocol, insurance bureaucracies, the press, and other processes that need and rely on categorization. So on the one hand, a trial needs a disease category in which all patients are similar enough to cohere into a group. On the other hand, cancer treatments in the last centuries or so have borne a conviction: that people with cancer will, and should, undergo pretty much anything. One physician has named this burden the "toxic cost of cancer."[31] This combination justifies the variance in control group characteristics that one so often finds. Let me explain.

In the eighteenth and early nineteenth centuries, before anesthesia and antibiotics, women with breast lumps frequently underwent extremely risky mastectomies. Prior to cellular pathology, which enabled physicians to distinguish between malignant and benign growths, all lumps were perceived as dangerous. Amputation for that groups of patients—those with lumps—was considered the only chance for survival. In the same way that we now know which patients are more likely to benefit from tamoxifen or trastuzumab, we now know that of those patients who survived the early surgeries, those with the benign lump were more likely to survive into old age. In other words, the early diagnostic category was so broad as to include people who did not need the treatment. At that time, though, the disease definition could not have been reduced from those with lumps to those with malignant lumps. Similarly, the too-large population category misled in the case of anthracyclines; a more finely calibrated study could and should have been done much earlier.

A rhetoric of aggression, namely the toxic cost of cancer, offers one avenue to defend treatment injury. Confusion between aggressive and efficacious treatment pervades the chemotherapy literature. When I asked an oncologist at the SABCS about the anthracycline news and how it would change his approach to treatment, he told me that he would immediately stop using anthracyclines except for patients with advanced cancers. For them, he said, he would want to "shoot from both barrels," even where the specific diagnosis did not fall into the category of those who were helped by the drug.[32]

This conflation of aggression and benefit reflects another treatment disaster, the use of high-dose chemotherapy (HDC) as a treatment for breast cancer. The procedure involved removing up to a quart of the patient's bone marrow before giving an otherwise lethal dose of chemotherapy, keeping the patient in isolation to prevent infection, and then replacing the marrow. Clearly, it was dangerous—in one Phase II trial, ten of the sixty-five patients died in treatment. No one keeps data on how many people undergo which treatments, but an estimated 23,000 to 40,000 women in the United States received the treatment, using drugs that had been approved by the FDA for other purposes. The completion of Phase III trials, delayed because so many people feared being put into the placebo arm of the trial, showed it to be of no benefit over standard chemotherapeutic treatments.[33] Some physicians believe that HDC treatment became popular because of its profitability. Patients also wanted the most aggressive treatment available. Several people explained to me that they wanted to know that they had done everything possible so they'd have no regrets on their deathbed. I knew what they meant: after all, I had chosen the red death. Aggressive treatment offers regret insurance.

As long as patients are understood to be living in a state of emergency, in some sense already dying, then the treatments are always already warranted, even when they kill the patients or when the physicians could have known better, sooner, with more carefully designed trials. The anthracycline example offers only one of many cases in which a too-diverse initial trial population has led to vast treatment injury. The formation of such treatment groups may be innocent, accidental, unavoidable, or it may be the result of greed, sloppiness, or unexamined protocol. Either way, the human and social costs are not separate from the so-called real science of which chemicals are produced, how treatments are used, and what cancer looks like in the collective of bodies that the treatment affects.

CONCLUSION: VITALITY EFFECT

"Why wage war?" asks Elaine Scarry in trying to figure out the centrality of injury in combat. A chess game, she suggests, could settle an international dispute as well as a war could, if all parties agreed on the terms. Despite the centrality of injury—indeed, of outinjuring—in war, she notes the key omission in most accounts. Just think of the Civil War dead. No one mentions the infected bayonet wounds in inauguration speeches. Acknowledged but justified as a by-product, treatment injuries, like war injuries, are explained away as "something on the road to a goal, or something continually folded into itself as in the cost vocabulary, or something extended as a prolongation of some other more benign occurrence."[34] In its parallel mission to "outheal," oncology literature glosses over injuries through narratives of hope and aggression or attributes them to new primary causes (leukemia becomes a standalone disease, rather than a radiation-based injury).[35] As in any war, no matter the winner, everyone loses something.

Themes of competition and war complement each other so well we hardly notice. Yet they disguise several questions. What is the ethical difference between treatment injury and cancer injury? How much time should elapse between distinctions in diagnosis and the continued use of prior categories in new trials? What can we make of the fact that treatments at least as promising as anthracyclines never make it to the Phase III trials, which cost so many millions of dollars to run? Where does responsibility rest for these injuries and false hopes amid so much profit?

Many patients do accept the risks of treatment injury over the risks of cancer, even when the chances of cancer death are low and those of treatment injury are high (though often neither alternative is well understood). In addition, cancer patients have long been used as guinea pigs for experimental treatments with radiation and chemical poisons—sometimes with their consent and sometimes not, sometimes leading to efficacious treatments but usually not, often producing enormous wealth for someone else. This history raises questions about dying humans as experimental subjects, as natural resources, and as health-care consumers in a capitalist economy. These questions cannot be asked if injuries and profits are explained away as side-effects of failed but valiant attempts to find a cure.[36]

I don't wish to argue that the RCT method has no role or that there is some better method out there. But we can trace a process—maybe necessary, but not without consequences—of shifting responsibilities: away from the stinking failing flesh of the patient (attitude is so important), from patient to doctor (here are yet more treatment options and promising trials), from doctor to pharmaceutical firms, from pharma to research subjects. RCTs present a bumpy route—often taking decades, mistaking diagnostic categories and groups, causing patients undue suffering, and rendering highly debatable results of unclear clinical value. In other words, cancer's default front line offers no clear path toward conquest.[37]

Three hundred years ago, a bite test may not have been the state-of-the-art method for testing currency, but it could divulge the softer lead that lay at the center of a counterfeit gold coin. In like fashion, an advantageously positioned nibble can reveal the sometimes shaky conjectures that buttress the evidentiary gold standard of cancer treatment.

CHAPTER 6

Inconceivable

Where IVF Goes Bad

As I sat in my cancer group wondering if it would be rude to reach across the coffee table for yet another scone clumped with clotted cream and strawberry jam, one of the women began talking about egg donation. In our meetings we take turns speaking about anything that happens to come up—treatment options, relationships, children, drugs, side-effects. That week, an informal tally of our smaller-than-usual group revealed that two women had been egg donors and two others had taken fertility drugs. Granted, the tiny gathering skewed 100 percent toward those with cancer. But research of any kind starts with an open question, and I had always wondered about a potential connection between the hormonal drugs I had taken in 2000 to enable my former partner to have children (I was on the donor side of the room) and the cancer that was found four years later.

In Vitro Fertilization (IVF) refers to a process of removing eggs from a woman's ovaries, combining them with sperm, and then implanting the resulting embryo into a woman's body.[1] In 1983, a live birth resulted by extracting an egg cell from one woman and implanting it into another, and the first donation program started in 1987.[2] For the donor, although the extraction of one egg doesn't require it, drugs are almost always administered to stimulate the production of extra egg cells (also referred to as ova or gametes). Hormones also stimulate the uterine tissue of the birth mother to encourage an implanted embryo to develop into a fetus. Donated eggs account for over a quarter of IVF live births, even though only about 12 percent of IVF procedures use them.[3] In other words, while donated egg cells account for a mere 3 in every 200 births in the United States, the practice underpins the very viability of a multi-billion dollar industry whose success rates would be too low without them.[4]

Despite (or because of?) the centrality of IVF to the formation of American families, my research into the long-term effects of hormone drugs on fertile women who have undergone egg extraction was in one way straightforward. Quite simply, no one tracks donors to try to understand the physical or psychological consequences of donation, and in the twenty-year history of artificial egg extraction, no one ever has.[5] No protocol or requirement mandates that clinics contact women after egg extraction, and no agency collects data on subsequent health issues that a woman may want to report. Therefore, this chapter can't be about proof, or even about uncertainty, which would imply that data have been collected and their relevance debated. Easy research makes for a difficult project. In the absence of data, all I can do is examine the array of reasons for, and deployment of, proof's opposite: ignorance about the health consequences of donorship.

The IVF industry portrays the procedure as generally successful and extremely safe. IVF advertisements peddling motherhood portray sweetly swaddled babies, and the IVF clinic welcomes would-be patients with pastel-pink-and-blue walls replete with large framed pictures of chubby little hands and feet (quite different from the screaming-bloody-murder babies used to advertise condoms). When I first considered donating my eggs to my partner, I asked Dr. Yuzpe at the Genesis Fertility Clinic in Vancouver about the risks of cancer from donation. He brushed my concerns aside with a smile: "It's worth the risk," he said as he walked away. He didn't tell me that six years prior, given the dearth of research, the Canadian government had recommended that women not undergo egg extraction for the benefit of another.[6] He definitely did not tell me about a generally demonstrated association between hormone drugs and cancer, nor that the drugs I would be taking had been approved for uses other than fertility treatments and were being used "off-label." He didn't tell me that long-term follow-up on egg donors had never been done. I vaguely wondered how donating an egg would be worth any risk whatsoever, but since he'd walked away, I had no opportunity to ask further questions. Still, I silently reasoned, surely a doctor would tell me of any risks. It felt cool to be able to do something for someone who wanted a child so desperately. The physical discomfort I anticipated seemed relatively minor.

The last thing I want to believe as I nibbled my scone was that the process that resulted in two amazing kids also led to cancer (though no one would want to think that for unamazing kids either). However, the lack of research puts everyone in a bind; without data, anecdotes and assumptions drive the conversation, and any position one can take on the issue becomes a personal one. Any of the players here might be dismissed as having too much at stake in the issue: perhaps one has an ax to grind with doctors, with medicine, with progress, or with children. Perhaps doctors or would-be parents don't want to consider that they may be agents within a cancer-causing industry. In any case, it's an unpopular move to seem to impugn the Child and people's desire for one. The lack of data on the hormones used in IVF as they relate to cancer creates ignorance and confusion. It is frustrating having to wonder at all, let alone have that wondering dismissed as if it were a simplistic search for a blame, when actually the situation could not be more complex.

The time lag and the inability to relate most cancers to a specific cause have led in some cases to endless debate about carcinogens, while in others the question of cause remains effectively unnoticed. The hormones used in IVF fall into the latter category, even though IVF hormones have been shown in not dissimilar circumstances, such as hormone replacement therapy (HRT), to cause cancer. The high stakes for young women and for the practice of medicine mar the issue even further. Until the last couple of years, virtually no research has focused on young adult cancers. Yet one in forty-nine women under the age of thirty-nine is diagnosed with an invasive cancer. Unlike for children and for older adults, survival rates for young adults have not improved. Given the inability of the medical system to access young adults (due to the often limited insurance coverage), diagnose this group (due to the belief that cancer is a disease of older folks), and treat them (given poor understanding of their cancers), even a small possibility of a medical procedure causing cancer in this demographic seems like a good moment to pause.[7] The dicey medical experiment of giving fertility hormones to the young, fertile women who are recruited to donate lays bare some of the mechanisms by which cancer remains shrouded in mystery.

The relationship between the hormones used in IVF and cancer would seem to be an obvious area of research. Hormones have been used in medicine and agriculture in the United States since the 1930s for everything from fattening livestock to stunting the growth of girls at risk of becoming offputtingly tall, from attempting (without success) to prevent miscarriages, to trying to reduce the effects of aging in women. The history of synthetic hormones includes the purposeful withholding of the correlations between hormone use and cancer by physicians when giving drugs to women in the 1960s so they would not worry.[8] Still, estrogen and progesterone, considered to be the core, natural "messengers of femininity and masculinity," have been the most widely used drugs in the history of medicine.[9]

Each live birth requires, on average, four IVF attempts. Each attempt (or cycle) requires several weeks of hormone use for either one woman or, in the case of donor eggs, two women. In the United States, clinics administer about 120,000 IVF cycles annually (no central agency collects data, so numbers are estimates). Despite the immense difficulty and expense of creating embryos, each year approximately 40,000 are discarded in the United States because people either do not want to keep them, do not want to pay for freezing them, or decline to donate them to other potential parents.[10]

Several commentators point out that the lack of long-term health data means that IVF remains experimental and thus precludes the possibility of informed consent.[11] Clinics and spokespeople uniformly communicate the lack of health data on egg donation and hormone use as evidence that no risk exists. For example, a 2012 study found that the risk of breast cancer for those who take hormonal drugs for IVF at a young age (precisely the demographic targeted by egg recruiters) actually *increased* by 59 percent after sixteen years—when most were still under forty.[12] A Reuters report on this study cited the American Society for Reproductive Medicine (or ASRM, a self-proclaimed interdisciplinary group of fertility experts that represents IVF clinics) as claiming that this should reassure women, since IVF *overall* is "not associated with an increased risk for development of . . . cancer."[13] As a result of this informational quagmire and the ongoing misrepresentation of data, many prospective clients and donors, as well as potential regulators, falsely assume that the hormonal drugs used in IVF procedures have been assessed by the Food and Drug Administration (FDA) for their safety in egg extraction.[14] I, too, made that assumption.

At first, the IVF story seems to follow the simple plotline of a profitable business in need of an extractive resource (in this case, eggs). To be sure, this oversimplification is not entirely wrong. Studies have shown that many clinics do not follow even the few unenforceable guidelines laid out by the ASRM.[15] In one of the very few instances in which the

FDA has been involved with IVF, it recommended against (but did not disallow) the use of a cell line created from African green monkey kidney epithelial cells that had been used to culture human embryos. The FDA warned that this xenotransplantation could result in cross-species infection of the sort that is believed to have caused HIV/AIDS.[16]

I needn't argue here that the data *should* be collected. That's obvious: they should. One doesn't need proof of danger, a personal history of cancer, or IVF-conceived offspring to know that such a lack of knowledge and research constitutes rotten business practice, let alone medical practice. The very lack of collected data on hormones and egg extraction seems to suggest that the data are still out there to be collected and that if a registry were set up, in thirty or forty years we would know any dangers. Then again, if I had been given a consent form asking whether the clinic could track me to see if there were long-term consequences—thus suggesting that they didn't already know—I would have dropped the whole idea. I didn't want to be a guinea pig. They would have been out a client and several thousand dollars. They also would have been out of seven eggs, four embryos, and two kids: a statistics-raising event with good publicity to boot. The very suggestion of a randomized control trial would have been enough to dissuade me (as would an honest answer from Dr. Yuzpe). The theoretical possibility of data collection doesn't lead to its practical possibility, as the last forty years demonstrates.

The intentional, years-long lack of research on egg extraction offers an example of a structured ignorance about cancer, its causes, and its acceptability, another stroke in the broader picture of cancer's everywhere- and nowhereness. The same combination of fear, power, and profit that underwrites so many aspects of cancer is present in the perpetuation of unknowing, the consequences of not knowing, and the cultural acceptance of ignorance around IVF. Given women's historically limited access to reproductive freedom, IVF epitomizes medical progress in theory. But women's rights and choices take place in a context that includes not only women's access to careers (and deferral of child-bearing), but also contemporary ideas about children, notions of health and its relation to the production of the Ideal Family, and the forces of private medicine.

BE ALL YOU CAN BE

Despite the fertility industry's ubiquitous ruddy-baby advertising, it is neither easy nor inexpensive to produce a baby. Fewer than 30 percent of IVF procedures result in a live birth, a statistic just large enough to prompt would-be parents to spend between $12,000 and $20,000 or more per cycle, often multiple times.[17] Contingent on age, success rates that hover at 40 percent for women under thirty-five plunge to about 10 percent for women over forty-two. However, if older women use an oocyte from a markedly younger woman, the chances of a live birth leap to just over 50 percent.[18]

Egg recruiters, sometimes as discrete agencies and sometimes as part of IVF clinics, represent the egg extraction process in various ways in their attempts to encourage young fertile women to undergo the procedure. One broker, for example, invites women to consider selling oocytes because Egg Donation, Inc., is "Where Dreams Come True."[19] Another program plays the gamete market as if it were recruiting models, calling itself "the Agency for Superdonors, known for representing the brightest, most beautiful and accomplished donors in the country."[20] This agency encourages young women to think of the process as giving a gift, telling women that "egg donation is possible through . . . the beauty of the human heart. Without angels like you, loving couples who are struggling to have a child would have little hope." One previous Donor Angel testifies to the pleasures of giving the "gift of life to a deserving couple."

These recruiting themes reflect dual psychological tactics: on the one hand—as in the promotional material of a company known as the Donor Source—young women are invited to help further the great march of humanitarian scientific progress, while on the other, websites uphold a conservative model of procreation reiterating that the donations are for couples. These sites use language that represents egg retrieval as itself a "medical procedure," drugs as "medications," and the doctor as "your physician." The Donor Source emphasizes, too, the importance of the potential donor's kindly nature, noting that "the journey of donation involves . . . most of all, willingness to help a couple struggling with infertility to realize their dream of a child."[21] The tone of recruitment blends scientific euphemism with moral superiority to conjure an irresistible call to participate.

Anthropologist Gaylene Becker interviewed one man who was going through photographs of women in inviting poses in order to select eggs for transplant. He said, "With the pictures, you start looking at them as people, and that made it more difficult. I found myself thinking, 'This is a really nice looking woman.' Then I felt like, 'What do I care? I'm not calling her up on a date!' But it was distracting from the birth data, from the genetic factors."[22] His dilemma is understandable: After all, the people selecting eggs and sperm are partaking in a highly intimate process, one that in the case of 98.3 percent of births results from a sexual encounter.[23] The precedent and cultural expectations for flirting, dating, and mate selection simply do not exist for gamete selection. As this man experienced, the selection of a donor inhabits an odd space ghosted with values and codes from a different set of practices. Gamete consumers half cruise, half mail-order their way through quasi-understood reproductive science.[24] Another ambiguity pervades the process of gamete selection: although the buyers purchase sperm more or less as a commodity on the free market, no regulations insist that clinics test the donors or the collected sperm for genetic flaws. In this *hors la loi* frontier, it's buyer beware all the way. But of what?

The recruitment sites actively palliate another unspoken anxiety about donation: the third parent. After the announcement that Dolly the sheep was cloned from three sheep ova in 1996, President Clinton withdrew federal funds for human cloning and called on private companies to do the same. The creation of a cloned sheep created much uproar, yet the similar processes involved in egg donation have barely been discussed. One reason may be that the cloning of Dolly required three egg cells, represented by sheep scientists and the press as "three mothers." Using sheep terms, a child produced with a donor egg cell has, in a way, three parents (two genetic donors and a birth mother). If we used to disparage a child with only one obvious parent by calling her a bastard, how might we legitimate a child with three? The translation from sheep to human reproduction seems to require wrapping the third "parent" in a ribbon of discretion and topping him or her with a gift card labeled "donation."[25]

The Pacific Fertility Center's ads target the serious crowd: gorgeous young women in graduation caps or thoughtfully posed with pencil in hand. The center's booklet offers nourishing imagery (fig. 14), while its website magically turns a frightening and intrusive event (making one's way to an office, sitting in a waiting room, dealing with strangers, being poked and prodded, giving self-injections, having numerous blood tests) into one that "many of our egg donors say . . . has been one of their most rewarding experiences."[26] It is almost impossible to believe that the carefully choreographed ads use actual testimonials, so perfectly do they address every possible hesitation a young woman might have. While one plucky testimonial claims, "It's such a neat feeling to know I have helped to give new hope to a childless couple," another implies that she gets to give something away at no cost to her, since "all those eggs would be wasted anyway." If a potential donor were concerned about the drugs, worry no more: "It was exciting to see my body

Realize Your Dream Of Building A Family
Pacific Fertility Center Egg Donor Agency (PFC EDA) understands there are times when a gift from another person is needed to create a family. We are proud to have been an integral part of over 2000 donor/recipient cycles. Let us assist you along this sensitive journey.

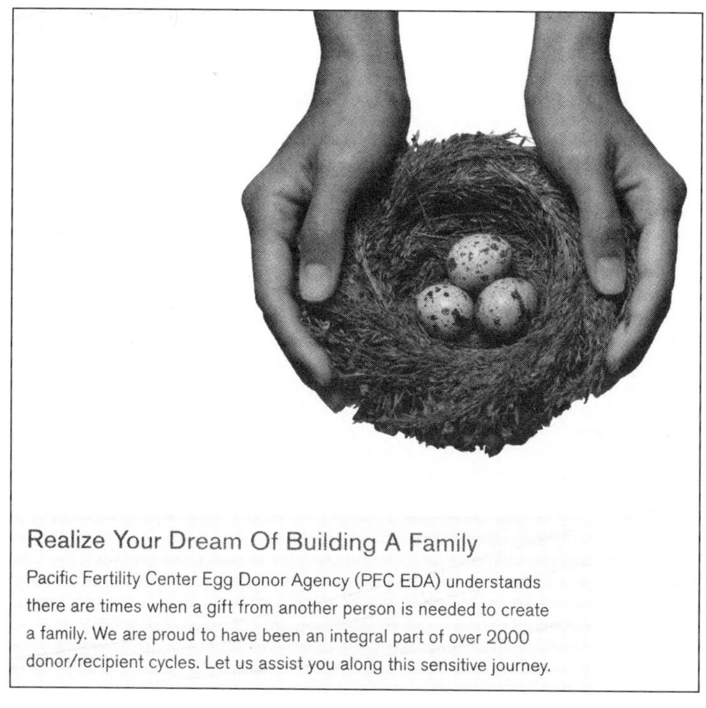

FIGURE 14. San Francisco's Pacific Fertility Center illustrates its 2012 informational pamphlet for its Egg Donor Agency with this image of manicured farmgirl hands proffering wholesome and presumably fertile eggs.

respond to the treatments as I daily got closer to giving my recipient the opportunity to bring a new life into the world."[27]

The donor who has chosen not to have children of her own provides a further insight. She found that the process gave her the existential benefits of actual children: "Since there are now three children in this world with my genetic endowments, I no longer have to feel that I have not participated in the greater meaning of life. . . . A little bit of my family heritage and myself will be passed on through them. This pleases me greatly. I also derive a great deal of pleasure thinking about the endless possibilities for their futures." It makes one wonder what social injunctions led this woman to feel that if she chooses not to procreate, she has not participated in "the greater meaning of life" and whether such loaded cultural judgment might be at issue for other IVF donors.

In another testimonial, aimed at young women who might feel guilty about cashing in, a donor offers a sympathetic spin, since she, too, was in it for the money until she spoke to an infertile couple. "After hearing their story, I knew that I needed to do something besides 'making some money.'" For another, "It was being a part of making a family's dream of parenting come true that was truly an honor." And the website's final pithy words of wisdom: "Don't give up this once-in-a-lifetime opportunity to truly make a difference in someone's life. The gift is immeasurable and the reward everlasting!" A cynical reader might well wonder if she were being exhorted to purchase a boxed set of Barry Manilow records or a pig for a Cambodian village.

In sharp contrast to the media representations of "welfare moms," who presumably should not have children at all, let alone support for those children through entitlement programs, egg-donation ads portray infertile couples as loving, deserving, struggling, and dreaming, a rhetoric that juxtaposes these victims of tragic infertility with hazy-edged photos of laughing babies and children. The noble and innocent goal of wanting a child tints the whole IVF infrastructure as similarly unimpeachable. Through alchemy, say these ads, we all can participate in the miracle of life.

Loosely extrapolating from the time involved for sperm donation, the American Society for Reproductive Medicine, in a report titled "Financial Compensation of Oocyte Donors," suggests that eggs should be priced at around $5,000. The price should not be so high that "women will discount the physical and emotional risks of oocyte donation out of eagerness to address their financial situations or their infertility problems."[28] The organization's concern implies that the physical and emotional risks are known and can be measured (and hence discounted), while this very group has consistently opposed tracking women after they've donated.[29]

Soft-focus nostalgia blurs a not so warm-and-fuzzy fact: the word *donor* actively misrepresents the exchanges at play in the gamete market. Of all the ethical and practical considerations attending egg extraction, the most vibrant ones fizz around the issues of reimbursement and payment, as we fret over the commodification of human life. Donor-payment structure reflects real-world salary distribution: Harvard donors make more than women from the University of Kentucky; straight-A students make more than C-average students. A recent report found that the price scale advertised for eggs correlated nearly exactly with SAT scores. To the young people who are the most coveted donors, even a small amount of cash can be a large motivator.

The label *donor* could more accurately be substituted with "person undergoing extraction," "seller," or "genetic parent." In addition to evading the financial issue, the euphemism *donor* bolsters the normative, heterosexual, nuclear economic unit of reproduction—ironically, given that the actual practice of IVF expands single people's and same-sex couples' ability to have children. The money doesn't discriminate; a cheap egg supply works for nearly everyone.

The following statement by an ethicist illustrates the typical divide between intent and commodification: "When people want to [provide an egg] for altruistic reasons, it's a wonderful gift. . . . When donation becomes commercialized, it raises all sorts of deep, philosophical questions about using humans as a means to an end."[30] The assertion suggests that altruistic intent in itself defers the "deep, philosophical issues," which surely range from coercion to eugenics, that a purely commercial venture might raise. This false distinction between gifting and commerce, common also in organ exchange debates, confuses a critical point. Even when the gamete is freely given, doctors, nurses, moneylenders, accountants, pharmaceutical companies, lawyers, and many others profit from commercialized, for-profit IVF.[31] Donation is anything *but* a "wonderful gift," regardless of a donor's intent and even if the donor herself never sees a penny, because it takes place within an already commercialized ethos.

Anonymity has also been used to assuage anxiety about both the Three Parent problem and the baby-exchange market. Many potential egg recipients insist on anonymity. Some others—recruiters, physicians, recipients, even donors themselves—also prefer donor anonymity. When the United Kingdom banned anonymous donation, donation rates in that country decreased by 25 percent. Anonymity is the primary reason the industry gives for not wanting long-term follow-up on donors, despite the fact that critical genetic information about the donor will not be accessible to the children. To properly track people over time, you have to know who they are.

The private, often anonymous nature of donorship can be both socially and medically isolating. Like many other donors, I didn't want to tell anyone about my plans (it's all so awkward to discuss at Christmas parties), and the family physician I saw for my required physical was not a reproductive medicine expert. There simply weren't options for getting second and third opinions, even from friends and family, on the physical or psychological aspects of what turned out to be a life-altering decision. Anonymity also leaves people exceptionally vulnerable in medical emergencies. One college student suffered a severe stroke in reaction to Lupron. Since her parents hadn't known that she was undergoing the extraction procedure, they were called in only after she was in the emergency room.[32] Medical settings often require full disclosure to ensure proper diagnosis or treatments, especially in emergencies, and secrecy or unease around medical history heightens risk.

Every once in a while I wonder why I didn't do the research myself, why I accepted Dr. Yuzpe's casual brushoff. Independent research is easy to do in the age of the internet, but in 2000 it was more difficult. Certainly email existed, but no cell phones unless you wanted to forgo the entire trunk of your car. My research that year, on cigarettes and car crashes, required me to look in old periodical indexes. Rather than simply entering search terms into a digital database, scholars back then still visited archives to round up imagery and documentation. Still, it would not have been so terribly difficult to find the harbingers of danger that had appeared by that time. My English professor friend reminds me fondly, "You were a pioneer," followed by, "and we all know what happened to the pioneers."

At that time, I had never been in the medical system aside from the odd physical exam, nor had anyone in my family been seriously ill. In my family myth, we came from strong stock. Because good health is required of donors, those considering selling or donating eggs have typically not had to deal with or understand the health system before, nor have they developed the skills to successfully negotiate the multiple demands of being a patient. At the time I embarked on the project, I thought of giving over an egg or two (or seven) as the equivalent of handing over some sperm—with injections in the place of magazines. In that trust—or naïveté—I was the perfect candidate.

In short, the system discourages young women with little or no medical experience from thinking too much about fair and legitimate payment, encourages them toward secrecy even at their own physical peril, and requires them to take untested drugs without any warnings of the decades-long history linking hormones to cancer. Often clinics underplay even the acknowledged health risks.[33] The industry represents all this as part of an innocent process in the higher service of the Family (or more accurately, specific Families). If Pacific Fertility had requested a blurb from me for their recruitment website, I would have written: "It's like signing that BMW in the showroom. Something seems fishy."

MORE IS BETTER

In 1978, British physicians announced the birth of the first test tube baby. Louise Brown's mother did not take fertility drugs, nor was she aware at the time of the procedure that IVF had not yet yielded a live birth. In this instance, the doctors removed the single egg produced in an ovulation cycle, fertilized it in a lab, and implanted it back into her uterus.[34] In the 1980s, doctors began injecting hormones to artificially increase the number of eggs produced in one cycle, enabling them to implant more than one egg at a time and thus increase the chance of pregnancy (as well as the chance of twins and triplets). Multiple egg harvesting also enabled the freezing of embryos, making possible several pregnancies from one round of superovulation. The number of women over thirty-five having children has increased twelvefold since 1970.

Central to the functioning of the endocrine system, hormones control growth, mood, and the messaging required for reproductive cycles. In the first phase of egg extraction, called hyperstimulation, doctors serially administer three potent hormonal drugs to encourage the development of extra eggs. The brain processes these synthetic hormones as if they had been produced by one's own body to magnify aspects of the reproductive cycle.

First, a gonadotropin-releasing hormone agonist (GnRHa, a.k.a. luteinizing hormone-releasing hormone, or LHRH) is self-administered daily for one to two weeks (yes, you give yourself a needle!). This blocks pituitary function and creates a temporary menopause that enables the physician to sync the donor's ovulation with that of the woman who will receive the embryo.[35] Lupron, a drug initially approved for the palliative care of prostate cancer, is currently the most popular of the GnRHa's, despite an ongoing criminal investigation into its fraudulent marketing, the falsification of data, numerous settlements for price fixing, and findings of significant and damaging irreversible effects.[36]

Second, gonadotropin is injected with Gonal-f, Perganol, or Clomid. Normally used to promote fertility in women who have a deficiency of the hormone, the overdose of gonadotropin in fertile women triggers the ovary via the pituitary to develop several egg-containing follicles. A third injection, this time of human chorionic gonadotropin, forces an extreme ovulation with the goal of producing several eggs at one time. By now you've swollen up and are doing your best not to get body-checked on the ice hockey rink.

Beyond these basic functions, the precise mechanisms of these drugs remain largely unknown. One of the main stumbling blocks for both studying and regulating hormone use is the fact that these notably finicky drugs can have opposing effects at low and high doses: low doses of Lupron, for example, "result in the ovaries producing estrogen or the testes producing testosterone; only after reaching a high dose is the drug's desired effect, inhibition of estrogen or testosterone production, achieved."[37] As a result, hypothesizing the effects based on assumptions about larger or smaller doses working in a linear, rather than opposing, way have missed the mark. Scientists' use of experimental animals that have greater or less susceptibility to hormones than humans also skews results.[38]

The Scottish surgeon George Beatson researched hormones and reproductive cancers in the 1890s.[39] His discovery that cancers contain hormone receptors that feed on the hormones either produced by the body or taken in by the body exogenously lay behind a whole series of twentieth-century treatments meant to "starve" reproductive cancers, including hysterectomy, removal of the pituitary gland, and ovarian ablation.

Despite the temptation to think of these hormones as safe because bodies already produce them, the contemporary use of synthetic hormones in no way augments a natural ovulation process. As is true with most supplements, including vitamins, just because a body produces a substance does not make it safe. A more "natural" state for women of reproductive age may well be that of constant pregnancy. In fact, the very idea of monthly menstruation is only about fifteen decades old, so in a way the cycles that synthetic hormones adjust and modify are remnants of the industrial revolution itself. Not giving birth is a known risk for breast and ovarian cancer, since the hormones released during ovulation overload the hormone receptors in those tissues. Pregnancy gives a break of nine months per child to these overloads, and over the course of two to four decades, the breaks add up. In other words, without the hormone vacations that pregnancy brings, the overloaded hormone receptors can create malignancies.[40] Most pregnant women don't think of their pregnancy as a holiday from anything except possibly tampons and taking out the garbage, but the link is clear.

The tie between hormones and hormone receptors also supports the recent finding that estrogen and progesterone hormone replacement therapy (HRT) significantly increases the risk of cancer and heart disease.[41] Many experts attribute the recent small decline in breast cancer mortality (from 178 per 100,000 in 1998 to 160 per 100,000 in 2008) to the decline in the use of HRT by postmenopausal women.[42]

Drug companies promoted HRT for decades for reducing hot flashes, weight gain, and heart disease and as a cure-all for the decreases in skin tone, muscle mass, bone density, and memory that come with aging, without any evidence that HRT could in fact fulfill such promises (fig. 15). In 2010, fifty years after the introduction of HRT treatments,

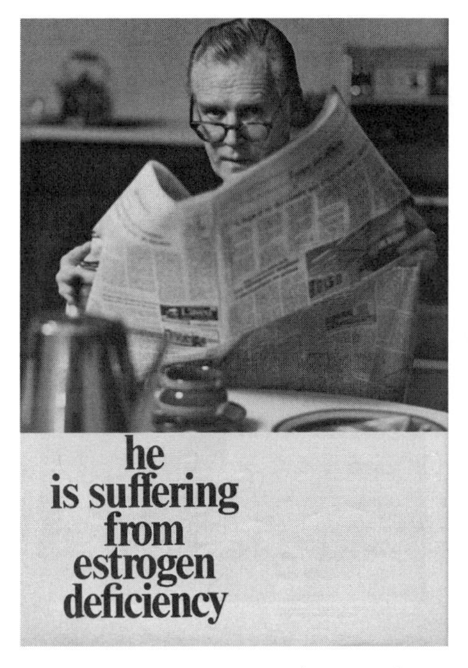

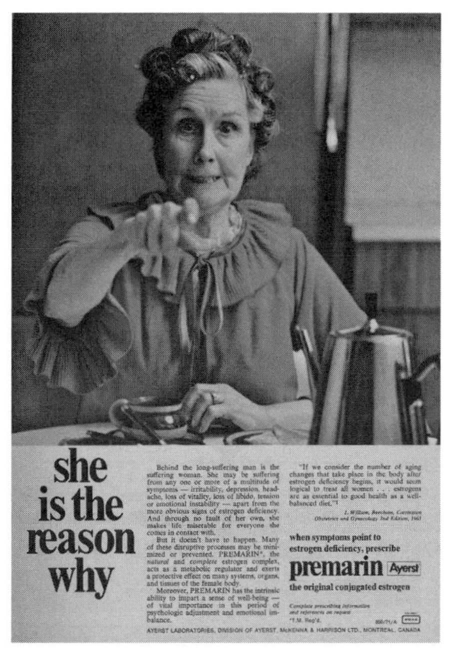

FIGURE 15. Hormone replacement therapy advertisement, circa 1960, suggesting that menopause will turn a woman into a nightie-clad lunatic who will strain the patience of her calm, professional husband. Proposing its own wet dream, the pharmaceutical company claims that "Premarin has the *intrinsic* ability to impart a sense of well-being" and should be used to "treat *all* women" (italics mine).

enough convincing evidence was found against Pfizer (the company that in 2009 purchased Wyeth, producer of the Prempro hormone replacement pill) that juries awarded millions of dollars in punitive damages to plaintiffs, indicating reckless disregard for women's health in selling the drug without warnings or adequate study. Since then, more than nine thousand other women with cancer have sued Pfizer.[43] Some plaintiffs who alleged their cancers were caused by HRT showed that Wyeth knew the dangers of hormone replacement therapy well before the Women's Health Initiative found that it caused increased rates of cancer, stroke, and other health problems; in other cases, however, Pfizer has successfully argued that cancer has many causes and therefore couldn't be traced specifically to its products.

HRT is one strand in a complex story of the way synthetic hormones have been falsely marketed as natural substances. It also illustrates how easily we assume that data are being collected and regulation is taking place as drugs become increasingly common. In fact, the opposite is

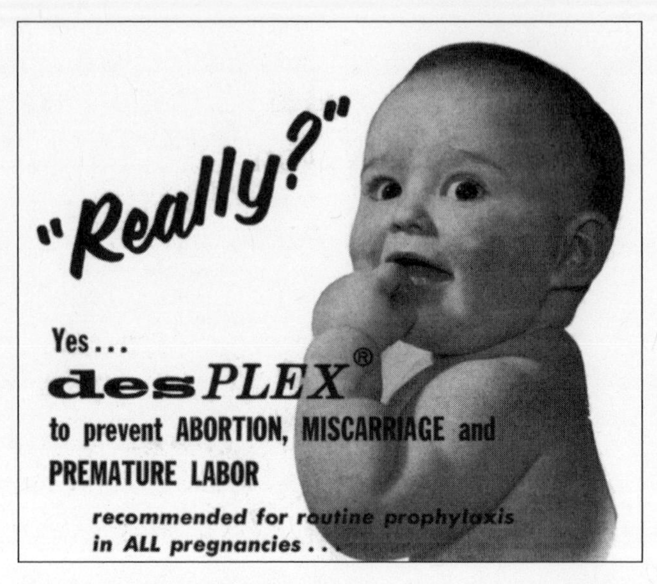

FIGURE 16. Advertisement for DES, circa 1957—"Recommended for routine prophylaxis in ALL pregnancies." (Courtesy of DES Action USA, www.desaction.org)

often true. The creeping normalcy of certain procedures and drugs in the medical field still renders invisible whole swaths of questions about drug safety. In another example of the ill-fated twentieth-century use of hormone therapies, physicians prescribed DES (diethylstilbestrol) to women for several seemingly conflicting reasons: to prevent miscarriages, suppress milk production, and, in the 1950s and '60s, as a morning-after contraceptive (fig. 16). Historian Susan Bell found evidence from the 1940s citing reasons that DES would be harmful to pregnant women. Only decades later did the true injury become evident: the *children* of those who took DES had high rates of cancer.[44] Only the rarity of the cancer types triggered further investigation; had the DES-exposed babies suffered from common forms of cancer, the correlation would almost certainly never have been made and these cancers would have been simply absorbed into the statistics.[45]

Oncologist Siddhartha Mukherjee notes that doctors have known since the 1960s that the estrogen and progesterone in HRT treatments act as pathological activators of breast cancer. He writes, "A more integrated approach to cancer prevention, incorporating the prior insights of cancer biology, might have predicted this cancer-inducing activity . . . and potentially saved the lives of thousands of women."[46] Despite this overall critique, Mukherjee doesn't press this observation to note any of the current medical, military, and industrial practices that would benefit from the integrated approach he advocates. Somehow the amount of time it takes cancer to present, so long after the possible triggering exposure, tricks us into a collective forgetting that sees us, each time for a new reason, continuing to use demonstrably dangerous drugs with nearly identical molecular form and biochemical effects.

The market for ova offers a nearly perfect example of the impossibility of enforcing, or even encouraging, better organization of the fields of cancer biology, drug marketing, and medical (or medical-like) protocols. As I mentioned in chapter 4, an injured patient cannot bring a legal suit for what the whole practice of medicine "should" or could have known, though she can sometimes bring a lawsuit against a drug manufacturer, asserting that it should have known or disclosed the dangers of a particular drug. As with any critique of large institutions, a delicate balance of power, money, class, and influence affects who gets to speak and who gets heard. The IVF industry offers a financial mainstay to many hospitals and clinics. And big money nearly always brings multiple conflicts of interest.

TERMINATED DISCUSSION

Anxiety about the relationships among birth control, IVF, family formation, and abortion has itself aborted the discussion about the status of embryos and fetuses. A full discussion of this mix would take entire libraries to address, but noting the peculiar alliances amid these interests reveals the complicated vectors of silence around IVF.[47]

By coincidence, the earliest attempts at IVF took place in New York and the United Kingdom in the explosive aftermath of the 1973 U.S. Supreme Court decision on abortion. In *Roe v. Wade,* the court balanced the government's two competing interests in protecting a mother's health and also in protecting a potential human life. Based on the Ninth Amendment's right to privacy, the court ruled that a woman can terminate an early pregnancy "in harmony with her own beliefs on the mystery of life," while states maintain the authority to limit abortions as fetuses become viable later in a pregnancy. Lawyers continued to debate the legal logic of the justices' arguments as IVF joined the miasma of discussion on how concepts of rights would relate to the many potential players in the reproductive process.

Many interests lead away from having the discussion at all. Pro-choicers worry that regulating IVF based on concern for future children's health would lead down a slippery slope by setting a precedent for valuing a fetus's right to life over a woman's right to reproductive choice: the issue at the very core of abortion debates. In this view, any public debate on IVF practices would reopen uneasy questions around abortion. Logically, if regulation of embryo implantation implies that embryos have a right to life, this right would also apply to abortion, which should then be banned. By this argument, pro-choice logic leads to a silently unregulated, yet potentially dangerous, practice. Similarly, a consistent pro-life position requires either that no freezing or destruction of embryos—a seemingly unavoidable aspect of IVF—take place.

Given the potential implications, perhaps the hush code over the three decades of IVF isn't surprising. The industry and the people who undergo the procedures have interests in this silence, and they wield considerable economic power. The average birth mother undergoing IVF is white, married, in the top 10 percent income bracket, educated, thirty-six years old, undertaking a highly visible, acceptable, and widely advertised procedure.[48] The gene pool represented by IVF participants is at face value one a nation would want to reproduce. (It doesn't take long probing cancer's underbelly to note the metastasis of some diseased social assumptions.)

A unique American politics of reproductive health offers one genealogy of IVF. Organ donation offers another. Medical anthropologists have written extensively on the unknown long-term health consequences for organ donors and the dicey ethical issues of a medical procedure which carries much risk and no benefit. Sharon Kaufman discusses the multiple pressures imposed by family on younger relatives to donate organs within kinship networks.[49] This practice puts families in the excruciating position of having to risk a younger family member's health as a trade-off against the possibility that an aging parent or relative may gain a small increase in lifespan. Complicated issues of gifting, marketing, caretaking, familial economics, inheritance, gender, and interfamilial relationship history play into these heartbreaking decision-making processes.

IVF clinics sometimes suggest that people ask sisters, relatives, and even friends and students for donations without suggesting safer alternatives. Alternatives include procedures, shown to be equally successful, that use fewer hormones or involve the extraction of the usual one egg cell produced each month.[50] These known-donor stories provide some of the most painful ones, because if the donor suffers from bad health afterward, nobody knows if it is related to the procedure. Price-fixing the gametes to make them seem more giftlike does not change the basic endangerment of actual kinship networks in the name of potential future ones.

The FDA regulates oocytes not as organs but as human tissue, encouraging the idea that egg cells and embryos are merely clumps of cells rather than personally invested objects produced with significant effort and technological infrastructure that may one day become people. Still, the egg market mimics the organ market in that, typically, older people covet the tissues of younger people (age-related fertility accounts for some 80 percent of IVF cases).[51] In that sense, IVF relies on—one might even say, requires—structural inequities among the generations as well as material differences in the bodies of younger and older people.

A recent book aimed at middle school students (yes, *children*) touted egg donation as a way to save for their college expenses.[52] (Imagine this one shelved between *Little House on the Prairie* and *Watership Down.*) Ironically, the increasing burden of educational expenses lead some women to wait until their mid-thirties and forties to have children, so they have time to pay off what they owe for their own education and to save for their children's future debts. All of these decisions take place in an economic structure downright unfriendly to the health and education of actual, existing children.

The confusion about how, exactly, IVF donorship should be envisaged—in the context of reproductive health? as organ donation? as tissue exchange? as commodity exchange?—has also led to confusing ideas about who should pay for it. Fifteen states currently require that insurers provide coverage for infertility, despite mixed research on whether having children actually improves people's happiness, life satisfaction, and mental well-being.[53] The notion of health that underpins the inclusion of IVF in health insurance seems to advocate for the notion that reproductive health means choice about whether (and when) to reproduce. The current formation of families reflects broader practices and assumptions about desire, technology, choice, health, economic stability, and consumption. Similar ideas have produced the possibility of IVF, and so it's virtually impossible to distinguish them.

The manic language of gifting and donorship muffles an even more serious issue rumbling just below the surface of fertility clinic waiting rooms and ultrasound equipment. IVF commodifies the desire to produce children in an economy less and less friendly to actual children.

The sentimental innocence of children themselves forecloses questions about the social and physical costs of how they are produced.

DATA DUMP

A recent report offers an illustration of how easily the lack of data can be manipulated to sound as though no correlation exists between hormones and cancer. In 2006, the California Institute for Regenerative Medicine initiated a $3 billion program to fund stem cell research, in which the main source of stem cells would be oocytes extracted from young women. Simultaneously, the institute convened a committee through the Institute of Medicine and the National Research Council (NRC) to examine the risks of oocyte donation. Although it acknowledged that the long-term effects of IVF are completely unknown, the committee nevertheless concluded: "The evidence to date . . . does not support a relationship between fertility drugs and an increased prevalence of breast or ovarian cancer."[54] The report cites a *lack* of evidence as evidence of *no* danger, rather than acknowledging that no data exist on the long-term effects of IVF drugs on young fertile women.

The scant research on fertility hormones and cancer has tracked infertile women, both those who became pregnant with IVF and those who did not.[55] Infertile women represent a completely different population than donors. They tend to be ten, twenty, and not uncommonly thirty years older, and often have age- or life-related hormonal imbalances related to their infertility that egg donors do not have. Generally, the first wave of research found an increase in cancers among those who took fertility drugs; this was followed by a wave of research that found no significant difference, and a more recent wave that found very significant differences. Most studies have used small subject numbers with short follow-up times to study a narrow range of cancers. To add to the difficulties of studying the effects of IVF on infertile women, the doses and types of hormonal drugs frequently change.[56]

While most studies of fertility drugs have focused on cancers of the reproductive organs, both normal and malignant cells in other parts of the body have estrogen receptors. For example, some types of estrogen have effects on the proliferation of normal and malignant colon cells.

One of the very few longitudinal studies tracking infertile women who had ovarian induction treatments found some dire results. Published in 2009, this study tracked 15,030 women who had given birth in 1974–1976 (before IVF) and found that those who did not get pregnant within twelve months of taking the ovulation-inducing agent clomiphene citrate, or Clomid (on which long-term animal studies have not been completed), had double the risk of cancer compared to untreated women thirty years after the treatment.[57] Furthermore, the median age at cancer diagnosis was 49.4, significantly under the median age of diagnosis for the average population. The results of this study may understate the issue, given the more aggressive treatments developed in the 1980s.

The authors of the study conclude that treatment exposure without subsequent pregnancy raises the risk of a variety of cancers, including uterine cancer, breast cancer, malignant melanoma, and non-Hodgkin lymphoma. This makes sense given the increased risk caused by hormonal exposure that is not offset by the "pregnancy break." The authors further point out that the few small trials that have been conducted have been inadequate to study cancer incidence. An adequate study of the cancer risk from hormone exposure would require a registry of thousands of women, which the reproductive industry has actively opposed and which the desire for anonymous donations further complicates. And then there's the money barrier: just who would fund such a study?

Clearly, a definitive answer to any association of hormone exposure and cancer would require more research, as several small studies suggest. For example, a 1994 study published in the *New England Journal of Medicine,* again of infertile women who took clomiphene citrate for more than a year, found that the women had over double the risk of developing invasive ovarian tumors compared with the general population.[58] A 2008 study advised further research on finding a connection between IVF therapy and breast cancer.[59] A 2011 Dutch study, the first to add a control group of fertile women, found that fertility treatments double the rate of ovarian tumors.[60]

Given these studies, combined with what we already know about hormones and cancer from historical examples such as DES and HRT, the connection between hormone exposure and cancer incidence seems utterly undeniable. However, consensus in the medical community is rare. Debate over the 1994 *NEJM* article on infertile women and clomiphene citrate brewed in the subsequent issue of the journal, demonstrating the differing opinions among physicians as to what constitutes adequate evidence. Several letters, criticizing methodological details of the study, dismissed the correlation out of hand, advocating for the continued use of the drug even without counterevidence of its safety.[61] In contrast, another letter cited anecdotal clinical evidence of a threefold increase in invasive ovarian cancer rates for patients who had taken fertility drugs, with a control group of 1,100. The authors of that letter concluded that, regardless of the control group size or other study details, legitimate grounds for concern exist regarding the potentially increased risk of ovarian cancer.[62]

In lieu of large randomized control trials, some medical studies focus on case-by-case clinical reports. Two British doctors, K.K. Ahuja and E.G. Simons, collected sixty such reports published in U.K. medical literature between 1992 and 1997 on a variety of fatal and life-threatening cancers that followed within a few years of ovarian stimulation.[63] The authors note the difficulty in systematically correlating these incidents to causation given a variety of factors, including the more potent drugs now used, the difficulty of tracking those who have undergone ovarian stimulation, and the requirement of physician interest in making the correlations, writing them up, and publishing them.

Because of the lack of a registry or follow-up, when cases of cancer pursuant to fertility treatment turn up at all, they do so most often in clinical case reports, blogs, documentaries, and magazine articles, venues that make the incidents easy to dismiss as individual and anecdotal, albeit tragic, cases. Although the lag time of cancer makes it difficult to attribute cause, single adverse outcomes have in the past occasionally led to the discontinued use of experimental drugs.[64] Indeed, in the face of negligible research or commitment from the medical industry, informal testimonies in the public sphere may be the only way to turn the tide from silence to disclosure.

The Ahuja and Simons report is a key document in this debate. One of the cases they reviewed involved the death of a thirty-nine-year-old British woman who had undergone oocyte extraction for her sister at the age of thirty-three. The patient file had been closed as a successful procedure after the birth of a baby girl. Five years later, however, the clinic made contact with the mother of the baby girl to inquire whether she wanted to continue to keep the embryos she had frozen at the clinic. At that point the clinic learned—only incidentally—of the donor's terminal colon cancer and death. (This is exactly the kind of information that formal tracking procedures would bring to light.) Upon researching that case and others, Ahuja and Simons concluded that these cases of cancer following egg extraction should not be discounted as insignificant, and that "empirical findings about the actual experiences of parents and children in families created by assisted conception should form the basis of future policy, rather than uninformed opinion."[65] Ahuja has since become an active proponent of compulsory embryo donation, a program adopted by several European countries that avails unwanted embryos to would-be parents, thus reducing the need for new rounds of fertility treatments.

Even one of the studies most often cited as evidence of no increased cancer risk with IVF concludes that "given the recent marketing of fertility drugs and the fact that exposed women are only beginning to reach the cancer age range, *further follow-up is necessary*."[66] The author of this study, Dr. Louise Brinton, discussed with me the virtual impossibility of tracking egg donors to find out the long-term risks. With no central registry, making the necessary correlations would require intricate methods, including finding the addresses of donors, figuring out names changed after marriage, and so on. Such a study would cost millions of dollars, though that would be a relatively small fraction of industry profits.[67] Even if a study or registry were to start now, it would take thirty to forty years to collect adequate data, by which time the drugs will surely have changed. Tracking data using population aggregates, as has been done to track the efficacy of population-wide cancer screening, will not work, given the low numbers of donors compared to the variation in potentially resulting cancers, spread among at least four or five types.

Until the correlations gain more research traction, we are stuck in our cancer meetings eating scones, hoping that future families will have more palatable fertility options. Then again, if hope is our strongest weapon against cancer, the party is over.

CONCLUSION: WAITING

A flurry of assumptions accumulate under the awning of reproduction: the idea that reproduction is a natural and healthy social and medical right, that science can help the process along, that the doctors who perform the procedure work primarily in the interests of health rather than out of intellectual curiosity or for financial gain, that egg cells should be free or cheap, that hormones do not pose hazards, and that unborn children will not have certain rights (to know their genetic parents, to not be put at risk for prematurity or other health risks).

This cluster of contradictory ideas can sometimes crowd out the active debate about each of these complex points in addition to an astonishing fact: neither clinics nor government in the United States track the main players in IVF—the genetic parents, the birth parents, or even the babies. Though couched in terms of the well-being of families,

IVF really is a barely regulated billion-dollar market. Unlike any comparable commodities-based system (the stock market, futures, meat production), this one exists without the usual legal or regulatory protections against injury or expected guarantees of the product's or contract's quality. Very few plaintiffs sue for egregious errors involving IVF; people find it galling to sue for a poorly designed product when that product is your baby.

These details of IVF, embodying the spectacular promise of science and technology and the extremes of marketing and profit-based medicine, make IVF a perfect contemporary case study for understanding the way cancer slips through virtually every means we have of making injuries visible, tracking them, compensating for them, and easing the substantial burden of future injuries. It also offers a diagnosis of how we have configured notions of choice, children, and health.

Aside from the posters of chubby baby knees and unblemished young mothers, the IVF clinic was not so very different from some of the cancer clinics I later haunted: same colors, same magazines, same distracting Muzak in the waiting room, the same brand of feminized sentimentality that sometimes keeps the queers away. (Though to be sure, I had my share of industrial, train station–like cancer clinics, too.)

Was it the first IVF waiting room experience that led me directly to the *Us* magazines at the cancer center? An untimely mushrooming of interests, from reproductive rights to free market healthcare and pro-procreation, maintains the impossibility of answering that question. Sniffing out the elements that have collaborated to maintain ignorance about the health consequences of donorship requires the painful recognition of the dearth in knowledge that may well enable the continuation of the practice. The outline of the blank space offers no more than a chalked-out remembrance, like those body-sized elegies that appear on the sidewalk each August 6 in rememberance of those who evaporated after an American pilot in a plane he named after his mother hastened away from Little Boy, the bomb that drifted gently down toward Hiroshima.

Postcancer, the dissonances gain a strange clarity. But before one lives in prognosis, before ruminating about the correlations and guessing about the intentions, the stakes somehow seem lower. All kinds of actions, even ones that in hindsight seem suspect (if not outright lunatic)—such as testing nuclear bombs in the American Southwest or giving hormones to perfectly healthy young women—can from a certain vantage point be made to seem as if they were the most normal thing in the world. Trust me.

CHAPTER 7

Can Sir

What Screening Doesn't Do

Grab your wellies: at least one guidebook recommends the large intestine as a pleasant, if mucky, place for an afternoon stroll. The Prevent Cancer Foundation's "Prevent Cancer Super Colon™," an eight-foot-high, twenty-foot-long replica of the human colon, slinks around the country with this inviting offer, while reducing the indignity of cancer symptoms by making the colon our friend. The Super Colon campaign aims to reduce the number of people who literally die of embarrassment, too ashamed to speak of the symptoms of "below the waist" cancers.[1] Another awkward one, testicular cancer, remains the largest cancer killer of guys between the ages of fourteen and thirty-four even though treatment can be very successful. Testicular detection ads focus on loving one's body, on the acceptability of touching one's privates (junk, jewels, nuts and bolts, whatever; fig. 17).

Bodies are mortifying. Then again, visits with the doctor, often a stranger, require etiquette, and one might be in a position of requiring moves that might give even a lover pause. Early detection campaigns aim to tweak relationships so that bodies can be a proper subject of conversation at the doctor's office.

Attention to the body in itself is not a guaranteed good. With breast cancer, the ethereal representation of the body part mixes oddly with a thudding materiality. Quite aside from pink ribbons, diagrams illustrating how breast cancer spreads tend to portray slim young women in

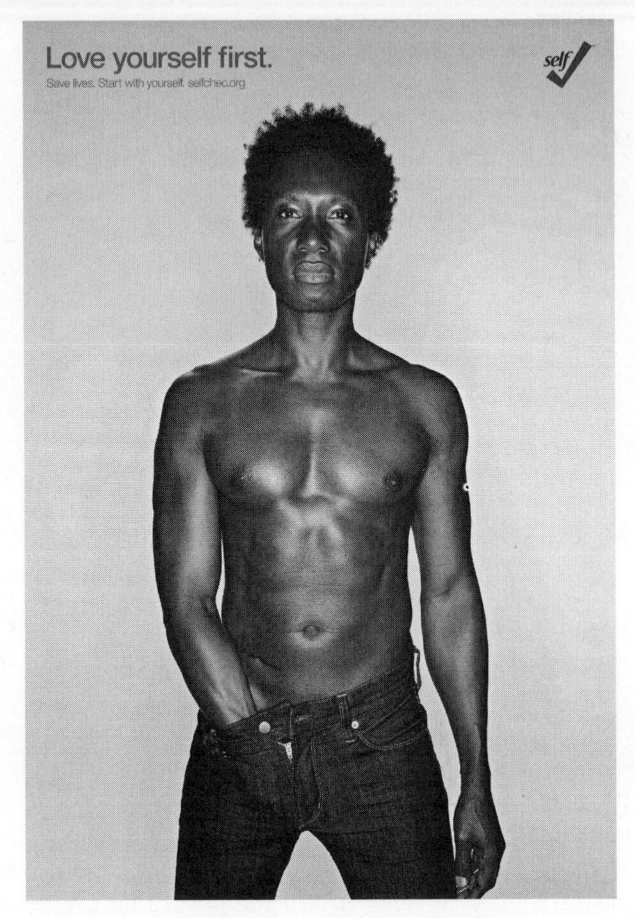

FIGURE 17. A rare ad representing a young, nonwhite person in an early detection campaign, circa 2012. (Courtesy of selfchec.org, © selfchec)

sexualized poses adorned with see-through breasts illustrating schematics of ductal and invasive carcinoma in syrupy brown pods and clusters (fig. 18). This kind of fantasized sexuality reflects a 2007 study which found that fewer than 20 percent of both male and female physicians complete the recommended two-minute manual breast exam on their patients for fear of seeming sexually motivated.[2] In these cases, propriety on the doctor side interferes with diagnosis. Regular screening with either a go-to technology such as mammography or a mandated and communicated standard protocol can at least in theory override awkward interactions and concerns about intentions.

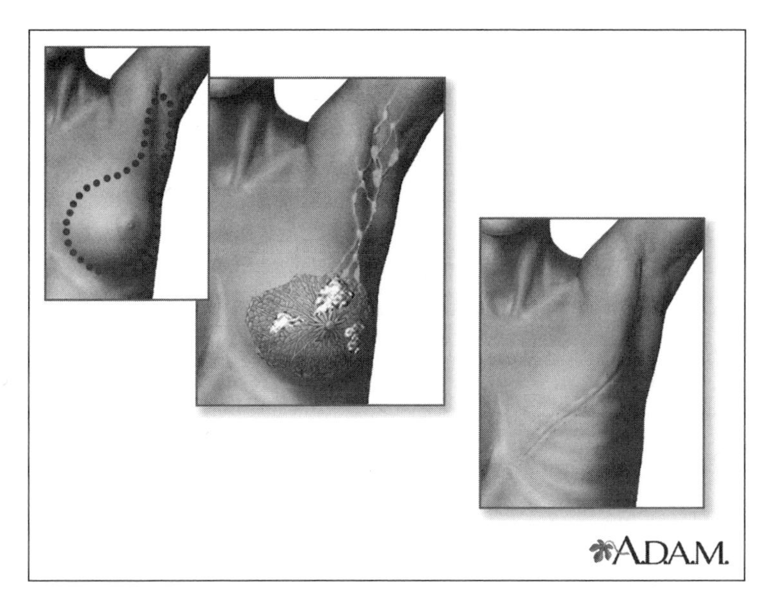

FIGURE 18. Medical diagram of modified radical mastectomy. Reprinted with permission of A.D.A.M. Images.

After a century of campaigns, Americans by and large accept screening, in which large swaths of the population are tested to see if they might harbor incipient, symptomless cancers.[3] Find a tumor early when it's small, and cut it out. This isn't just magical thinking: screening policies do correlate to stage-based survival data. The "stage" at first diagnosis predicts the five-, ten-, and twenty-year chances of recurrence, recurrence-free survival, and overall survival. The bigger the tumor or the farther it has spread when found, the lower the survival rate. Consider the five-year survival rates averaged among colon, breast, prostate, and lung cancers: Stage I, 98 percent; Stage II, 74 percent; Stage III, 45 percent; Stage IV, 5 percent. Cancers immune to early detection techniques, such as pancreatic, have higher death rates, since less than 20 percent of them are discovered before metastasis. Screening in itself does not prevent cancer; it merely detects potential cancers, at, one hopes, treatable stages.[4] This theory of a progressive development of cancer combined with stage-based survival data drives the screening industry.[5]

One early screening debacle led, eventually, toward a search for other screening methods. At the beginning of the twentieth century, the largest cancer killer of women took aim at young women, such that the *New York Times* claimed it a disease of young families.[6] By 1928, the American physician George Papanicolaou found that the "Pap smear," a diagnostic test of exfoliated cervical cells, could detect asymptomatic cervical precancer. He presented the results of his further research on 10,000 smears in 1943, in a publication explaining the technique and potential benefits of universal screening.[7] Some fifteen years after that, the American Cancer Society (ACS) began promoting the test[8]—although one physician told me that until the recent adoption of the human papillomavirus (HPV) vaccine, virtually no young women who came into her office were aware that cervical cancer was caused by a sexually transmitted virus. About four thousand people per year now die in the United States of cervical cancer, the vast majority of whom do not have access to Pap smears.[9]

With the widespread adoption of the inexpensive test by the 1970s, forty-odd years after Papanicolaou's discovery, cervical cancer mortality dropped to less than a third of previous rates. Historian Kirsten Gardner attributes the nearly half century delay between the discovery and implementation of the test to a lack of infrastructure for universal testing as well as to a lack of financial and political clout for women's cancers.[10] Sociologists Adele Clarke and Monica Caspar suggest that institutional practices had to be reorganized before the Pap smear could be widely adopted, including determining classifications of precancerous cells and training technicians.[11] Epidemiologist Devra Davis suggests that the delay resulted from physicians' interest in maintaining control over profitable surgical biopsies and cancer treatments and from a resistance to "the notions that public health agencies and nurses could conduct tests, train experts to read them and screen large numbers of people for signs of illness."[12] According to Davis, physicians understood this move as a step toward socialized medicine—and indeed, the question of who, exactly, should pay for screening remains open. These few examples only begin to show the complex stakes in screening, ones that become more slippery still for the vast majority of cancers for which the effect of screening on mortality is much harder to ascertain.

The population diversity and the decades-long follow-up time required to link screening to mortality account for some of the difficulty in gathering data. But most centrally, the screening bind reflects an intractable reality of contemporary science: knowledge about tumor characteristics remains rudimentary. Despite much talk of the potential of tumor biology to pinpoint treatment options, that science is still in the very early stages. No one knows how and when cancers spread, why and when they will grow, if they ever shrink on their own, or why some large tumors never return after treatment while other small tumors do. All this creates a major problem for oncologists, one whose many dimensions make up this book. Since we don't know how cancer will grow and spread, and when it does it's both expensive and deadly, what do we do?[13]

Well, as I've shown, we have to rely on population data—but that has led to some unique issues in the screening debates, and these issues reflect back on both the problems of uncertainty and how we understand and treat cancer. Specifically, two fundamental questions underlie, and to some extent undermine, contemporary screening debates. First: *What is being detected with screening?* Second: *Is "it" cancer, and how do we know?* In other words, the screening debates get to the very heart of some fundamental ethical issues about cancer, since once a set of cells is named cancer it opens the door to the arsenal of treatments used on late-stage disease. Whether aggressive treatment for early cancers signifies caution to the point of recklessness remains an open question. The broad ineffectiveness of these treatments even for late-stage cancers compounds this impasse and may even lead to a situation in which the treatment to some extent defines the disease.

The terms of contemporary screening debates miss these critical points by relying on evidence from randomized controlled trials (RCTs) or population data, rather than on undertaking more expansive studies of doctor-patient interactions, examining the quality of screening equipment and technician skill, and understanding how multi-pronged approaches to cancer detection might work together. The screening debates epitomize the attempt that I've been tracing in *Malignant* to locate lines of knowledge and make policy under conditions of extreme uncertainty, resulting in both over- and undertreatment. When nobody knows how to proceed (and nobody wants to admit that), certain kinds of knowledge claims come to seem most logical and therefore guide thought and action.

Internet- and newspaper-reading Americans crave boiled-down information. Many of us have been well trained to accept the kinds of everyday data that separate statistics from the material they are used to describe. Just turn from the health-section page of the *New York Times* telling you to drink more green tea to the business page with news of the Federal Reserve's attempts to regulate the economy through another set of aggregated statistics. The store of gold bullion or the marks on a ticker tape are to the economist as dividing cells are to the oncologist: a material thing that anchors a series of practices and strategies.[14] Since World War II, the fields of both economics and oncology have justified the contents of their expertise as much or more through their ability to represent, aggregate, abstract, manipulate, and advise as on their ability to cure. These experts focus not on individual circumstances but rather on separating out a series of indicators from the conditions of everyday life, as I examined in chapter 5.

Screening debates offer one site at which these processes of separation gain force as modes of knowledge and production of expertise. In essence, the recent cottage industry in screening-efficacy studies can be valuably revisited to better understand how at its crux lies a confusion about what role cancer's uncertainties should take. What good screening entails is not an easy calculation, but simple solutions ruin the problem. Refocusing attention on what we don't know—rather than trying to generate knowledge that obfuscates what we don't know—could change the terms, for the better, of these high-stakes debates.

DEBATE

Both mammography and PSA (prostate-specific antigen) testing, the main screening tools for breast and prostate cancers, have spurred sprawling, vibrant, and sometimes vicious debates about what constitutes sound science and what evidence supports the efficacy of screening in reducing cancer mortality.[15] The debates have generated a fair amount of confusion among generations of patients and doctors alike about which screening methods work and, primarily, about whether and how often one should be screened. A vocal minority of doctors has recently claimed that screening for breast cancer and prostate cancer doesn't, in fact, save lives. Furthermore, they argue that a significant number of people who are told that they have cancer undergo treatment—treatment that is in fact needless—since their cancers would not have spread. These doctors dub the slow-growing cancers "indolent" cancers.[16]

Pressing this argument further, some doctors dismiss the entire theory of early detection behind screening. In their view, most cancers *could* only be caught at the stage and size at which they actually are detected by screening. While screening advocates believe that a late-stage cancer could hypothetically have been caught earlier with adequate screening, the critics offer a two-pronged conclusion. First, screening would not have led to a late-stage cancer being caught at an earlier stage. Second, even an early-stage cancer would not necessarily develop to become dangerous. Proponents of this argument thus claim that, on the one hand, screening does little good for the people whose cancers would kill them anyway, and on the other hand, it actually injures people who undergo treatment for very small malignant tumors.

Small tumors, they further claim, may even regress on their own. These experts have influentially lobbied that policy should be changed and screening cut back.

One of the most prominent advocates of this view is Dr. Laura Esserman, an oncologist and MBA-holding businesswoman. In 2009, she and two coauthors published an article in the *Journal of the American Medical Association* suggesting that screening for breast and prostate cancers is of little use.[17] Discussion about mammographic and PSA screening raged in the media after Esserman et al.'s publication, and the debate continues.[18] A close reading of Esserman et al.'s "Rethinking Screening for Breast Cancer and Prostate Cancer" can shed light on the production of expertise in oncology.[19]

Esserman et al. claim that population data from the last two decades support the conclusion not that screening leads to the earlier detection of curable cancers, but rather that screening can generally *not* catch fast-growing tumors at earlier stages than they would otherwise be discovered. They call these deadly cancers, which emerge and grow quickly *between* screenings, "interval cancers," as opposed to the "indolent" cancers that would not have spread and would not have caused illness and death had they been left alone.[20]

Their argument can be summarized as follows: The incidence of prostate and breast cancer increased after the introduction of screening, and never returned to prescreening levels. An increase in early-stage cancers accounts for the higher incidence rates, but they find no reduction in "regional" (later-stage) cancers (specific stage-based data are unfortunately missing from the argument). They claim, logically, that if screening were effectively locating and treating early cancers, then we should be witnessing a decline in the incidence of later-stage cancers. They cite here the success of colon cancer screening in following this pattern.[21]

Esserman et al. explain the pattern they observe with the following claim: Screening does not significantly reduce cancer mortality, but it does substantially increase the diagnosis of cancers that would not kill people if they went undetected. Physicians are therefore uselessly treating indolent cancers; that is, they are "overtreating" these cancers.[22]

On the face of it, the article offers a logical argument, though it does seem to shift from offering a simple (if controversial) observation about the population statistics to a strong declarative conclusion: screening generates expense and morbidity for cancers that pose minimal risk.[23] On the one hand, the article implicates two key questions of oncology. How aggressively should cancer be treated (or, does a potentially indolent cancer need chemotherapy?), and when should many people be treated for the benefit of a few (that is, should everyone with a similar stage disease be treated when only a small percentage of those treated will benefit?)? They imply a negative response on both of these, though the debates have been key to the broader adoption of chemotherapy for treatment of both early- and late-stage disease.[24] The article offers a frustrating oversimplification of screening dilemmas by sidestepping these questions.

Five issues make the thesis logically seductive: the reliance on population statistics, the use of diagrams, the lack of discussion about screening and mortality, the lack of data on spontaneous regression, and a reliance on a cost-benefit model. Each of these can provide insight into how the debate has been structured to privilege certain kinds of knowledge claims.

The Population

Esserman et al.'s points rest on the assumption that national cancer statistics reflect an unscreened population before the mid-1980s, and a screened population after that time. This belief enables them to compare historical eras as if they represented different populations and render conclusions about screening and mortality.

The cleanest, or most objective, approach to gathering data would adopt the RCT method described in chapter 5. A study of this sort would compare a large screened group with an unscreened group, controlling for factors such as age and exposures to carcinogens, and then track both groups for the natural course of their lives. Neither incidence nor five- or ten-year survival rates alone in this case would constitute evidence for or against screening, since screening may lead to earlier diagnoses with no reduction in mortality. That's to say that an earlier diagnosis may lead to a longer period between diagnosis and death, but not necessarily to a longer life overall, thus increasing five-year survival rates without reducing overall mortality.

Because RCTs require enormous amounts of time and money, examining population data for historical patterns presents a compelling alternative. Looking at specific populations for patterns essentially involves comparing time periods as if the time periods were control groups. One finds many such examples of this approach. For instance, before the introduction of PSA screening (a blood test that measures the prostate-specific antigen), surgeons most often discovered prostate cancers while completing an unrelated surgery. This surgery started to lose favor by

1994 when the Food and Drug Administration (FDA) approved the use of the PSA test in concert with a digital rectal exam to screen asymptomatic men, so it's difficult to delink the statistics from the history of seemingly unrelated events. Still, the broad adoption of PSA screening in the 1990s correlated with a spike in prostate cancer incidence, presumably due to the wide adoption of the test, resulting in a burst of cancer diagnoses, rather than to a sudden, short-lived increase in the absolute number of prostate cancers. Those who advocate prostate screening, in the midst of controversy, tend to agree with the observation that since the initiation of screening prostate cancer mortality has decreased—from 38.2 per 100,000 in 1994 to 23.5 in 2006: as one letter-writer observed in *JAMA,* "It is not clear to us what factor or factors other than PSA screening could be driving this decline."[25] A look at the age-adjusted death rates from 2011 reveals that the death rates now are roughly two-thirds of what they were between 1950 and 1990, before the screening era began.[26]

Clear as the correlation seems between the introduction of the PSA test and the spike in incidence, the use of population data in making such general conclusions comes with perils. To illustrate, imagine an extreme hypothetical. Say the United Kingdom widely adopted a new procedure in 1920, the aim of which was to reduce the number of arm amputations. To determine the efficacy of the procedure, a researcher might compare the number of one-armed people in 1910–1919 with that of 1920–1929. He would, though, have to figure out a way to control for the amputations resulting from World War I, a virtually impossible task. The inability to retrospectively account for such "background" differences (in this case, the war, together with the rise of dangerous mechanized industrial labor) renders such historical comparisons virtually useless.

Screening studies relying on population data most often use the National Cancer Institute's Surveillance Epidemiology and End Results (SEER) database, which offers the most comprehensive cancer data registry in the United States. Collecting data from about 25 percent of the population, it collates the results with legally mandated case reports submitted to the Centers for Disease Control (CDC).[27] For each cancer case, the registry records demographic data such as race and age at diagnosis as well as type and stage of cancer, histology, and treatment. Collated each year, the data enable researchers to track changes in incidence and mortality rates. The most recent available data are generally five years old.

The SEER dataset offers complex, but also markedly incomplete, information. It does not, for example, include such information as method of detection; whether a cancer was misdiagnosed, and if so, for how long and why; whether screening was available or was done, and if so, what type, how often, of what quality, and at what intervals. Using the dataset proves complicated, as there is no way to control for these variables, let alone for the vast demographic differences of the U.S. population, such as geography, class, vocation, access to care, quality of care, diet and exercise, exposure to carcinogens, and morbidity. When scrutinizing a population defined as "the American public," these data would support only the most obvious cause-effect relationships. To illustrate with another extreme hypothetical: If one exposed a local population to a nuclear bomb, the effects would be observable without the need for an unexposed group, since the effect would be immediate, unique, and complete. But expose the global population to a nuclear reactor meltdown in Japan or Chernobyl—let alone hundreds of aboveground nuclear tests in the U.S. Southwest, the South Pacific, and Kazakhstan—and the effects become more difficult to track with pre- and post-exposed era data.

Prostate cancer has been linked to environmental toxins. Endocrine disruptors have been used since the 1930s in prescription drugs and meat, as well as plastics and other durable goods. Their effects on the U.S. population have been virtually impossible to document, since regulatory agencies do not track the amount of drugs in meat, let alone pesticide residues. The small amount of research done since the 1930s suggests that well over 50 percent of the meat eaten in the United States contains hormones significantly over the rates allowed by the FDA. Nancy Langston has traced the political and economic history of drug additives in the U.S. food supply, comparing these to the more cautious approach of other developed nations. (Europe, for example, despite the best efforts of the U.S. government, has not imported American meat that has been fattened with hormones since 1989.)[28] A population feeding on carcinogens *will* suffer an effect, even if research doesn't track it. Echoing the problem with IVF statistics, or the lack thereof: no data does not equal no effect. This adds a complicating factor, not just in the effort to account for cancer rates, but also in making sense of international comparative studies, even though mainstream oncology literature rarely raises the issue.

Combined with the SEER data, Esserman et al. rely on data about the prevalence of screening. They write, for example, that "50% of at-risk men have a routine PSA test," and "70% of women . . . reported having a recent mammogram."[29] Defining neither "at risk" nor "recent," Esserman et al. imply that the "screening eras" for these cancers adequately cover a large enough percentage of the population to allow general conclusions to be reached.

Such an assumption encounters immediate problems. A recent study found that only about half of American women over fifty have an annual mammogram, while 25 percent of women over fifty have not had a mammogram in the last four years.[30] Esserman et al. bumps up against into the problems of retrospective comparisons, without offering information on methods of premammogram or pre-PSA screenings that would bear on the diagnosis of early- and late-stage cancers. What they refer to as a "prescreening" population may be a *differently* screened population or a population with a different set of carcinogenic exposures. This matters because both PSA and mammography have become standard referents for a diagnostic process that most often requires a multipronged approach.

The definition of screening for chronic disease remains unclear and heterogeneous. Studies suggest that the quality of colonoscopies varies considerably, such that "screening" can describe several different standards of care. The length of the test in minutes has been shown to affect the number of polyps (precancerous lesions that require removal) found and the accuracy of diagnosis. Similarly, the length of a manual breast exam matters to an accurate diagnosis.[31] Another study found that charts that include a photograph of the patient receive more scrutiny by radiologists than those that do not.[32] Even for the same type of test, interpretations are inconsistent. Equally as confusingly, the protocols for what age to start various screenings and how often they should be recommended varies. It's nearly impossible to control for screening when practices fluctuate so greatly, which is one reason the trial results for screening vary so dramatically. Nevertheless, in medical articles "screening" has come nearly exclusively to indicate a black-boxed mammography, PSA test, or colonoscopy.

Making all of this still more convoluted, diagnosed illnesses that seem similar because they initially present in the same organ may in fact be separate diseases with different behaviors. For example, in 1968 the reporting codes for heart disease mortality were changed, resulting in a significant drop in mortality rates from hypertensive heart disease, with a concomitant increase in ischemic heart disease. Although the total number of heart disease deaths remained static, the changed categories altered mortality data, treatment plans, and the correlation of demographic factors to disease patterns.[33] A similar issue arises in the case of breast cancer. Mammograms are nearly useless for women under forty, in whom almost 7 percent of breast cancer diagnoses, and disproportionate mortality, appear. Indeed, as the go-to technology, mammograms can do more harm than good for this demographic, as they seem to produce evidence of a negative diagnosis rather than being recognized as a test that simply doesn't work well on younger women because of the greater density of their breasts. Distinguishing breast cancer as it appears in different-aged women, even by giving each different names, could have a dramatic impact on the conclusions reached about screening, disease behavior, and diagnostic practice.

The variety of the population compounds the diversity in cancer biology. To begin with, the notoriously piecemeal medical system results in a large un- and underinsured proportion of the population, patients making frequent changes in medical insurance providers, and people decreasingly having one physician overseeing continuity of care. Just because a procedure such as a recommended screening is a standard of care does not guarantee that even a small majority of people will get it. As we've seen in other chapters, aggregates that are too diverse have not much explanatory power.

Trials that attempt to measure the efficacy of screening by using population data without a control group are, as one epidemiologist put it, "impossible even to meaningfully design."[34] Several reasons can be pointed to. Where population data can be useful in epidemiological methods originally developed for infectious disease, chronic diseases such as cancer present different challenges. An infectious disease is often immediately diagnosable (think of a strep test), whereas cancer more often requires multiple diagnostic tests to find. In practice, the more tests required, the higher chance of false negatives, false positives, and delayed diagnosis because of the sheer number of places a misstep can occur: the tests need to be prescribed, paid for, adequately completed, well interpreted, coordinated, and reported. What seems like a problem with screening itself may rather be a problem with screening delivery.[35]

The history of tobacco use offers a final example of the difficulty in extrapolating from historical population data. We now confidently link lung cancer to inhaling tobacco smoke. Graphs comparing smoking rates with lung cancer rates throughout the twentieth century essentially present the same-shaped line twice—one upward stroke following the increase in smoking rates, and an identical line following twenty years later with the rates of lung cancer mortality, so closely do the numbers correspond. This causal association was not always so transparent, however.

Medical researchers debated the cause of lung cancer as incidence rose from nearly zero in 1900, to 13 of 1,000 males in 1940, to over 30 in 1,000 by 1950.[36] Some physicians hypothesized that a late manifestation of tuberculosis (TB) and influenza caused the higher rates of lung cancer, since the vast increase in lung cancer toward the 1940s and '50s roughly correlated with the surge in influenza during and after WWI. Others attributed the escalation to new early-detection or treatment methods, including bronchoscopy and antibiotics. The early twentieth century also witnessed a dramatic decline in the major killers of the previous century: measles, scarlet fever, typhoid, whooping cough, diphtheria, TB, and influenza. (TB spurred the foundation of the American Lung Association, now associated chiefly with lung cancer.) The declining rates of these diseases provided opportunities, as it were, for diseases with longer incubation periods. People who weren't dying sooner of scarlet fever could die later of something else, like cancer.

Other researchers attributed the higher rates of lung cancer to automobile exhaust, industrial pollution, tar used in road construction, and smoke from domestic fires. (Much smoke, but no tobacco smoke.) Still others just threw their hands in the air, noting the difficulty in general of locating causes of death.[37] Looking back at these debates, one sees that the population statistics in and of themselves did not yield enough information to pinpoint the mechanism behind the rising rates of lung cancer. A prospective cohort study in which researchers followed British physicians' smoking habits and causes of death between 1951 and 2001 more closely tracked the culprit, as did animal studies and, finally, increased understanding of the biology of lung cancers.

The fact that comparative study worked in the case of cigarettes does not, alas, lead us to conclude that *any* carcinogenic cause-and-effect relationship will be so obvious. Indeed, because the relationship between smoking and lung cancer in long-term studies was eventually so clear, it set the evidentiary bar high enough that few other carcinogens have been able to meet it.

Population data present some insurmountable, potentially disastrous problems for studying any medical cause-and-effect relationship, especially with regard to cancer screening, whose effects may not be apparent until decades later.

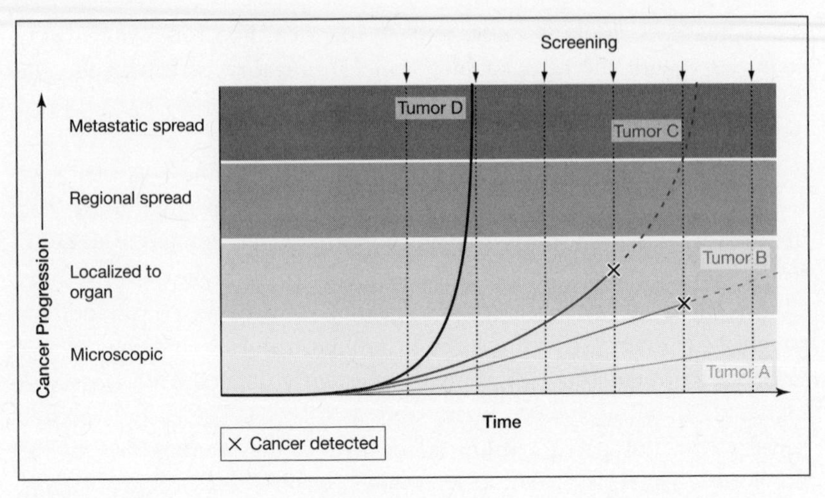

FIGURE 19. Esserman et al., in "Rethinking Screening for Breast Cancer and Prostate Cancer," *JAMA* 302 (2009), speculate about the progression of cancers and their coincidence with screening.

Abstraction

Esserman et al. illustrate their article with a series of figures. These abstracted charts and graphs, portraying theoretical situations, play a key rhetorical role in their argument. None of the graphs specify amounts of time, note details of tumor growth, or refer to individual cases. In one figure, for example (fig. 19), they juxtapose four hypothesized tumor types with a screening scenario. They claim that the graph demonstrates that the imaginary tumor D will ineluctably grow into a metastatic cancer in between screenings, with no symptoms. They further claim that since tumors A and B are indolent (though the graph seems to suggests that they will spread within a decade or so), "only the patient with tumor C benefits from screening."[38] The reader cannot tell from this graph what percentage of tumors the authors believe to be in the tumor C category.[39]

Aside from the oversimplification, this abstraction defies common sense. Esserman et al.'s graphs correspond with a "natural history of disease" model, with the disease progressing in one of several predictable ways. However, they offer no evidence that actual diseases correspond to such ideals. For example, in the real world, tumor growth rates can be spurred by exposure to carcinogens, and thus an untreated tumor A or B may morph into the tumor D category. It is as if one were to draw four pictures of a face, each representing a single ethnicity, and then deduce that all humans would look like one of them.

The natural history of cancer—firsthand knowledge about its behavior—remains an utter mystery for two key reasons. First, all cancers behave differently. Second, it's unethical to observe cancer "in its natural habitat"—that is, developing in someone's body, untreated, from beginning to end. Although cancer patients have been popular experimental research subjects, there has been no cancer experiment, as far as we know, that mirrored the U.S. Health Service's withholding of syphilis treatment from black men for several decades simply to see how the disease would progress.[40] (This is a relief. To add insult to insult, those data were worthless.)

In the conclusion to their article, Esserman and her coauthors offer a flowchart of their recommended screening process (fig. 20), in which they advise that only those with a "susceptibility biomarker" be screened.[41] The article does not previously discuss such a biomarker, so the flowchart, presented as a "framework for advancing screening and detection," appears as something of a non sequitur.[42]

The three outputs at the end of the chart include: "no further screening," "less invasive curative intervention," and "high likelihood of cure." Anyone with a low risk of cancer receives no screening; all cancer treatments are targeted, and anyone who has a poor response to therapy receives more tailored screening. No one receives excessive screening, everyone with cancer gets the perfect treatment to match his or her disease, and best of all, no one dies. We *love* this version of cancer!

Such assumptions give the chart a graceful simplicity: cancer itself virtually disappears, hidden away in the codified circles, rectangles, and hexagons of the flowchart. Indeed, nothing about cancer, or even screening, drives the form of the graphic. By offering a diagnostic and treatment plan that, with a few changes in word choice, could be mapped onto *any* disease category, Esserman et al. erase the specificities of cancer as a disease, namely: the high and unstudied rates of misdiagnosis in screened and unscreened populations, the dearth of knowledge about what causes cancer, the notion of an "adequate biomarker" (the lack of which defines their "no further screening" alternative), the huge expense of genetic screening versus relatively inexpensive imaging and blood-test screening, and the fact that not many targeted treatments exist.[43]

Unlike other graphic practices, such as music notation or time-lapse photos that depict a process unfolding through time, diagnostic charts aim to represent nodes at which distinctly different futures might ensue. The differently shaped boxes are symbols for some action or reaction related to the flow. The diamond, for example, depicts a "conditional,"

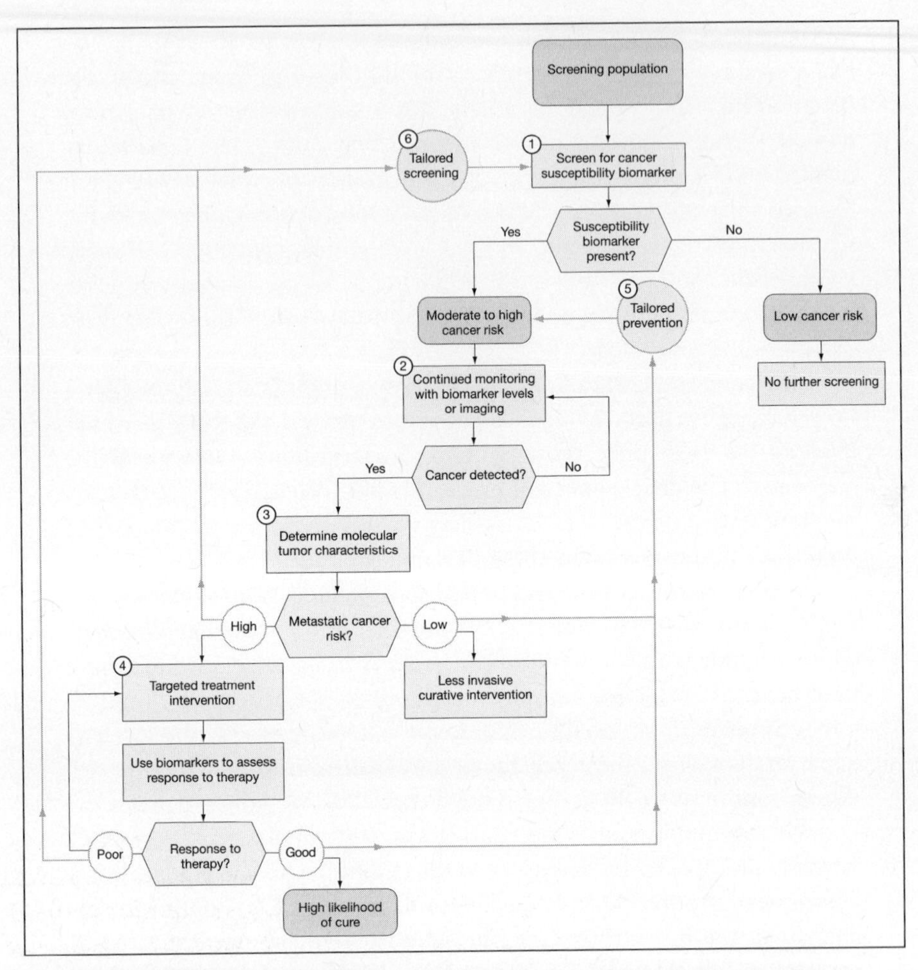

FIGURE 20. A flowchart illustrating a model process for cancer screening—though it does not specify what "tailored" screening means. (*Source:* Esserman et al., "Rethinking Screening for Breast Cancer and Prostate Cancer," *JAMA* 302 [2009])

in which a decision is necessary. In Esserman et al.'s chart, these appear as questions: "Cancer detected?" "Metastatic cancer risk?" "Response to therapy?" According to flowchart protocol, these must be yes/no questions; only with a clear answer can one proceed to the next stage.

Charting threatens to render invisible the places at which errors are most likely to occur. The most critical conditional boxes in this flowchart are subjective: high or low risk of metastatic disease, and good or poor response to therapy. Meaningful individual prediction can't be definitively calculated for an individual until *after* one has, or has not, had cancer, at which point the chance will have been either 100 percent or 0 percent. Such explanatory charts have the ironic effect of making the complexities of the actual flow more baffling, rather than less, by oversimplifying the roles of doctor, patient, and decision. Anything that muddies this flow would be counted as "noise" or be dismissed as an exception to the general rule of the flow.[44]

The chart highlights a paradox inherent to Esserman et al.'s argument. While on the one hand they claim that we do not know enough about the natural history of cancer to diagnose and treat all cancers as if they were life threatening, on the other they replace uncertainty with a model of knowledge that requires a kind of pretend certainty: *if only we had such a biomarker, we could screen properly*. We need, they suggest, a change in "mindset," not knowledge (!), and "screening should follow a multi-decision path such as the one shown in [figure 20]."[45]

Just close enough to current medical knowledge, the chart poses as a real set of choices, despite the vast amount of hypothetical knowledge it calls for. Focusing on "susceptibility biomarkers" entrenches an already problematic categorization of "risk" in oncological research and practice. Even though fewer than 10 percent of breast cancers are related to known genes, and fewer than 30 percent of those diagnosed have any of the commonly cited "risk" factors (such as age at menses, breastfeeding, gene profile, cancer in the family), the language of risk dominates the discussions of early detection.[46]

The idea of a susceptibility biomarker also negates any possibility of chemical, military, industrial, or medical carcinogenic exposure, harking back to the days when the tobacco industry claimed that certain individuals were "genetically susceptible" to lung cancer, tracing cause to individual constitution rather than to the carcinogen itself. Basing an entire system of screening on such debunked logic is certainly not a forward step into the new research on epigenetics and environment.

Another form of abstraction bears noting here in regard to the authors' selection of breast and prostate cancer, as the two cancers that have the highest incidence rates for men and women, respectively, and the second-highest mortality rates for each gender after lung cancer. Age-adjusted rates for annual mortality hover at 28,000 for prostate cancer and 40,000 for breast cancer.[47] Both cancers have been causally linked to common carcinogens and both have undergone an explosive rise in incidence rates (as opposed to simple numerical increases) since the 1950s.

Despite the tendency to conflate the two cancers in both Esserman et al.'s article and much of the media discussion, critical differences between them must be acknowledged and accounted for, since the specificities of the disease inform the costs and benefits of screening. The median age at death for prostate cancer is eighty, twenty-two years higher than for breast cancer, at fifty-eight. A quarter of those who die of breast cancer are under the age of fifty-four, whereas 70 percent of prostate cancer deaths occur in those over the age of seventy-four. For Americans between the ages of twenty and forty-nine, there are fifty breast cancer deaths for each prostate cancer death, and while women have a 1 in 46 chance of developing an invasive breast cancer before the age of thirty-nine, men in this age group have a 1 in 8,499 chance of developing cancer of the prostate.[48] For American women under forty, the incidence rate of late-stage breast cancer has doubled in the last two decades.[49] While prostate and breast cancers are often reported as comparable "men's" and "women's" cancers, this could not be further from the truth in light of costs, numbers of people affected, and years of lost life.

Mortality

Esserman et al.'s case against screening would make sense where the reduction in mortality was nil or minimal. However, in one of the most flummoxing dimensions of the article, they note the opposite, citing seven randomized trials that found a 20–30 percent reduction in mortality due to screening. Their interpretation of this decline is unclear. At one point they write of an "uncertain" reduction in mortality, claiming that the "absolute incidence of aggressive later-stage disease has not been significantly decreased."[50] Elsewhere in the article they attribute an acknowledged decrease in mortality to "both screening and adjuvant therapy."[51] Then they claim that the "decrease in incidence . . . is attributable to [hormone replacement therapy], not to [very early, precancer] removal."[52] On the same page, they claim that "there is evidence and agreement that screening saves lives."[53] That such a widely cited study should contain so many seemingly basic contradictions of logic and data interpretation seems mind boggling.

While claiming that several reasons could account for the fact that "screening has not led to a . . . significant reduction in deaths," they take only one seriously: "tumor biology dictates and trumps stage."[54] This critical point, had it been explained, might have offered insight into a problem that has been the central plague of oncology: namely, how to match the limited treatment options appropriately to the array of tumor biologies, given the impossibility of knowing which cancers will spread.

Looking more carefully at their turn of argument, one notices that Esserman et al. move from a proposition (screening likely misses the most aggressive cancers) to a declaration (tumor biology trumps stage), and then an assertion (cancers caught at late stages would be deadly even if they had been caught earlier). In support of their argument, Esserman et al. cite a report finding that tumors larger than 6 centimeters have a poorer prognosis because of their aggressive biology.[55] In so doing, they neatly bypass any discussion of other data—indeed, a vast amount of data collected over decades—that suggest not only that stage, grade, and method of detection offer independent predictors that together form a prognosis, but also that tumor biology can change quite dramatically, becoming more aggressive (faster growing) over time.[56]

The fact that larger tumors may be more aggressive does not in itself mean that they have grown more quickly than those that are caught when they are smaller. For example, studies have found that the argument that African Americans tend to have more aggressive tumors than whites (due to their higher mortality rates and to the fact that their cancers are more often caught at later stages) evaporates when African Americans are offered screening and their tumors are diagnosed at earlier stages.[57] This research suggests that demographic access to medicine can easily be mistaken for biological explanations about tumors. Epidemiologist Nancy Krieger likewise has found that the reduction in breast cancer mortality is demographically specific rather than evenly distributed throughout the population.[58] More finely calibrated data could be used to better understand whether certain subcategories of Americans are more likely to have "interim cancers" with social rather than biological roots and what relation screening has on that.

In real life, what looks like a tumor D cancer in Esserman et al.'s analysis may well have been a misdiagnosis. A recent federal study estimated that 70,000 cancers are missed by mammograms due to faulty radiological readings, improper positioning of the breast in the machine, and poor oversight of the machines.[59] Add the estimate that 30 percent of women with abnormal mammogram results do not receive follow-up notification or treatment, not to mention the high rates of missed or delayed diagnosis, and one has convincing enough explanations for the sluggish decrease in mortality rates that some more evidence from Esserman et al. seems warranted.[60]

Attention to individual cases, as opposed to population-based averages, can be revealing. One group of physicians, aiming to better understand the reasons for missed and delayed diagnosis—both because of their prevalence and because of the "especially severe outcomes" that result—found that such cases tend to be multifactorial: that is, arising from more than one glitch in the process and involving multiple providers. These doctors highlight the "challenge of finding effective ways to reduce diagnostic errors."[61] Such analysis makes clear that diagnoses are missed for complicated reasons—reasons, in general, other than aggressive interim tumors simply surging up between diagnostic tests. The missed-diagnosis angle is a major component lacking in the study of cancer mortality.

As I've mentioned elsewhere in *Malignant,* I've interviewed many young adults diagnosed with cancer. Their answers made evident the far-reaching failure of early detection for this age group, which may well have statistically relevant consequences.[62] Carolyn, diagnosed with Stage III breast cancer at thirty-four and with a family history of cancer, told me about her experience with her doctor:

> She gave me a hand exam that must have taken fifteen seconds. I was kind of shocked and asked her if that was it. I mean, it was totally ridiculous. She basically whipped her hands across my breasts and then was done. It was almost as if she was in a time trial or something. But I felt embarrassed asking her to do a more thorough job and figured that I should just drop it. . . . I did find my own lump in late October (almost exactly three months later) and got a mammogram the next day. The rest is history.[63]

When I asked an administrator of the medical group that Carolyn was insured through about their policy on breast exams, she told me: "[Our] MDs . . . do the exams if the patient wants it and spend about 30 seconds on it."[64] A thirty-second exam falls well below the two-minute standard for clinical breast exams, which itself falls below the three minutes per breast required to do a thorough exam.[65] In following up with me, Carolyn said: "[The doctor] is outrageously beautiful and very nice. I wish she would use her good looks and charm to become the poster child for giving good breast exams."[66]

Later, in an effort to encourage that very thing, Carolyn spoke to her doctor. She explained that the exam had been very brief and that the tumor might have been caught earlier had the doctor done a more thorough exam or encouraged her to see someone who was willing to do so. She also explained her embarrassment at asking for a longer exam, and said that she didn't know at the time what a thorough exam really was. She described feeling nervous and worrying that the doctor would shut down in anticipation of being sued, and so she worked into her conversation that she had no intention of suing and that of course they would never know if a better exam would have given a different result. Initiating the talk involved careful strategizing and management of her doctor's potential fear, even though ultimately the doctor said she would take her comments into account.

Regression

Esserman et al.'s argument that many early cancers do not need to be located and treated hinges on a controversial Norwegian study which found that 22 percent of breast cancer tumors spontaneously regress (no comparable study for prostate cancer is cited).[67] Tracing Esserman et al.'s use of this study offers an example of how data, shorn of their context, can gain new life when buried as a key tenet of another argument, one that in this case has continued to have international policy implications and a whole new citational network.

The Norwegian study that Esserman et al. rely on was not a randomized controlled trial, but rather offered a comparison of the six-year cumulative breast cancer incidence in two groups of Norwegian women, aged fifty to sixty-four, from before (109,784 women in 1992) and after (119,720 women in 1996) the broad adoption of screening, respectively; in the latter group, the majority of women had screening, while in the former most did not (two-thirds of the women are in both groups). After a single "exit" mammogram for the unscreened group at the end of the study, researchers found that the unscreened group had significantly fewer cancers (stage was unspecified)—a surprising result, given the authors' expectations.

The authors speculated that the 22 percent "excess" cancers found in the screened group would have regressed spontaneously.[68] This conclusion was based not on observation of any regressions, nor on a longitudinal study of the subjects tracking mortality, and for those reasons their results generated significant controversy.

Letters in response to the Norwegian study suggested reasons other than spontaneous regression for the hypothesis not being borne out. Two physicians, for example, wondered why the researchers expected twice the difference in incidence than "one could expect according to the rate observed in 1992–93," noting that given the number of women who participated in both the groups "there would be little argument for spontaneous regression."[69] Another observed that the single mammogram received at the end of the study by those in the unscreened group might have missed tumors that would have been picked up in a second, third, or fourth test in correspondence with the known error rates; yet another response suggested that because the groups were not randomized, women who had no reason to seek mammograms (in particular before screening was routine, but also after) might simply have been at lower risk. A further critique notes that no data were included on the mammogram machines, which may have increased cancer incidence.[70]

Women who had access to screening likely had access to better medical care, including, ironically, hormone replacement therapy, which in Norway has been found to have increased breast cancer incidence by 58 percent. This observation was used to critique both the Norwegian and the Esserman et al. reports.[71] This point about HRT is exacerbated by the separation of the study cohorts by time. Juxtaposing the historical annual sales of HRT with the first and second groups, three commentators accounted for the full difference in cancer rates as due not to screening or spontaneous remission, but to the reduced HRT use by the latter group, after the widespread reduction in its use.[72] Subsequent follow-up of the Norwegian data has stirred similar debate.[73]

Dr. Barnett Kramer of the U.S. National Institutes of Health told me that spontaneous regressions of some "preneoplastic lesions" have been reported in several cancers, though not in breast or prostate. He pointed out that "regression is not equivalent to spontaneous cure, since at least some lesions can also subsequently recur."[74] Esserman et al. cite the Norwegian findings as though they were authoritative, although follow-up was insufficient to determine the efficacy of screening in light of its primary endpoint: neither incidence nor subsequent recurrence, but death.

In stating that "many early cancers go nowhere," Esserman et al. do not discuss any of the possibilities or ramifications noted by the broader medical community for alternative explanations of the Norwegian screening data. Nor, for that matter, do they discuss differences between the Norwegian and American context of heath and healthcare. Rather, in this paper and in subsequent publications, they repeat the Norwegian study's shaky speculation about spontaneous regression as fact.

Cost

Esserman et al.'s foundational assumptions—that the SEER data correspond to a screened population, that screening does not catch deadly cancers but does catch indolent cancers, and that physicians are treating indolent cancers too aggressively—lead to a seemingly straightforward argument: screening requires too much hassle for too few lives saved. Turning again to breast, rather than prostate, cancer data, they reason that "for every breast cancer death averted, even in the age group for which screening is least controversial (age 50–70 years), 838 women must undergo screening for 6 years."[75] Such screening, in their view, generates "thousands of screens, hundreds of biopsies, and many cancers treated as if they were life threatening when they are not," the upshot being that early detection has increased "costs and morbidity due to overtreatment of non–life threatening cancers."[76]

Their argument is twofold: (1) screening overburdens the population, which spends time, money, and energy on it, with little chance of averting a death, and (2) oncologists overtreat some cancers. These keystones of cancer screening debates need teasing out, as they are not self-evident.

Benefit

Measuring "quality of life" against time and money is perhaps one of the most recalcitrant problems of our modern lives. On the one hand, such a trade makes utter sense, echoing the decision making we do many times a day *(Is this soda worth $3? Do I want to drive all the way across town to run one errand?)*. On the other hand, cost-benefit thinking in medical policy literature requires a uniquely conjectural notion of mortality.

Extrapolating from Esserman et al.'s statistics, we find that one deadly cancer detected and successfully treated requires 5,028 occasions (838 scans × 6 years) on which a test finds either no cancer or a cancer of the "indolent" variety. This fact presents as a straightforward calculation. However, anyone living in prognosis knows that numbers can't fully be trusted.

While "number of tests" and "number of lives" initially seem to offer a tidy equation, further scrutiny reveals that a test differs quite significantly from a life. An unambiguous comparison needs similar entities (apples to apples, dust to dust—not tests to lives). For the sake of precision, then, let's use time as the common denominator. For the moment, we can accept the calculation of scans and lives, and assume that each of the 5,028 mammograms takes on average an hour, including time in the waiting and changing rooms. Using cancer data, let's say that finding one deadly cancer requires retesting 10 percent of the initial group (a further 503 hours), biopsying 10 percent of the retested group (50 hours), and treating three of those early-stage cancers with a lumpectomy and radiation (2 months' treatment, or 1,440 hours × 3 people = 4,620 hours).[77] In this search for cancer, one unlucky (or, in a way, very lucky) person will have his or her life saved.

Some cancer deaths take only weeks, while others take over a decade and many recurrences and rounds of treatment. The average cancer death results in eighteen years of lost life (157,248 hours), but for the sake of argument, since we are comparing hours spent in active medical care, let's say that the one cancer death averted by these 5,028 scans would have required five years of active and palliative treatment, which translates to 42,484 hours of illness. So, again using time-in-healthcare as the common denominator, averting one cancer death would actually *save* over 30,000 hours, in addition to several thousand more hours of caretaking and the physical and emotional disruption for families and communities that a cancer death implies. Even in this calculation, the hours of the nuisance of screening do not readily compare to hours of the physical illness.

Even as we get closer to an analogous comparison, such equations miss a key social fact that frames nearly every aspect of cancer detection and treatment: the calculations that craft the worth of a "statistical life."[78] The worth of any given person in America varies greatly—indeed, this is a founding principle of the nation. Institutions such as law frame these values through damage claims that can calculate the cost of an injury because we know exactly who has been injured (the plaintiff) and their worth (their salary). Medical equations at this level ignore questions of monetary value, using instead statistics generalized from speculations about quality of life or risk avoidance. Still, for a highly paid banker or doctor those lost hours might add up to millions of dollars, whereas the illness hours of a nonworking or low-wage person would be relatively inexpensive. At any rate, an adequate cost-benefit calculation in the U.S. healthcare system would require some specificity around *whose* cancer death is averted, a fact that these statistics don't account for, although actual access to healthcare in some measure does.

Alternatively, we could frame the question in personal terms, asking each of those 838 women if they were willing to undergo a mammogram a year for six years to save, say, their favorite celebrity, or someone they had gone to high school with, or a friend of a friend. Having a mammogram under this framework would become akin to giving blood, which many people do for no apparent personal benefit, or to participating in a charitable event such as a race for the cure. If there's one thing we've learned in the last decade of cancer walks, runs, marketing, and sponsorship, it's that many people will go out of their way to do something about cancer. Including making a U-turn to drive a BMW.

It may matter if you've seen someone die of cancer. It may matter if you have a family history of cancer. It may matter if you think you are saving yourself or someone else. It may matter if you have a religious or ethical commitment to altruism. When human motivations puncture cancer data, some sobering questions spew out. What cost is worth what benefit, and to whom? When? Why? No one considers these issues, if we take the objectivity of cost-benefit equations for granted.

Treatment

The treatment for breast "precancer" and Stage I cancer ranges from lumpectomy, simple mastectomy (as opposed to the radical mastectomies of a bygone era), and lumpectomy and radiation to a double mastectomy (both breasts, even when one is cancer-free), chemotherapy, and full reconstruction. According to medical historian Robert Aronowitz, the option of mastectomy for even these precancers has become increasingly popular, up from 4.1 percent in 1998 to 13.5 percent in 2005.[79] Medical anthropologist Ilana Löwy has found that the percentage of patients opting for mastectomy varies greatly by medical center, ranging from about 3 percent to more than 50 percent. She hypothesizes that such differences reflect the opinions of the physicians involved in the patients' cases.[80]

In addition to the medical counsel they receive, the reasons that motivate women to undergo invasive surgeries for early-stage diagnoses vary greatly and include: fear of losing medical insurance and thus the ability of being closely screened in the future; not wanting to be in the medical system either as someone being constantly screened or later as a cancer patient; worry over future misdiagnoses and so eventual diagnosis with advanced cancer; the opportunity to have breast reconstruction, with its promise of physical improvement, covered by insurance; and the raw, naked fear of recurrence itself.[81] One piece of advice given to a young woman trying to decide whether to undergo chemotherapy for a Stage I breast cancer went this way: Write two letters to yourself in which you justify your decision. In one letter you imagine that you suffer from the long-term effects of chemotherapy and write a justification of your decision to undergo it. In the second letter, write of your decision not to have the chemo and imagine opening it after having been diagnosed with a recurrence. In other words, a mix of ideas about cancer, treatment options, economic access, and attempts at insuring against regret determine decisions about surgery.

Controversy surrounds not only what counts as legitimate treatment in the use of toxic chemotherapy for small tumors, but also how much further surgery, unrelated to curing the cancer per se, will fall under the treatment umbrella. Since passage of the Women's Health and Cancer Rights Act of 1998, federal law requires most group insurance plans that cover mastectomies to also cover breast reconstruction, as well as surgery and reconstruction of the remaining breast to preserve symmetry after mastectomy. This act followed from litigation brought by a woman after her insurance refused to cover the cost of reconstruction, claiming that it was purely cosmetic rather than part of the treatment.[82]

Surgeons commonly suggest that women already considering a mastectomy consider a double mastectomy or additional cosmetic surgeries for the sake of "evenness." These surgeries have high complication rates. As one former patient who eventually had to remove an implant altogether wrote, "In retrospect, I wish I'd considered the choice of no reconstruction at all, but it was not something that I even thought to discuss with the plastic surgeon, nor did he mention it to me."[83] In the end, studies find that 50 percent of women are unsatisfied with the surgeries after ten years because of discomfort, contraction of the flesh around the implants, pain, and loss of feeling in the area.[84]

The literature that recommends against screening, in part because of the risks of overtreatment, surprisingly does not address how the range of treatment options and the inclusion of extensive reconstructive surgery play into the definition of overtreatment. Perhaps oncologists don't want to acknowledge the vested interest that their surgeon colleagues have in aggressive treatment. Whatever the explanation, various components need further exploration if the category of overtreatment will determine screening policy.[85]

CONCLUSION

Make no mistake, screening efficacy is worth questioning. Cancer history leads one to be suspicious: I've already mentioned the extreme surgeries of the mid–twentieth century, the experimental injections of radioactive substances, and the bone marrow transplants, all of which were eventually found to have no medical benefit. Dr. Claudia Henschke found in 2006 that 80 percent of lung cancer deaths could be prevented through widespread use of CT scans; it was later disclosed that her research was underwritten by $3.6 million in grants from the parent company of the Liggett Group, a cigarette manufacturer.[86] In addition, screening, as defined in these debates, requires a procedure—a scan, or a blood test, or a biopsy, say. These procedures can be made less expensive through offshoring or, as we saw in the case of cervical cancer, the feminization of the technical work. Standardization makes it cheaper; it also makes screening a highly profitable paramedical growth industry.

The money connection triggers further skepticism. The financial gain represented by certain treatments provides incentive that may influence how diagnoses are made; some oncologists gain 90 percent of their income by administering chemotherapy. Several authors have carefully traced the difference in findings depending on whether industry funds their studies or not.[87] On the other hand, securing insurance coverage for follow-up testing can take hours of a physician's time. No one would be so crass as to suggest that doctors purposely overtreat in exchange for a briefcase of bundled hundred-dollar bills, but as in any financial transaction, a wise consumer follows the money and looks for subtle allegiances concealed by protocol. No matter which question you ask (are there too many diagnoses, or too few?), suspicion has a legitimate genealogy.

Like the rest of us, Esserman et al. are stuck in a medical system that wants a more mechanistic—and less and less expensive—means of diagnosing and treating cancer. For that reason, their paper has relevance for more than just screening and early-detection protocols; the issues refract across the whole cancer conversation. For example, linking these issues back to those raised in chapter 4, if doctors can convince one another that early detection is not of much value, and that cancers that kill will have killed whenever caught, then what is a doctor's responsibility in terms of diagnosing? The screening debates need to be read in the context of the current political moment of medico-legal responsibility, an era witnessing not only the erosion of patient rights and access to healthcare but also a swollen bureaucracy that increases work for each doctor or patient considering a diagnostic test.

These combined burdens erode the possibility of good medical care on many levels. Yet they have a history. Cancer historian Ilana Löwy points out that "cancer research, diagnosis, and treatment were at the forefront of the development of 'big medicine,' a multi-level, science-grounded endeavor," one that "favored the homogenization of diagnoses and outcomes, while the use of expensive substances and instruments, such as radium and cobalt bombs or high voltage radiotherapy machines, promoted the centralization of cures."[88] It has become clear that research based on the catch-all disease categories favored by the protocols of big medicine comes with major public health drawbacks, such as mass-produced industrial screening, trials, and overtreatment.

We all wish cancer could have a mathematical, sterile elegance, or if not cancer, then at least the institutions that administrate it. We want something to be done, too, and screening (or wearing a yellow wristband) may fill that need. At the same time, who really wants to have someone's finger up their butt, a stranger pinch their testicles, or have their boobs squashed by a machine? The major source of confusion in these debates lies not only in the inability to answer the fundamental question I raised earlier—what is cancer?—but also in the overall hesitation to clearly define the core ignorance about cancer and its role in the debates. This structural unknownness of cancer can't be resolved through higher-resolution data of the same type. Even the most objective-seeming analysis (what could be more clear cut than a cost-benefit equation?) requires a variable of fudge, no matter how detailed the accounting. Precision does not equal accuracy.

In an era of medical mass production, it makes business sense, at least, to spread icing on the fried dough around the empty hole at the center of the problem. But I still prefer those mouth-popping donut holes.

CHAPTER 8

Fallout

Minuets in the Key of Fear

Have you ever wondered why the phrase "You're the bomb" offers a slangy compliment, whereas "You are the gas chamber" would not go over well in a romantic situation? (Clearly, I have.) This translation of nuclear imagery into benign, even sexy, language is not uncommon. When the word *bikini* crops up, most Americans think of the swimsuit rather than radiation sickness. Though perhaps not the intent in naming the bathing suit, it would be difficult to think of a better way to diminish the significance of the Bikini Atoll's annihilation by the twenty-three nuclear tests carried out on the South Pacific island by the American military between 1946 and 1958, collectively seven thousand times more powerful than the atomic device dropped on Hiroshima. In the very definition of obliteration, a single bomb vaporized three of the islands and sprinkled them, in the form of radioactive dust from 100,000 feet in the air, onto inhabitants of islands farther north, forcing them to evacuate. Almost seventy years on, the islanders have not been able to return to this lethal paradise.

The name Bikini Bottom for the home of the popular children's cartoon character SpongeBob SquarePants may seal the insult. If not, the fact that UNESCO recently declared the Bikini Atoll a World Heritage Site surely does. Of the five sites that were exposed to one megaton of open-air tests prior to 1963, including Nevada and two in the former Soviet Union, the atoll was selected as representative of the role that atomic bomb testing "played in shaping global culture in the second half of the 20th Century."[1] Over five hundred atmospheric nuclear weapons tests were conducted at various sites around the world between 1945 and 1980, but UNESCO claims Bikini Atoll as "an outstanding example of a nuclear test site," stating that the "authenticity of the material elements constituting the property is unquestionable." Why? Because "human presence there has remained very limited because of the radionuclides produced by the explosions." In the event that the area ever becomes inhabitable again, conservation must "include the protection of the land-based military remains."

Specific state programs assisted in the U.S. domestication of terror about nuclear war. The post-WWII images of bomb tests that saturated American media, for example, choreographed a sterile, fungal sublime that many still associate with the bomb. American researchers scrupulously documented the effects of radiation on the Japanese, but these images were not released in the United States.[2] Americans of a certain age can still hum "Duck and Cover," the song that instructed people to hide under desks or in doorways to save themselves from evaporation. The innocuous ditty perfectly connotes the Cold War promised difference of zero when it came to the balance of terror, with the American nuclear stockpile as the minuend and the Soviet arsenal as the subtrahend. It's natural to forget that real terror was at stake, as easy as it is to miss the fact that "premium-plus" soda crackers really are top-notch. Rote phrases have a way of desensitizing one to their meanings.

Polished images of bomb blasts, combined with spectacles such as mass evacuations, placed the potential for nuclear disaster in the realm of the everyday, posing the idea that nuclear war, similar to other kinds of disasters, was just another facet of quotidian life while at the same time eliciting support for national defense spending. The government harnessed the same rhetorical methods, if on a rather grander scale than it had used to transform traffic fatalities into "accidents," in its efforts to conceal and refashion the new forms of illness and death purveyed by a nuclear culture, such as radiation poisoning and cancer.

Anthropologist Joseph Masco traces the enormous effort undergone by government to convince the public that a nuclear crisis could be "incorporated into everyday life with minor changes in household technique and a 'can do' American spirit."[3] This occurred, for example, when the government converted nuclear *terror,* a paralyzing emotion, into nuclear *fear,* which Masco describes as an affective state that would still allow citizens to remain calmish and able to act during a catastrophe. This emotional management required a two-pronged approach. First, government advertisements asked citizens to "take responsibility for their own survival" by knowing what to do in the case of a nuclear attack. Second, campaigns directed people to fear widespread panic, rather than nuclear war itself, thereby defusing the bomb as the main threat. Even with the release of radiation with atmospheric bomb testing, the discovery of high levels of radioactive strontium in American flesh and teeth, and the corresponding increase in cancer rates along fallout routes and among nuclear workers, the government created an image of the nuclear threat as coming from the outside, never as the predictable and calculated consequence of *American* programs. News media and government spokespeople often described antinuclear activists as communists, lesbians, or hippies—not fully American.

Only recently have governmental agencies emerged with more information, now warning people who were children, drank milk, and lived along fallout routes before 1963 to be aware of their heightened risks of thyroid cancer and leukemia as a result of their exposures.[4] Current recommendations by the Environmental Protection Agency (EPA) and Food and Drug Administration (FDA) would have seen the removal of milk from U.S. supermarket shelves throughout the 1950s and early '60s for months at a time.[5] Millions of gallons of milk would not have been sold, and millions of children would not have drunk it. Despite the refusal to study the health effects on Americans of nuclear fallout at the time (American studies were ongoing in Japan), the Atomic Energy Commission (AEC) acknowledged the physical effects of radiation by agreeing to alert Eastman Kodak in advance of nuclear tests: radiation caused unexposed film to fog.[6]

Cancers caused by military activities aside, the disease and the military served as perfect foils for one another. As a disease horrific enough to warrant virtually any treatment in the search for a cure, from plutonium injections to massive doses of radiation and chemotherapy, cancer enabled the government to demonstrate the humanitarian potential of nuclear technology. Amid much controversy in medical spheres, the military funded experimentation with large-scale, brutal, promising "weapons" against cancer, while the disease was so feared that doctors more often than not did not disclose the diagnosis to their patients.[7]

That cognitive dissonance between the horror of the thing and its transformation into a banal everyday occurrence reverberates in contemporary cancer culture as well. Bad enough to warrant atomic-level treatment; how can the social narrative of cancer possibly be reduced to pink bracelets, pamphlets, and BMW test drives? A *New York Times* article suggests that people returning to work after treatment will find that wearing "a wig or hat and makeup that conceals a pale complexion will put colleagues at ease and make you feel better about yourself." Or "Try a little humor, such as asking whether people like your wig, and maintain a positive attitude."[8] Many of the ways we are asked to think about cancer fit all too well with Masco's observations about government strategies during the Cold War, which transformed "an unthinkable apocalypse into an opportunity for psychological self-management, civic responsibility, and ultimately, governance."[9]

Just as fear incontrovertibly shapes our understanding of the bomb, so it is a central, understudied aspect of cancer. Fear of cancer starts early. If you are educated and middle class, you likely eat organic food, wear your sunscreen, and get your colonoscopy. If you take an active part in the medicalized and marketized socialization around cancer, you probably feel at least vaguely self-congratulatory as you do your bit to avoid it. Witness the shock so many people experience upon diagnosis ("but . . . but I did everything *right!*").

Cancer stands in ill repute, and its bad rap precedes it. Thus, little-understood assumptions about fear (and fear of fear) pervade the interactions around both early-stage and terminal cancer. For instance, the American Cancer Society's deputy chief medical officer Len Lichtenfeld discusses the valid problem of how (and if) doctors should manage fear in the diagnostic procedure, where the very word *cancer* may prevent a patient from absorbing important information about monitoring symptoms.[10] Screening debates acknowledge that diagnostic procedures carry the "risk of negative emotional consequences" and that this emotional fallout should be considered when attempting to make a cancer diagnosis.[11]

Even early-stage cancers that require relatively simple surgeries to remove and have virtually 100 percent survival chances can carry huge emotional burdens. Science historian Steven Shapin writes of two women, one of whom has cancer and goes through treatment and the other of whom has been tested and is negative. He notes that "their experiences eerily resemble each other."[12] This description of a similarity between a fear and a treatment could *only* be accurate in a world that takes fear of cancer as definitive of the experience of it (and even then it requires a rather significant disavowal of the intensity of cancer treatment).[13] Yet the publishability of this idea—that being-tested-for-a-disease-you-don't-end-up-having resembles cancer treatment—shows the extent to which fear has become a powerful, and problematic, current in the very definition of cancer.

From another angle, who can blame a doctor for being disinclined to give someone what is basically a death sentence, or for worrying that a patient will break down in her office? One nurse told me about a patient who was removed from a doctor's office in a straitjacket after being diagnosed with metastatic disease. Little literature addresses, head on, the question of precisely how fear should be considered in the mix that we call cancer, from screening policy to physician training, from supporting caretakers to pamphlet design, from the period of survivorship to replacing a plastic bottle.

No matter how innocently, the attempt to assuage the fear can trigger misinformation. Cancer patient literature, with its ubiquitous photos of smiling patients and competent, relaxed caretakers, offers another example of a place where fear might benefit from acknowledgment and more careful analysis. In a memoir about his mother Susan Sontag's death from chemotherapy-induced leukemia, David Rieff writes about the infantilizing language of an informational pamphlet: "The gap here between language and reality is simply too great [to convey useful information about cancer], and is actually a disservice to most patients and their loved ones, and, I suspect, even for physicians and nurses as well. . . . It may be appropriate to 'redirect' a small child who is upset about something. It is not appropriate to 'redirect' an adult cancer patient."[14] These insulting misdirections have become an inside joke in survivor cultures, as I continually witnessed in retreat discussions. Miriam Engelberg, a cartoonist whose book ends abruptly after she has been rediagnosed with metastatic disease, captures this misdirection perfectly in her book *Cancer Made Me a Shallower Person* (fig. 21). Reading this laugh-out-loud book on cancer ephemera tickles that now-familiar comfort-terror-solidarity spot of chemoflage.[15]

When I spoke to a former nurse about the sanitized patient information, she said that if brochures and doctors adequately described the procedures—if, for example, people really understood what a bone marrow transplant entailed—they might well opt out of the treatment. In this light, the fear management approach makes sense at one level, but it comes with costs: being treated like a child or an idiot has its own psychological ramifications. As much as the grief of losing his mother constituted Rieff's experience of cancer, so did his fury at the way the process of cancer was misrepresented.

I noted in the introduction that the twentieth- and twenty-first-century definition and management of what we call cancer tracks with the institutions that have come to define America—the military, postwar

SOMETHING UNPLEASANT AND YOU
FOR ALMOST EVERY MEDICAL PROCEDURE THERE IS AN EDUCATIONAL BOOKLET.
DON'T BE AFRAID - THIS WILL EXPLAIN EVERYTHING!
SOMETHING UNPLEASANT... AND YOU!
THE COVER OFTEN FEATURES AN ILLUSTRATION OF A NATURE SCENE.
CHEMOTHERAPY... AND YOU!
I WAS DREADING CHEMO, BUT NOW THAT I CAN ASSOCIATE IT WITH THIS LOVELY BEACH SCENE I'M LOOKING FORWARD TO IT!
OR SOMETIMES THE COVER SHOWS IMAGES OF INSANELY CHEERFUL PATIENTS...
BREAST CANCER SURGERY ... AND YOU!
I ALWAYS WONDER WHAT THE PATIENTS ARE DISCUSSING SO ANIMATEDLY...
I LOVED HAVING SURGERY!
ME, TOO!
PLUS WE GET ALL THESE GREAT PRESCRIPTIONS.
THE TONE OF THE BOOKLET IS ALWAYS COOL AND CALM.
YOU MAY EXPERIENCE SOME NAUSEA DURING CHEMO.

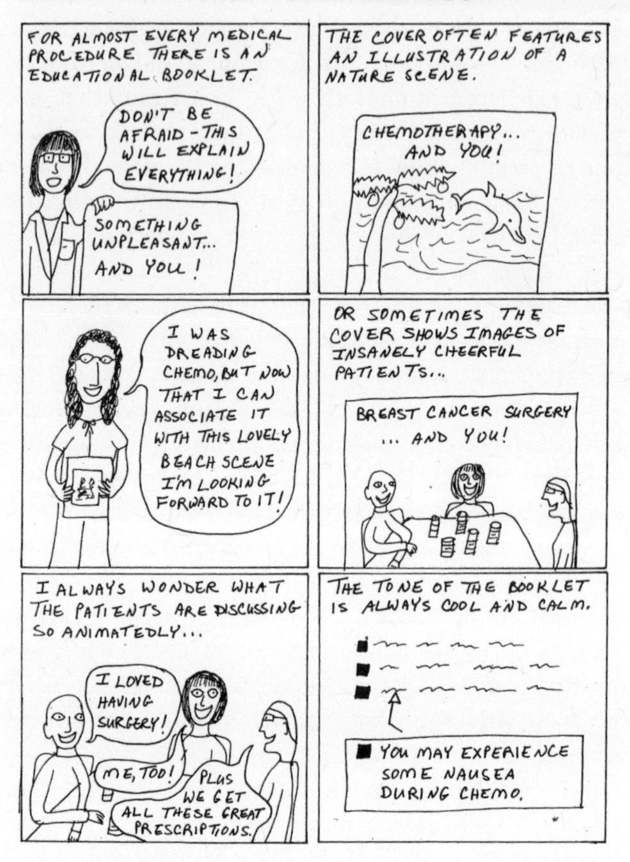

FIGURE 21. Miriam Engelberg, in her book *Cancer Made Me a Shallower Person,* comments on the patient who is always smiling in cancer pamphlets.

big medicine, technology, advertising (imagine the swelling orchestra in a Made in America commercial). But one of cancer's biologically defining features—the lag between exposure and symptom—enables us to clearly (and misleadingly) separate it from these industries. As I mention throughout this book, it is virtually impossible to prove that a particular exposure has led to a specific injury by cancer. This latency partly accounts for cancer's everywhere- and nowhereness. If cause can't be shown, how can cancer be located? Is it in the body or in the culture around it? Does it arise through practices such as smoking, or through screening that potentially detects too much of it? Everyone knows some-

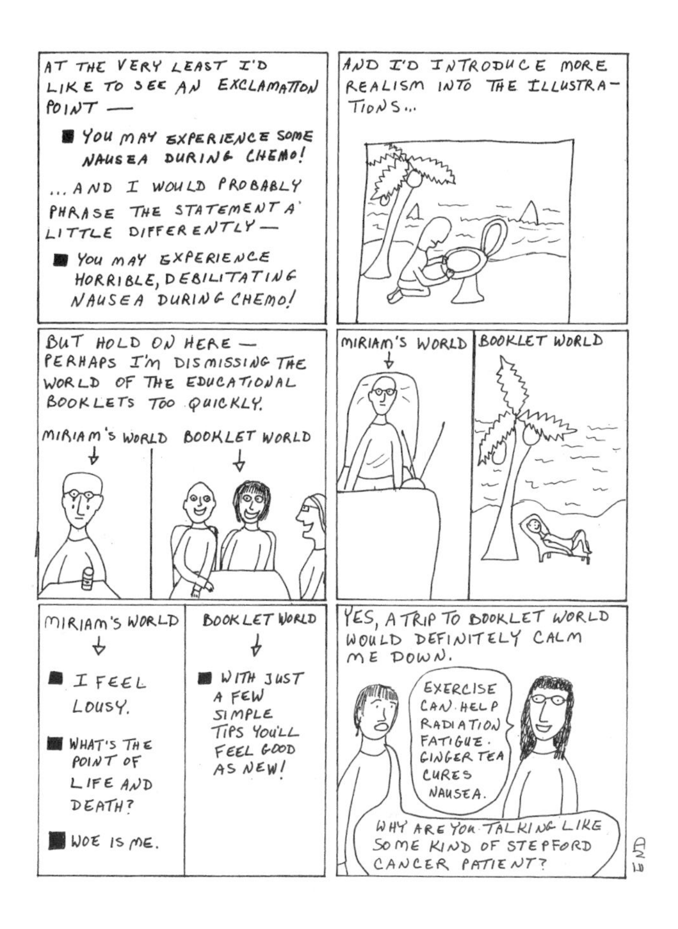

one who has or had it, but where is the thing we can point to, the evidence that Something Is Being Done? American laws and regulations for the most part are built around immediate and provable causation, not a death fifty years later, and thus the debates about how many cancers are environmentally caused are likely to continue for many more decades.

On the one hand, many Americans realize that carcinogens buttress the American economy. On the other hand, we rarely consider the actual people living with and dying from cancer as being a sacrifice to, and a structural result of, our use of these toxins. Some of this disjuncture results from campaigns (think pink) that divert attention away from the links between chemical exposures and the disease. Framing survivorship as a personal accomplishment further separates cancer causation from its manifestations. Cancer becomes a passively occurring hurdle to be surmounted by resolve rather than the direct effect of a violent environment, as incongruous a substitution as a lisp versus a gunshot wound.

Even if we did consciously decide (rather than simply fail to collect the data) that the injuries resulting from the daily use of proven carcinogens are a worthy trade-off for a certain standard of living—one that includes chewy toys, spray cleaners, and cheap cherries—the injuries would neither go away, nor would they be evenly distributed among those who made the decision. Unlike lead exposure through gas and paint or mercury exposure through dental amalgams and tuna fish, which can subtly decrease coordination and intelligence in whole swaths of a population without attracting notice, cancer signifies a specific, diagnosable, singularly borne disease. Cancer may be widespread, but it strikes clearly individuated victims. Environmentalist advocates suggest that we could get rid of cancer if only we could get rid of the carcinogens. Whether that's true or not we may never know. In the meantime, the languages that justify cancer at the individual and social levels reveal valuable information on who we are.

A minuet is a social dance. Partners mutually agree on the cadence of the steps. The rest of this chapter examines the underpinning choreography of some of cancer's dissonances and the languages that squash these dissonances into a strict cadence. In searching first for the everywhere- and nowhereness of environmental exposures, I'm not particularly arguing that the environment should be cleaned up (although I think it should) or that such a cleansing would eliminate cancer (maybe it would, maybe it wouldn't). Rather, I want to examine the broader costs of accepting the general lack of proof, despite serious suspicion, about cancer's causes. This sets the stage for the second act of this chapter, where I analyze the virtual eradication of cancer and carcinogenic exposures as legally compensable injuries through "fear of cancer" lawsuits. The government's attempt to use graphic warnings on cigarette packaging serves as the chapter's denouement. Somewhere in each of these episodes, we've been interpolated as partners, asked to accept a logic of cancer that both piques and diminishes the fear.

EXPOSURE

In 1971, Congress charged the newly constituted President's Cancer Panel with monitoring the multibillion-dollar National Cancer Program. Each year, this panel of two to three experts writes a report to the U.S. president on cancer-related topics. Reports generally cover noncontroversial aspects of cancer, such as diet, survivorship, racial disparities, insurance, and drug development. However, the 2008–2009 report, written by two members appointed by George W. Bush, examines the use of industrial, military, and agricultural carcinogens. Making the case that cancer programs have grossly underestimated the real costs of environmental pollutants, it details the true burden of environmentally caused cancers. The report notes, for example, that of the eighty thousand chemicals in daily use in the United States, only a few hundred have been studied for carcinogenicity. Ultimately, the report "most strongly" urges the president "to use the power of your office to remove the carcinogens and other toxins from our food, water, and air that needlessly increase health care costs, cripple our Nation's productivity, and devastate American lives."[16]

The report offers a succinct and straight-talking overview of cancer causation in the United States, pointing out that U.S. rates of cancer remain higher than those of other industrialized nations. It also lists the primary challenges faced by Americans, as follows: limited, underfunded, and scattered research on the environmental causes of cancer; reliance on animal studies (whose subjects can be bred to have higher tolerances for chemicals); a lack of data on low-dose exposures and combinations of exposures; ineffective regulations; medical radiation exposures that are often underestimated by physicians; and hazardous, unmeasured, and concealed exposures by the military (in weapons testing and development, for example).[17] The report further notes that the medical community has not taken seriously clear correlations between environmental exposures and cancer. Although less than 5 percent of cancer diagnoses can be linked directly to inherited genetic traits, the primary focus of medical cancer research has consistently honed in on the genetic causes of cancer.[18] Physicians rarely ask about exposures to carcinogens in patient interviews, even though rates for certain types of cancer can be clearly correlated to occupational exposures.[19]

Using well-known examples such as lead, asbestos, plastics, and other common household and medical materials, numerous authors have detailed the political barriers to regulating dangerous chemicals and products.[20] Unlike European regulations that tend to rely on a precautionary approach, in the United States "a hazard must be incontrovertibly demonstrated before action to ameliorate it is initiated."[21] In other words, while European governments regulate chemicals based on initial evidence of toxicity, the U.S. government allows even chemicals ranked as "likely," "potential," and "actual" carcinogens to be produced and used for many years until adequate proof of danger has been gathered (the passive voice is appropriate here, since it isn't clear, often, who would collect the data). Industries maintain unique access to political power through well-funded lobbyists who work to keep ingredient lists off product packaging and ensure that manufacturers need not disclose the carcinogens in proprietary ingredients.[22] Commonly used known carcinogenic chemicals such as cadmium, phthalates, asbestos, chromium, diesel fuel, mercury, and formaldehyde require no federal labeling or warnings.[23]

The report identifies numerous hazardous materials in our everyday lives. For example, agricultural industries pour eighty million pounds of the herbicide atrazine, an endocrine disruptor and possible carcinogen, onto U.S. soil each year, though the chemical was banned in Europe in 2004 because of its toxicity (despite its being manufactured by a European company, Syngenta).[24] Often these chemicals linger in the environment. The pesticide dichloro-diphenyl-trichloroethane (DDT; see fig. 22), banned in 1973 thanks in large part to the work of Rachel Carson, remains ubiquitous in American bodies, foods, and environments forty years later.[25] A recent study of randomly sampled foods found DDT metabolites in 60 percent of heavy cream samples and 28 percent of carrots,[26] while another study found a five-fold increase in the risk of breast cancer among young women who as girls had been exposed to DDT.[27] Similarly, polychlorinated biphenyls (PCBs), slowly degrading carcinogens banned in the late 1970s, are still found in human flesh, soil, water sources, and the walls of buildings.[28] The EPA classifies approximately forty registered chemicals used in pesticides as known, probable, or possible human carcinogens.[29] Over 75 percent of food in American grocery stores has residues of one or more pesticide chemicals.[30]

Bisphenol A (BPA), used in the manufacture of plastics, is found at biologically active levels in 93 percent of Americans, and 130 studies have linked BPA to breast cancer, heart disease, and liver abnormalities.[31] Despite much recent attention in the media, BPA is still legal and commonly used in food packaging; it requires no labeling or warning. It has only recently been banned in children's chewable toys

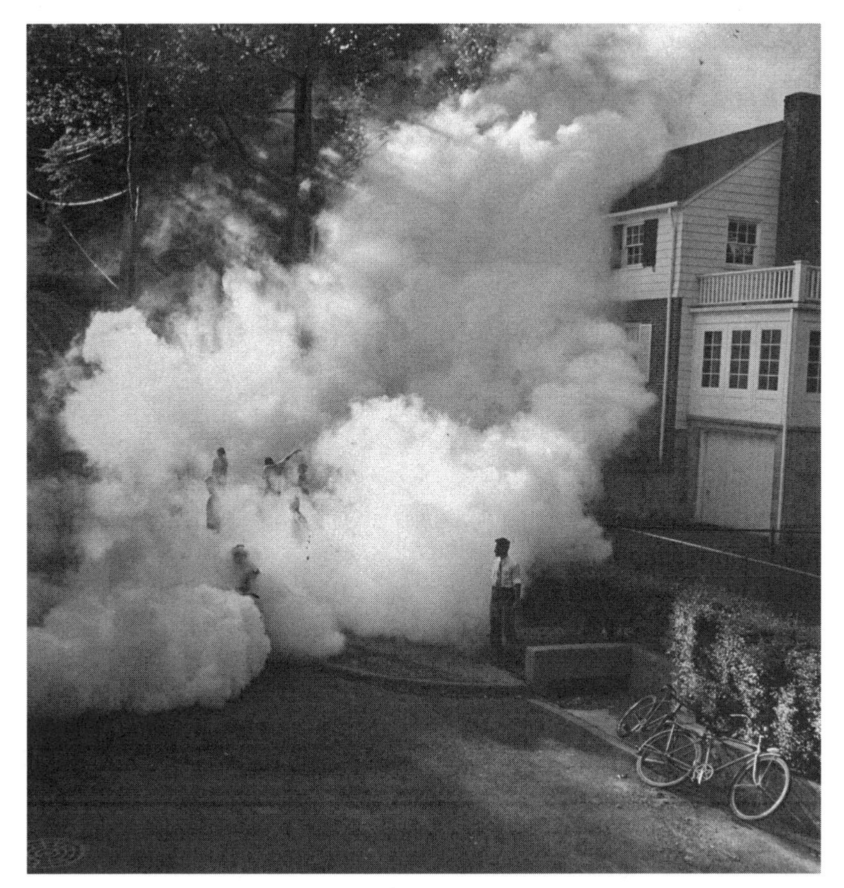

FIGURE 22. Photographs and films in the 1940s and 1950s often featured children playing in DDT or being sprayed with the chemical while eating lunch. None of these children were followed to gain a long-term understanding of the effects of DDT. (Photo by George Silk, 1948; reproduced by permission of Getty Images)

and bottles—just because the popular Nalgene water bottles are now BPA-free doesn't imply an industry-wide level of regulation. Even when a particular carcinogen has garnered press, most Americans remain ignorant of most known carcinogens, and low-income people are more likely to suffer exposures due to working conditions and geographical stratification.[32]

The Cancer Panel Report, at nearly 150 pages, details the hazards of living and dying in America and the ways and reasons that these risks continue to be underestimated, unknown, and covered up. From this exhaustive document, two critical points emerge for thinking about toxic exposure. First, we simply do not understand toxic body burdens. Studies have shown that virtually all Americans are now born with body burdens of known toxic chemicals.[33] However, well over a decade after the EPA was mandated with identifying human exposures to endocrine disruptors, it has yet to develop screening tests.[34] Not only do we have no frameworks to understand exposures, but the "pure" body that underlies so many ideas of cause simply does not exist. When it comes to toxic exposure and humans, there is no such thing as a blank slate.

A second problem arises from the fact that U.S. regulatory agencies tacitly permit the use of toxic chemicals if their benefits outweigh the risks they pose. The EPA allows chemicals that do not pose an "unreasonable risk to man or the environment, taking into account the economic, social, and environmental costs and benefits of the use of any pesticide."[35] (Atrazine, for example, increases agricultural productivity by an estimated 3–6 percent.) Obvious contaminants pollute this logic. For one thing, citizens unequally absorb the risks, costs, and benefits depending on factors such as their occupation, gender, race, age, and geographic location, such that the categories used by the EPA—"man," "environment," "costs," "benefits"—bear no necessary overlap to enable comparison.

Whole libraries of books have been published detailing all the ways that American industry and the military have produced deaths, fear, and uncertainty. We don't need more proof of that. Rather, I'm struck by the seeming inability to bring this production of cancer (with the notable exception of cigarettes) to the fore of cancer research, law, and history. There is a pervasive social taboo—an uncoolness, so to speak—around recognizing cancer production, opposing that production, or expressing genuine fear about living in this chemical cesspool. This cultivated inhibition plays a key role in the making of cancer.

The most powerful culture-makers—industry, government, medicine—have been slow to recognize, let alone advocate for research into, the connections between environmental toxins and the disease. If fear results in part from the unknown, then keeping things unknowable contributes to the circulation of an unattributable anxiety. Ask anyone whose heart has pounded when a kindly doctor responded to her questions with a shrug and a sad look in his eye.

FAUSTIAN BARGAIN

As we saw in chapter 4, tort law offers an awkward and expensive cost-sharing ideal. Theoretically, the law protects citizens from the dangers of products or actions.[36] A plaintiff must prove, in launching such a suit, that, first, he has an injury, and second, the injury has been directly ("proximately") caused by the product or action of the defendant. Historically, tort law ensures that all costs of production—including the costs of injury—remain visible and taken into account. However, in the case of exposure to a carcinogen, such proof is virtually impossible to provide. Thus, exposing people to carcinogens carries virtually no risk of lawsuits from injured parties.

The delay in the onset of some kinds of injury—such as cancer—has led courts to accept a claim for "toxic tort," which enables someone to bring a suit long after the statutes of limitations would normally have run out. Some cases have successfully been brought because a cancer was rare enough to be directly related to an exposure (asbestos and mesothelioma, hairspray and angiosarcoma of the liver, cigarettes and lung cancer), even past the usual one- or two-year statutes of limitations. But most generic, common cancers have no demonstrable cause. Perhaps they resulted from multiple exposures, or perhaps only one. Perhaps none. Who knows?

People who have been exposed to carcinogens have two practical legal choices, each of which differently juggles the problem of proving an injury and proving its proximate cause.[37] In the first scenario, a potential plaintiff can wait to see if she develops cancer and then attempt to prove proximate cause in a toxic tort. The necessary delay in bringing this kind of complaint will run several risks: the company may no longer exist when the suit is brought; the cancer may not be linkable to the exposure; the patient will have to front the costs of the cancer screenings and treatments.

Alternatively, a plaintiff can open a case immediately after exposure under standard tort rules. Since the plaintiff will not yet have developed cancer, she must claim that the injury is emotional rather than physical. In "fear of cancer" cases, injury refers not to cancer itself, but to the plaintiffs' fear that they may, in the future, develop cancer as a result of their exposures.[38] These suits have proven practically impossible to win. Consequently, the tort system has failed to render cancer into a legible injury.

One such "fear of cancer" suit that set the standard in California and most of the United States came before the state Supreme Court in 1993. In *Potter v. Firestone Tire and Rubber,* the court acknowledged the legitimate nature of fear-of-cancer claims; nevertheless, for reasons discussed below, it reversed a lower court's award of punitive and general damages and remanded the case for retrial.[39] The court acknowledged the legitimacy of the plaintiff's fear-of-cancer claim; yet it found for the corporate defendant. In its decision, the California Supreme Court set an extremely high bar for the plaintiffs to meet in order to recover damages under a negligence theory. One could reasonably argue that the intent of the *Potter* decision was specifically to prevent further fear-of-cancer lawsuits.

The facts and allegations presented in the case were as follows: Between 1967 and 1980, Firestone disposed of toxic chemicals and known human carcinogens at the Crazy Horse dump in Salinas, California, despite having been required to abide by environmental standards for disposing of hazardous waste because of the dump's proximity to local residents' drinking-water sources. In 1984, benzene, toluene, chloroform, and vinyl chloride were found in local wells, in a chemical fingerprint later found to be identical to that of the chemicals dumped by Firestone. About 6,200 people within three miles of the site had consumed contaminated drinking water, and in 1987 the City of Salinas bought the houses in the affected area and bulldozed them.[40] Two families sued Firestone.

Because internal Firestone documents revealed that plant managers knew that the company had been illegally dumping the chemical wastes from its vulcanization processes since 1977, the plaintiffs were awarded over $1.3 million in compensatory and $2.6 million in punitive damages. When Firestone appealed, the California Supreme Court reversed the decision on the grounds that the plaintiffs had failed to prove that they had a legitimate fear, which would require establishing the following: (1) that Firestone's conduct was specifically directed at them and (2) that the exposures were more likely than not to result in cancer.[41] The court remanded the case for retrial to allow the plaintiffs to prove that the defendants were "aware of the presence of these particular plaintiffs and their use and consumption of the water." They chose instead to settle out of court.[42]

The state Supreme Court interpreted the law as requiring plaintiffs to prove that their fear of cancer stems from knowledge, corroborated by reliable medical or scientific opinion, that they are more likely than not to develop cancer in the future due to the toxic exposure. Plaintiffs, the court stated, could avoid this high standard of proof only if they are able to show that the defendant acted "recklessly" or "outrageously." In that case, they would only have to demonstrate that the "actual risk of cancer is significant." (Though just what "significant" means is not clear.)

Meeting this burden of proof would require nothing less than a randomized controlled trial, and one that exposed a population to a similar panel of chemicals and compared it over time to an unexposed group—both unethical and impossible given the short span of human lives and the newness of many of the chemicals. Practically speaking, the court made it impossible to bring a complaint against a person or company who knowingly exposes others to carcinogens.

The pseudoscientific language of a "more likely than not" threshold makes it appear sensible. Yet closer scrutiny suggests that this threshold would allow a chemical exposure that kills off 20, 30, 40, or even 49 percent of a population—as long as the company does not directly target individuals. If, after an exposure, forty-nine in a class of one hundred sicken and die, the more-likely-than-not threshold will not have been met. Even after an actual cancer diagnosis, each *individual* would initially have been more likely to *not* have developed cancer. The levels of cancers caused would have to be stunningly high—and provable in advance—for these cases to be won.

Ironically, one of the court's major concerns in finding for the plaintiffs was the vast political and economic problem of carcinogenic exposures. The court stated: "All of us are potential fear of cancer plaintiffs, provided we are sufficiently aware of and worried about the possibility of developing cancer from exposure to or ingestion of a carcinogenic substance."[43] In the early 1970s, scientists found that one such substance, vinyl chloride, at low doses causes cancer in animals. Yet this ubiquitous chemical continues to appear in hairspray, saran wrap, car upholstery, shower curtains, floor coverings, and hundreds of other consumer products. As a chemical supervisor wrote in 1973, if lawsuits were brought over vinyl chloride, the industry would have "essentially unlimited liability to the entire U.S. population."[44] While the California Supreme Court recognized the depth of the problem, at the same time it refused to take on the role of adjudicating the justness of such exposure.

In making its policy claims in the Firestone case, the court relied heavily on an article by Robert Willmore, an attorney who, according to his website, "supervised the defense of over $100 billion in tort claims against the federal government involving such areas as asbestos, Agent Orange, radiation exposure, environmental and toxic torts, and aviation disasters."[45] Willmore states that allowing fear-of-cancer claims would "make it much more likely that a person exposed to small amounts of a carcinogen will sue rather than shrug off the risk as one more of the numerous small cancer-causing risks to which we are all constantly exposed."[46] Willmore, in other words, asks us to wave off all exposures as equivalent, everyday occurrences. In his analysis, the Firestone exposure would be no different than using a microwave.

Rather than demonstrating that large awards may act as a deterrent to companies like Firestone, Willmore worries about plaintiffs. He claims (without grounds) that large awards are more likely to increase the number of plaintiffs who are willing to deceive. "They may feel, after all, that they are entitled to something for having been exposed in the first place." He further argues that "the understandable fear of a surge of cancerphobia liability was one of the issues that led to the ultimate defeat by filibuster in 1988 in the Senate of a Worker High-Risk Notification Bill (S. 79)," a bill that would have required employers to inform workers about their exposure to carcinogens.[47]

Potter v. Firestone represents just one of many instances of litigation in which the court has justified erring in the defendant's favor with the argument that a finding for the plaintiff might lead to a landslide of claims about dangerous exposures. The Cancer Panel Report, meanwhile, indicates that fear-of-cancer claims (and the judicial fear of such claims) would in some cases have validity. Turning claims about exposures into claims about fear or a platform for potential deceit at once diminishes legitimate fears and concerns and prevents cancer injuries from gaining traction as compensable injuries. This legal logic increases the ability of some people and companies to expose populations to carcinogens without incurring any costs, while decreasing the ability of those exposed to those chemicals to challenge such exposures. For anyone living with exposure, fear, cancer, or all three, such logic increases cognitive dissonance to a near-toxic level.

PRODIGAL SON

Tobacco, now the most politically acceptable object of anticancer awareness, history, and activism, offers the most visible representation of disease and death. With cigarette warnings, the government has attempted to manage behavior through a unique combination of awareness about the inherent dangers of tobacco products and negative provocations about the consequences of using it. Because of its extreme lobbying power, the tobacco industry has dodged regulation by the

FDA, Occupational Safety and Health Administration (OSHA), and other federal agencies and so legally produces one of the few products that regularly and predictably injures and kills its consumers as a matter of course. We've now reached a stalemate: governments rely on the taxes that sales generate, and many smokers have been unable or unwilling to quit.

The first health warnings appeared on cigarette packages in 1966. They resulted from a great deal of negotiation between the Federal Trade Commission and industry, and read: "Cigarette smoking may be hazardous to your health." The industry soon came to see this warning as positive, since it bolstered their assertion in litigation that consumers knowingly accepted the dangers when they opened a pack of cigarettes.

The peculiar legal, regulatory, and marketing history of cigarettes eventually led to the partial regulation of tobacco products through the FDA (a result of the 2009 Family Smoking Prevention and Tobacco Control Act). In an effort to undo the age-old image of smoking as a glamorous, sexy, daring, pleasurable habit, the agency chose a set of warnings for 2012 release based on their ability to stimulate strongly negative emotional responses. The proposed cigarette warnings attempt to overcome the lag between smoking and injury by illustrating the potential consequences of smoking directly on the box. These images can't be mistaken for the Lance Face.

The FDA aimed to scare people away from smoking—in their words, to elicit "strong emotional and cognitive reactions to the graphic cigarette warning label," to enhance "recall and processing of the health warning."[48] These graphic warnings would offer—as they do in Canada, Australia, and other countries—one of the few places in the public domain where realistic images of cancer appear: no sanitized, patronizingly pretty pictures here. (Early detection ads also aim to instill a fear of cancer and of the consequences of delay, but more often they convey a stylized or sentimental notion of cancer, which is no image of cancer at all.)

In selecting a warning for the tagline "Cigarettes Cause Cancer," the FDA studied a series of images. These included one used in Canadian labels, which depicts a former model who was photographed as she was dying of lung cancer (or being killed by cigarettes?). Cropped down from a larger photo that includes a nurse and hospital IV equipment, the image (fig. 23) clearly portrays a young woman (young to be dying of cancer, anyway) in an angled hospital bed, her gender evident

IMPORTED FOR/
IMPORTÉ POUR:
IMPERIAL TOBACCO
CANADA LTD./LTÉE.
MONTREAL, CANADA
H3C 3L6
Tobacco smoke contains benzene, a chemical
that causes cancer.
Health Canada
La fumée du tabac contient du benzène, un produit
chimique qui donne le cancer.
Santé Canada
©The Edmonton Journal
WARNING
This is what dying of
lung cancer looks like.
Barb Tarbox died at 42 of lung cancer
caused by cigarettes.
You can quit. We can help.
1-866-366-3667
gosmokefree.gc.ca/quit
Health Canada
20
V
VICEROY
V 20
CIGARETTES
KING SIZE

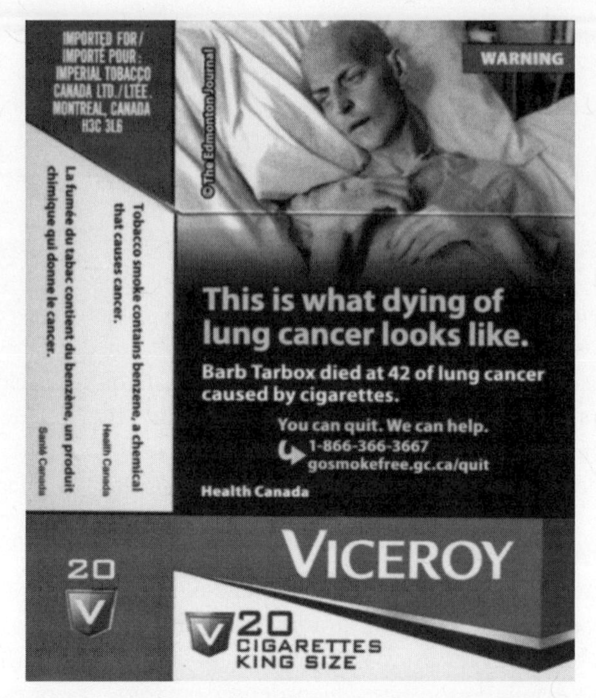

FIGURE 23. This image of the late antitobacco activist and smoker Barb Tarbox appears on Canadian cigarette boxes with the warning, "This is what dying of lung cancer looks like." The Canadian warnings take up three-quarters of the surface of the package.

only from the painted fingernails—perhaps the final gift of a friend, family member, or lover. The Canadian warning depicts consequences by naming this person and stating her age at death: "Barb Tarbox died at 42 of lung cancer caused by cigarettes." The warning itself—"this is what dying of cancer looks like"—poses as both information and fear factor, though it could be read with a hint of sarcasm—*You still want to smoke?* The ad then gives encouragement ("You can quit") and an offer ("We can help"), followed by a phone number and a website URL.

The FDA ultimately found that an image of mouth cancer (fig. 24) better met the ability of viewers to remember and respond to it, and so chose it over the Tarbox image and several others. The studies that the FDA relied on suggest that disgust provokes more of a physiological response in individuals than does fear (though both are related and difficult to measure), accounting for the greater recall success of the mouth

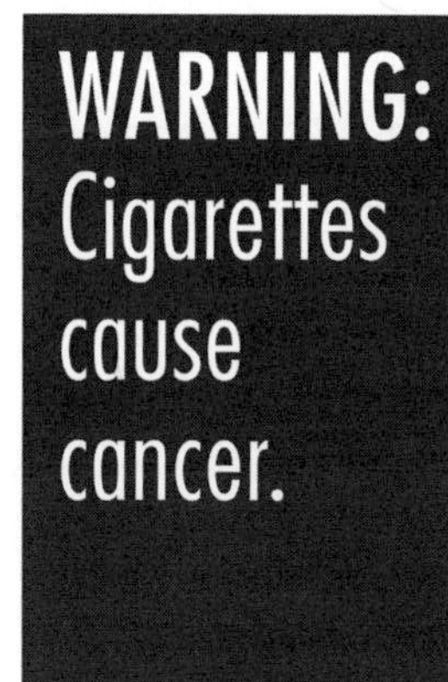

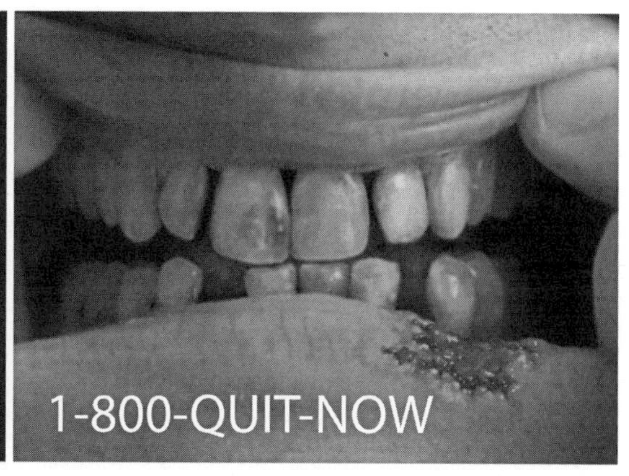

FIGURE 24. In 2009, the FDA, authorized to regulate the manufacture, distribution, and marketing of tobacco products, proposed graphics intended to cover 50 percent of each cigarette package. In 2012, a Washington, D.C., federal judge and a federal appellate court both ruled that the requirement was unconstitutional, as it compelled specific kinds of commercial speech. In the FDA's defense, the government claimed that the warnings offer legitimate public-health messages. At the time of writing, the Supreme Court has yet to decide whether to hear the case. (Courtesy of the FDA)

cancer image.[49] Arguably, it matters whether cancer is represented as something to be avoided because it is disgusting or because it is scary. Still, the negative affect differs from the airbrushed visual iconography of cancer hospital brochures, patient pamphlets, or pharmaceutical advertisements, which aim at encouraging affective attachment to an HMO, reducing the fear around a potential treatment, or plugging a chance of survival.

At the date of this writing, a U.S. Court of Appeals in Washington, D.C., has upheld the tobacco companies' claim that the warnings violate their First Amendment right of free speech, since the warning requires them to engage in advocacy on the government's behalf. A Cincinnati Federal Court of Appeals upheld the FDA, leading many to speculate whether the Supreme Court will hear the issue. The graphic warnings signal an ambiguity. While unwilling to take cigarettes off the market, even though they present many dangers and no benefits (the standard cost-benefit model for other products), the government at least aims to provoke a physiological and psychological response at the moment of purchase and consumption. The cigarette warning conveys the message, "If you smoke, a bad thing will eventually happen, so choose not to buy this package." In other words, the images *imply* governmental and regulatory protection against the dangers of cigarettes, even as the addictive qualities of cigarettes continue to go unregulated. Something Is Being Done, the warnings seem to say. And to be sure, regulations now control such issues as where people can smoke and where and how the product can be advertised. But the physical design of the product remains in the hands of the manufacturers.[50]

Cigarette development, consumption, epidemiology, and litigation offer an extreme exception to environmentally caused cancers, rather than an exemplary case, despite the prominence of tobacco and cigarettes in many mainstream cancer histories. The product remains, now, much easier to "expose" to a mainstream audience than, say, the military or medical causes of cancer. Antitobacco advocates and governmental health agencies represent tobacco as the "leading cause of preventable death"; however, a more accurate description would portray tobacco as the substance most easily correlated with cancer. Although the initial epidemiology making the link between smoking and lung cancer was anything but straightforward (as chapter 7 examines), the rarity of lung cancer prior to cigarettes and the solid science that has proven smoking's addictive and carcinogenic aspects have led to an accepted causal connection. Despite the unique aspects of the smoking issue, one might well ask why the so-called *leading* cause of death attracts so much governmental attention (albeit an attention focused solely on product use rather than product design), while other potential causes (as outlined in the Cancer Panel Report or the chapter on IVF) attract practically none. And not only do they garner no attention, but anyone who dares consider these forms of causation risks being labeled a paranoiac. Only dorks *worry* about environmental toxins. After all, they're everywhere.

In his ethnography of New Mexico, *Understories,* Jake Kosek captures the specter of cancer as pervading the environment, hovering beyond explanations of cause. Kosek relays a conversation he had with a woman about her husband, a blue-collar worker in Los Alamos whose job required him to scrub the radiation out of worksites. After he died of cancer, she said, "He [knew] where the cancer came from—we all do—but it's hard to admit you were wrong and it's hard to bite the hand that has fed us for over thirty years. Besides, . . . it's hard to know for sure."[51]

Perhaps the creation of the special case, such as cigarettes, gives an impression of controllability and causality, as opposed to resigning ourselves to the fact that we all live in a general cancer universe. When cause *seems* clear, shame, fear, and the diminution of fear build a social and biological paradox of uncertainty.[52]

CONCLUSION: FALLOUT

When I see the obituary of someone who had a cancer recurrence after two decades, I panic, thinking that someone close to me will read it and, reminded of my tenuousness, not want to be my friend. I dread seeing friends and family get skinny and old-looking and bloated; I'm frightened of what the people who take the corpse will say as they lug it down the stairs and out the door, of what my own dead face will look like. Fear, that sticky, primal emotion, cements so many unspoken elements of the cancer conglomerate.

The advice in the *New York Times* article mentioned earlier in this chapter *(just tell a joke and wear a wig!)* turns cancer survivorship from an emotional and physical state into an ability, a private trait rather than a communal effort and responsibility. Such advice instructs the cancer survivor to position herself in a socially acceptable role as an ennobled survivor who has undergone a personal tragedy, bravely shrugging off the failure of the state to regulate carcinogens, to provide healthcare, to control medical costs. This self-help literature rarely addresses the material needs of survivors. Nor does it recognize a system that often ejects patients without educating them on follow-up care, the symptoms of recurrence, or even, often, the basic details and potential consequences of the treatments they have already received.[53] None of the literature acknowledges another aspect of being a survivor: that feeling of sacrifice, of having taken the fall for all those others who now don't have to enter life in prognosis. I've never seen a scrap of oncology literature address the "why me?" question—not the existential "why me?," but the real, causative question of why, specifically, *me?*—though most cancer patients or survivors I know speak of how excruciating it is to try and piece together an answer.

There's nothing wrong with trying to pass, with wearing a wig so as not to be stared at. There's nothing wrong with turning inward to one's family in times of struggle. It's like the bomb shelter images from the 1960s, which, as Masco describes, confer the normalcy of gender roles onto cement-walled living rooms, where mom prepares a meal while dad reads the newspaper or fiddles with the radio, protected from the dark cloud outside (fig. 25).[54] But there may be other responses as well

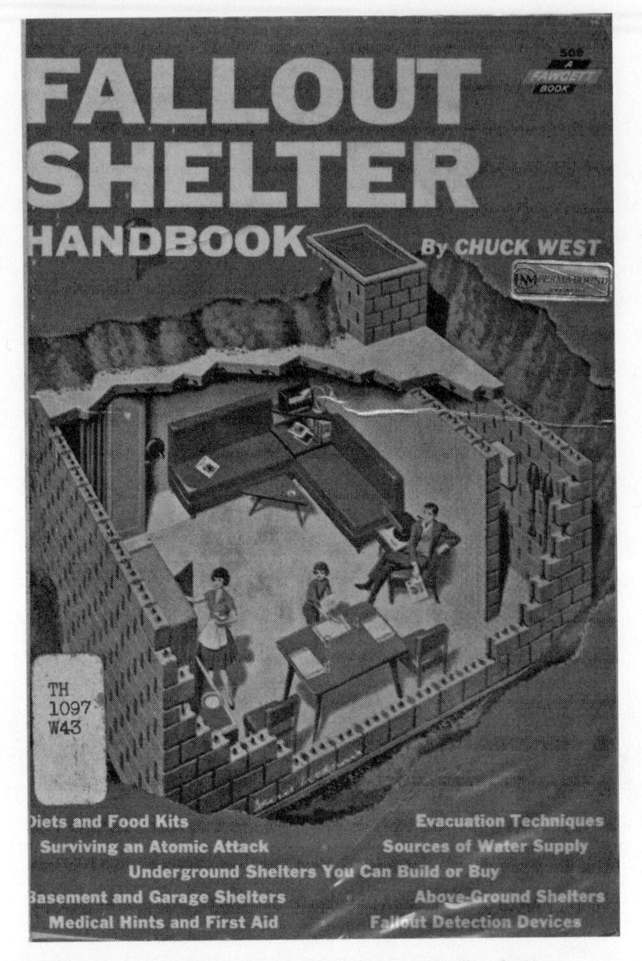

FIGURE 25. In the popular *Fallout Shelter Handbook* (New York: Fawcett, 1962), Chuck West describes how to build and stock a bomb shelter. The cozy space replicates a midcentury living room, complete with an aproned housewife preparing dinner as Daddy finishes reading a magazine. One does not find in this booklet information on the military's role in creating cancer, even though one in ten Americans today lives near a toxic military site.

as taking comfort in the structures we know so well, especially when it isn't clear that they serve us well.

One study found that "hospice in-patients who had witnessed the death of other hospice patients were significantly less anxious and depressed than those who had not."[55] Sometimes we die in the way we predicted, sometimes earlier, sometimes capriciously. Dancer Isadora Duncan died when her hand-painted silk scarf tangled with the open spokes of a car in Nice. Sometimes a cancer patient dies of a stroke, and sometimes someone who would eventually have been diagnosed with cancer dies in a terrorist attack. But we will all die. And when added to all the other levels of perpetuated fear and unknowing—cultural, chemical, legal, emotional—denying looming death only increases the frightening cognitive dissonance.

As any kid on Halloween knows, even a fun wig can make things scarier.

CHAPTER 9

Rubble

Bakelite Bodies

Whenever I move house, around midnight on the final day of the lease I end up with a little pile of things in the middle of my furnitureless place, things that don't really belong in any of the labeled boxes and yet that don't quite seem like trash: a jar of pennies, a Niagara Falls keychain, a sentimental Christmas ornament.

After my cancer treatment, as I packed up to leave my parents' home, the dreaded mound accumulated in my closet. In this case, I had bottles of pills I could sell on the street for hundreds of dollars. I had a couple of round cloth envelopes, each stuffed with an adjustable fake cotton puff and fastened with Velcro. A huge gel prosthesis drooped over the edge of the shelf. Other items had come in mortifying circumstances, but the acquisition of the prosthesis had been as straightforward as sizing a pair of sneakers. Next to the prosthesis sat a case of Ensure protein drink we had bought for my then-partner's sister just before she died. The tidy, cloying labels *(Complete Balanced Nutrition! Protein to Help Build Muscle Mass!)* belied Jane's last few days in a wheelchair, when she was barely able to talk. A used wig, which I had selected at the cancer center from a massive mound but never really wore, poked out from a manila envelope like a squirrel sniffing for danger. The cancer fracas had curated this tiny, now anachronistic, collection.

The objects in this uncanny heap had served not merely as isolated stand-ins for a body, but as crucial conduits for some semblance of a social life, for a normalcy that was by no means assured. They deciphered me. They enabled me to partake in life among friends and strangers—or at least to imagine the possibility of doing so. In some ways, they mimicked the role of the pathology report in its translational project between cells and physicians. With my pathology report, the material of my body (that me and not-me tumor) seemed to be literally lifted out of my self and into data. The objects in the closet, unlike the data that represented parts lifted *out* of me, and been plunked *into* me in order to rebuild a prior, or recognizable, or acceptable self. Or that was the intent, anyway.

Italo Calvino wrote about the simple act of taking out the garbage: "My relationship with the *poubelle* [trash can] is that of the man for whom throwing something away completes or confirms its appropriation; my contemplation of the heap of peels, shells, packaging and plastic containers brings with it the satisfaction of having consumed their contents."[1] My knoll of scraps wasn't quite debris in this sense, but it still embodied a sense of uncertainty, of viciously shifting value. Should I need them again soon, I would cherish those pills. If not, eventually they would expire, worthless. The most priceless situation would be not to need them, ever. These cusp objects were either imperative or meaningless, but nothing in between. The whole concept of worth took on a distorted quality, with me happiest when these valuable goods were totally useless; disgusting, even.

Had I fully consumed or appropriated these items? Was I ready for them to be junk? If they were trash now, what had they been to begin with? My cancer stuff had offered me opportunities, both ethnographic and otherwise, including a gateway to performing normalcy. Even the Port-a-Cath—yes, that's the real name for the catheter opening affixed to one's chest—had made me into a favored patient. In having it excavated I finally trashed that patient role, just as refusing the cheap warmed blankets in the freezing-cold chemo room felt in some pathetic way like rebuffing the part of helpless object. Only patients have blankets on their laps: one blanket + one gown = one patient. No blanket, one might want to think (or at least I did), disrupts the equation.

Hospital staff generally seemed to like an implanted, semipermanent orifice for chemotherapy, since it meant they wouldn't need to locate a new vein for the IV each time. I had two choices of ports, and as I was reminded several times by the nurses, whichever device I selected would make the nurses' job easier. The staff lobbied for the first device, a PICC line catheter, which inserts into a vein in the forearm, with a mechanical contraption hanging out that is taped to the arm when not in use. The drawback to that one was that I could not lift more than five pounds with it in, and, eager to tough it out, I wanted to get to the gym and work out a couple of times a week. I also wanted to be able to pick up my little kids, one and three years old and still in need of adult arms. Out went the PICC idea. The other option was the Port-a-Cath, which, placed under the flesh in the chest, required a general anesthetic to implant. When I requested it, the nurse looked at me as if I were crazy. "But, that's permanent," she said, as if nothing else about cancer would leave a trace. I asked if I could have it removed after the chemo regime was over: "Well . . . yes." So it was less enduring than many other scars would be—but those scars are harder to talk about.

I had the Port-a-Cath implanted one morning immediately before being shipped to the chemotherapy treatment. During the transit from surgery to chemo, someone lost track of my clothes, and after my partner strode from one department to another for two hours with no luck, I went home in the Canadian winter in just my hospital gown. The Port-a-Cath was a pretty loaded device, both in what it signified and in the experience of having it, so getting it removed was a key aspect of "finishing up" treatment—an optimistic finale. The doctor gouged away for a long, long time with his scalpel and finally told me that it was embedded as if in concrete and don't let anyone tell me that I wasn't good at healing. My body, evidently, wanted to absorb the port as much as I wanted to get rid of it. In the culmination of treatment, they did finally get it out, and when I walked out of the office in search of my waiting dad, I used my Game Face to crush an urge to weep.

When thinking about discarded items, anthropologists always cite Mary Douglas, the noted British social theorist who wrote of waste not as something inherently dirty, but as a society's decision about what would be considered as "matter out of place," or the stuff that does not fit within categories.[2] In my parents' house, I certainly didn't know how to categorize those newly useless objects. But something physical pervaded my interaction with the bits and pieces. They were revolting to me; they posed as evidence, as Milton might say, that I had fallen to the "lowest pitch of abject fortune." But something more animalistic underlay my relationship to them, like the grotesque paradox of eating miniature toasts with tapenade at a funeral organized by a heartbroken widow. Douglas famously said, "Where there is dirt, there is a system." Surely my feeling of disgust—in response to the possibility of one or three breasts, or of hunger in the midst of death—might provide insight into that system.

The discarded items on my cancer shelf had once enabled me to pass as normal and healthy (or at least to fake it to myself, if no one else). I already had something of an uneasy relationship to this act of passing: Did I want to? And if so, why? For me? To protect others? In that sense, I had an advantage: for decades I'd figured out strategies for living as a queer person and in my twenties eventually found communities that uneasily repaired some of the economic and social damage of homophobia.

Still, even used as I was to boundaries around "normal," cancer seemed extreme. I wore a prosthesis for a job interview the day before my chemo started, though I wouldn't have considered doing so in many other circumstances. Did it help me? Not that time, at least: I didn't get the job. (Even a prosthesis can only help so much.) And I gawked just as eagerly as the straight women did when two weeks after my surgery, an older woman at a lymphedema workshop pulled her prosthetic breast out of her bra to show us how it worked and to assure the sea of stunned faces that you really couldn't tell. (True, you really couldn't.)

Despite its awkwardness, the prosthesis, like the other cancer objects, offered me a gateway to a cancer community, a community of people who learn to use these props because they need to, who talk about their exploration of them. These conversations even offered a behind-the-scenes peek at how women buttress themselves with makeup and other devices, practices to which I had never been privy.

Cancer brought with it a makeup bag, and cosmetics were enlisted to help me—finally—acquire a true femininity. The cosmetic industry collectively sponsors the "Look Good . . . Feel Better" program to "help" women with cancer solve beauty problems introduced by chemotherapy. The program, "created from the concept that if a woman living with cancer can be helped to look good, her improved self-image will help her to approach cancer and its treatment with greater confidence," already boasts 700,000 female participants at 3,000 locations in the United States, and 1.1 million worldwide since its inception in 1986. They recently initiated a program for men as well.[3]

Even from outside the female paradigm, I already knew that the deeply ingrained attachment to looking better and thus feeling better gains more force when coupled with any chance that the messy, biologically functioning body might display itself. Educational videos from the 1950s, for example, exhort young girls to dress up just a teensy bit more during their menstrual periods, to look that speck more put together than usual. Airplane stewardesses had strict codes of appearance—including wearing contact lenses instead of glasses—well into the 1980s. While many of these gendered regulations have been sloughed away by the feminist movement, study after study has shown that both women's and men's looks have a major bearing on their job success, income, social lives, and quality of life.[4]

Beauty-discrimination seems patently unfair (unless, of course, you happen to be beautiful). Many researchers have observed that starting from childhood, good-looking people are more likely to be considered intelligent, friendly, and capable, while unattractive children and adults internalize the opposite assumptions.[5] Still, for virtually everyone, the pursuit of beauty requires expense and time. In one legal suit, *Jespersen v. Harrah Operating Co.*, a bartender sued her employer for discrimination when the employer, Harrah's casino, instituted a new policy requiring women employees to wear makeup. Jespersen had worked for twenty years at Harrah's with an exemplary record when the new requirement was adopted. Makeup conflicted with Jespersen's self-image, and wearing it felt like a personal indignity; when she declined the mascara and lipstick, the casino fired her.[6] Omitting potential queer identity issues, law scholar Deborah Rhode commented that in upholding the employer's double standard, federal judges demonstrated their lack of understanding of the time, effort, and expense that cosmetics, hairstyling, and manicures require.[7]

More immediately injurious aspects of feminine beauty include high-heeled shoes, which eventually cause back and foot problems for 80 percent of wearers, not to mention the risk of breaking an ankle trying to catch a taxi. Other secondary effects of constructed femininity can take years to develop, such as the angiosarcomas of the liver that some women have only now developed after heavy use of hairspray in the 1960s and '70s.[8]

The cosmetics industry rakes in $18 billion in the United States, and the global investment in grooming totals $115 billion.[9] While 7 percent of that figure goes into ingredients, most of the rest is rolled into packaging and marketing, not just of products, but of the feminine beauty standards that cosmetics can help each consumer attain. I'm as susceptible to a woman's beauty (high heels and all) as any guy, but when a powerful industry with such an obvious interest sets the standards, it warrants a closer look.

I'm not suggesting that people refrain from looking good. That isn't it at all. But Look Good Feel Better demands something nearly absolute.

Although it doesn't take its participants to be dupes, its advice that women with cancer "face the challenge of a lifetime" with the help of the cosmetics industry seems a bit tone deaf. The workshops aren't talking about the real challenge—cancer—or about what exactly is being faced and by whom and at what cost. They aren't informing people about cancer and treatment risks, nor do they lobby for better treatments; even the Online Resources page doesn't include any activist groups. The campaign focuses on looks alone. In other words, the Look Good Feel Better pamphlets and images offer one more version of the happy Stepford cancer patient. Again, nothing is wrong with smiling, feeling good, feeling hopeful, but given the dearth of other options, the hegemony of these feelings needs to be unmasked.

The PR around Look Good Feel Better hammers home the message that this program is a legitimate and fundamental part of cancer treatment itself. Doctors' and nurses' urgings to attend a Look Good Feel Better workshop, the slick pamphlets, and the endorsement and involvement of the American Cancer Society (ACS) all create an aura of respectability. No simple vanity trip, the program's website states that "significant data suggests a strong link between women's participation in these programs and their rates of recovery." What does "rate of recovery mean," though? It seems to suggest a cure; however, no research substantiates this claim.

Started by the Cosmetic Toiletry and Fragrance Association in collaboration with the ACS and the National Cosmetology Association, the Look Good Feel Better organization now has a budget of about $2 million (which it raises through large publicity campaigns), and each year the cosmetics industry donates $10 million worth of cosmetics to the program. Nowhere in the publicity does one learn that the industry has spent millions on political lobbying to prevent regulation, or even labeling, of the known and possible carcinogens commonly found in its products, such as phthalates, parabens, and other estrogen mimickers. The Environmental Working Group has found that over five hundred cosmetic products sold in the United States contain ingredients that are illegal in Japan, Canada, or the European Union, and that roughly one of every thirty products sold in the United States fails to meet one or more industry or governmental cosmetics safety standards. The industry's own safety panel (the Cosmetic Ingredient Review, or CIR) has, in its thirty-year history, assessed fewer than 20 percent of cosmetics ingredients.[10]

When I called to sign up for a Look Good workshop, the receptionist said excitedly, "And we give you $140 worth of free cosmetics!!" Sure enough, at the class that I attended, each person was given boxes of cosmetics as well as books on makeup application. When I walked in, the other eight participants of the class were busily applying foundation. The women didn't look so good, after all. One had an obviously fake red wig and brightly colored cheeks, the others looked old and depressed. I was the only dyke by a long shot, and about three decades younger than the other participants. (I chivalrously thought my relative youth might make them feel better about their own situations. At least they'd gotten oldish before they'd gotten sick. But then that doesn't sound very considerate.)

I told the exuberant volunteer that I had never worn makeup, and wondered aloud if perhaps this workshop was not for me. She cheerfully assured me it would be *fun!* I should just *try* it! But eventually she wandered away, murmuring that she could be more useful to another client. (Right she was.) Despite the poor fit, I stayed in the class. The anthropologist in me was interested in seeing how the disease might be mediated, even if just for an evening, by "look good" rhetoric. We learned, for example, that "lipstick can brighten your looks and lift your spirits."

As research or not, the whole experience struck me as quite contrary to feeling good, let alone looking good. The smells of the makeup, the time spent in front of a mirror, just sitting upright—it was all a challenge. Personally, I felt crappy. The previous day I had had my head shaved; the barber, after telling me it was illegal for him to do a clean shave with a razor and that he only had clippers and no shaver, left my head looking like some mangy rat in an Art Spiegelman comic. Later, my friend Jo shaved it for me, nice and clean, in preparation for the Look Good class. As everyone else at the workshop gamely applied various strata of powders and creams, I patted moisturizer on my bare scalp rather than penciling in an eyebrow. The instructor stubbornly refused to look my way. No Good Patient designation for me this time.

The fissures in the room were fascinating and terrifying. The fake-looking-wig woman talked about the trauma of losing her hair, while another laughed herself to tears relating how she'd lost her wig at a local shop when she leaned over to pick something up and it got caught on a hook. She finished the story by saying, "You have to laugh, otherwise you'll cry." Even in this gathering of like souls—people newly diagnosed with cancer—you still *had* to laugh.

When the wig demonstrator complimented one woman's long strawberry blond hair, the woman replied that she would be starting chemo the next day. The crowd let out an audible murmur; without missing a beat, the wig woman responded by whipping out a $600 long-strawberry-blond wig, which she began to lustily brush and shape as if bewitched. She placed it on the bald mannequin and the other women gasped at the wig's apparent beauty. It *did* look a lot like the other woman's hair. For a strange moment, the idea that this woman's hair was replicable pressed against all our fears: of chemotherapy, hair loss, disposability. If the wig, full of color and vitality, could replace her hair, perhaps that white, faceless Bakelite mannequin could replace her entire body.

Several of us in that room faced futures that would include not just losing hair for a few months, but losing everything to cancer, including identities as healthy people who look well, feel more or less fine, and are able to move through the world. Those presents and futures would sandwich some unspecified length of time between them during which we would be unrelentingly sick and awful-looking. If the wellness could not be faked, however, the "femininity" could. If we couldn't help ourselves get well, we could help ourselves look good. To what better use could cosmetics be put than this attempt to undo illness? No wonder the cosmetics industry gives so much makeup to this charity. What looks like benevolence merely extends the beauty industry's project: to enable people to pass in a world obsessed with looks—in this instance, with a humanitarian spin. No one cares more than they do, even when—especially when—you look terrible.[11]

I lost my hair in two stages. First, I had it cut short. This I didn't mind; I've had it even shorter by choice. My three-year-old daughter, Kahlo, was with me, and she sat very quietly in the too-big chair waiting. When it was over, she didn't want to touch my hair or look at me. Luckily, I could chase her outside in the cold sun and make her remember the me under the new cut. After a few days, she loved to touch it and let me scrub her belly with it and rub shaving cream into my head while we were in the bath.

To prepare Kahlo for my complete shave, I showed her pictures of Lance Armstrong. For about two weeks I told her that I would be getting my hair cut like his. When the hairs started falling out all over my hands and the bathroom, and when I could feel each follicle shivering on my head, I knew it was time. When the moment finally arrived, Kahlo exclaimed in a torrent of thrilled observation: "I like your hair, Mima—I like the back of it. It's spiky! I like touching it. You're *bald!*" And then, confidently: "I'm going to get my hair cut like yours." Kahlo had no problems with the hair. The same was not true, though, of the missing "nursie," which she asked me about every few days, assuring me that no one would take hers since hers was "full of blood." For years she asked if the breast would grow back as my hair eventually did.

Not everyone took the changes in the easy stride of a three-year-old. In the complete absence of gender signifiers, assumptions were made. For example, every time I ran into the resident doctor in the hallway during my treatments at the oncology clinic, she said to me: "You know, you could get a wig; they make really good ones and you can't even tell." When I'd go for a medical appointment, the nurse would invariably say: "Oh, you've done the 'hat thing,' not the 'wig thing.'" The first few times I didn't really notice, but after I was in chemotherapy for some time, I started to take the remark personally. I wanted to say to her, You know, I'm a dyke from San Francisco (true), I am not ashamed that I have cancer (not true), and I don't mind being bald (medium true), so quit it already with the wig comments! One friend suggested I respond that I *did* have a wig on, it was just very short.

Instead I just nodded politely at the resident, the nurse, and everyone else. I suppose the fact that baldness is a "medical side-effect" is supposed to drain the remarks of their personal nature. I can't help but notice when I survey the general population that an enormous number of people walk around unabashedly with various shades of thinning hair. For women, baldness has become a signifier of either illness or aggression. Though a shaven head, and even breastlessness, is a completely conceivable choice for a person like me (queer, out, athletic, relatively confident), the fact that I was bald from cancer supplanted using baldness or a flat chest to express identity. When my oncologist noted my lack of hair, she was making a general comment in the cancer framework; she genuinely couldn't distinguish what might have been, at another moment in my life, an expression of my specific selfhood.

Right before my diagnosis, I entered the academic job market. I was offered a bunch of interviews, all but three of which I gave up, not seeing how I could do a good interview while on chemotherapy. One I really wanted to try for. The department was stacked with amazing scholars and the old graystone campus made you feel like part of a bygone era when scholarship mattered. But I couldn't seem to fit the interview in between my various treatments. I requested the last possible day for the interview, and they set it for late March. As the time grew near, I wrote saying that I was under "medical watch" (I didn't want to mention the c-word) and so could not travel after all; was there any chance that they could change the interview date? Yes, they would postpone it by four days to the first week of April. Damn, that wasn't very much. So I lobbied my radiation oncologist for an early start to the daily treatments, and he doubled them for three days so that I would be finished in time. I did the interview with about three eyebrow hairs, radiation burns barely hidden by my collar, and 3 millimeters of hair on my head. I arranged the three-day interview such that I had the mornings to refamiliarize myself with my work, then meet with faculty and students in the afternoons and evenings before dropping exhausted into bed. Despite my weariness, it was fun, the perfect way to celebrate the end of that set of treatments. (If this doesn't clinch my qualification as a dyed-in-the wool academic, what does?)

Before I left home for the interview, I took a verbal poll on whether or not I should wear my wig. When I was completely bald, I had worn one to a previous interview—utterly abjectly, after having it styled by a gay hairdresser who specialized in drag queens. My friend Jode, who introduced me to the hairdresser, warned me that he might not do a great job, but the stylist made me laugh, so I was glad I went. When I finally decided not to wear the wig to the later interview, the same stylist very sweetly met me at the salon early and shaped my sprout before my morning flight.

A certain intimacy pervades the academic job market: for two long days you give a fully public performance, and whether or not you get the job, these people will be your colleagues in some way for the rest of your career. So in a way, wearing a wig, as several people had recommended, seemed to me like starting off with a lie. Then again, the job description didn't mention hair, so perhaps wearing a wig might be excused as merely a sin of omission. Then *again,* knowing I was a queer San Franciscan, perhaps the interview panel would take my sartorial decay as an intentional aspect of my gender identity.

But this kind of coming out was different. I wasn't worried about my sexual orientation; rather, I feared outing myself as a sick person. Surely no one, *no one,* in his or her right mind would hire a person just completing cancer treatment.

In the end, I realized that I had made the right decision, even though I didn't get the job. On the first day, a warm spring night, a few graduate students and I were on our way out for a Costa Rican meal when a leafless tree branch caught the cap I was wearing and, like a slingshot, flung it backward about twenty feet. Realizing that it might have been the wig on the ground, I managed to maintain my composure in front of the students and even laugh along with them.

The whole experience of cancer—attending the Look Good workshop, wearing the wig and not wearing the wig, having the port put in and having it taken out, trying on the prosthetic breast and taking it off—was a process of figuring out how and where and when to pass within a slew of identities and communities: as whole, as gendered, as job-seeking, as nonthreateningly queer, as healthy. In a way, such tensions mirrored life as usual. In another way, I had to come to terms with the full force of the work that all cancer patients do, each day, to stay within their various social crowds. Social lives depend on these norms, and people maintain the norms by everyday acts of passing. So if looking good might be dismissed as superficial, using precious energy to put on lipstick can also be understood as an act of intense resistance to the social exclusions that many people with cancer suffer.

Look Good Feel Better reflects the scramble to remain hot and healthy-looking in an imagistic society. Even without cancer, women, men, and everyone in between disguise themselves as young until it just can't be done anymore. If consumption makes you a better person—literally, a more beautiful person—the coping mechanism carries risks, creating confusion when you just can't hide anymore. One friend with advanced colon cancer told me just before she died, "No one in my cancer group will even look at me." She was the walking embodiment of what everyone feared most, and in order to manage, members of the group socially, if not literally, expelled her. One had to have cancer, but not too much cancer, to be in the group, simply because no one knew where to rest their eyes.

I think here of moments: of my friend's ashen—as in pure, titanium-zinc white—face two weeks before her death from leukemia. Or of being shown the lopsided reconstructed breasts of a woman a month before her death from breast cancer. Of Ann's mother's large body being dragged down the stairs of a three-story walk-up by two swearing, sweating paramedics; of Buddy's body stiffening and swelling as her partner kept her for an extra day in the living room. Or even of my friend's cursing of the woman whose estate she had bought at a discount after this woman died of cancer, for having left the drains clogged with the refuse of her illness. What do we call this clash between the no-longer-in-use tools, and how they continue to signify the *physicality* of it all?

Calvino says, again about taking out the trash: "This daily representation of descent below ground, this domestic municipal rubbish funeral, is meant first and foremost to put off my own funeral, to postpone it if only for a short time, to confirm that for one more day I have been a producer of detritus and not detritus myself."[12] Each day, we catalogue ourselves by this decision: what to keep, what to throw away. And through that appraisal we maintain our very selves. Today, will it be the bald head or the synthetic hair that becomes "matter out of place"?

Finally, I gathered these leftovers of my former person, reminders of my decisions about how to connect and refuse to be let go of, into a box. My little collection of detritus, I decided, could attend the next person enduring the rituals and expiations of treatment. I hiked into the hospital one last time with my two inches of jet black hair, shoulders square. I entered the building to leave it behind. My absurdly confident descent to the rubbish funeral mimicked the banal efforts to save ourselves that each of us makes everyday. If only for a jiffy, I succeeded.

Conclusion

Shameless

I bought [the journal] for the marbled covers and the thick creamy pages and ever since then the thick creamy pages have been saying, Piss off, what could *you* possibly write on *us* that would be worth reading?

—Pat Barker, *The Ghost Road*

Tell me what it is you plan to do
with your one wild and precious death?

—Derek Simons, in a reworking of Mary Oliver, "The Summer Day"

There is scarce any thing that hath not killed somebody; a hair, a feather hath done it; nay, that which is our best antidote against it hath done it; the best cordial hath been deadly poison. Men have died of joy, and almost forbidden their friends to weep for them, when they have seen them die laughing.

—John Donne, *Meditations*

Several years ago, well before my diagnosis, my family visited the Commonweal Center in Bolinas, California. My mother, a physician, wanted to find out more about the cancer therapies used at the famous retreat center. My family commonly undertook such medical expeditions; years ago we visited the barracks in Hawaii where lepers had been sent until Hansen's disease largely disappeared in the 1940s. There, too, we wandered amid the sheer natural beauty, though the cliffs and ocean had served as prison bars rather than comfort for those who had been sent there. I enjoyed the novelty and splendor of Bolinas and Moloka'i, but I didn't give the larger meaning more than a passing nod.

My mother's insatiable empathy for the ill did not seep down. To me, ill people were not well people who had had some misfortune; rather, ill people fell into another category: they went to, and were sent to, the sorts of places that sick people go—like Moloka'i, like the Commonweal Center. People with cancer seemed like a different genre of person. I guessed I would die mercifully fast in a car crash, or upon meeting a bear in Banff National Park and forgetting whether to play dead or climb a tree. In the end, I never really thought about it that much.

Maybe that's why during my doctor's uncomfortable avoidance of the Bad News Experience—"umh, do you know what this test shows?"—I felt as though she turned me into a pitiable blister beetle. Probably everyone's cancer diagnosis feels Kafkaesque. Therein lies the point: how can we possibly, in any imaginable world, understand something so exceptionally ordinary as cancer diagnosis and treatment—more commonplace than a college education—as in any way remarkable? And yet, when it happens to us, how can it not be noteworthy?

Still flush with the shame of diagnosis, I wrote anonymously (scared to link my name to the query) to a Vancouver retreat center called Callanish. They wrote back immediately, a gentle letter letting me know about their weeklong retreats for people dealing with and dying of cancer. They were forthright, did not shy away.

People dying of cancer? I thought. I wasn't dying of cancer. I wasn't metastatic. Deeply lonely, I was just cruising, sussing out the retreat experience like a swinger at a bar. Seven months after my initial application I received a call from Callanish's head retreat person, Janie: they had a cancelation. I asked to be placed in a retreat with others in their thirties. Still without making a full commitment to either Janie or myself, I booked my flights for "cancer camp." Only later—after having attended several other retreats—did I realize my luck. I might have been stuck for a week having to talk about how to beat the odds or remain cheerful; instead, we did actual in-depth work.

Retreat brings together a group for no other reason than this: we all had some cells in our bodies that split in natural but potentially lethal ways. We had been brought to our knees by a common disease, a more or less shared understanding of that disease, and a bunch of specific ways that we were medically and socially treated by people and institutions. And we gathered in that space to figure out what it all meant.

Janie later characterized people's motivation to attend a Callanish retreat as a compulsion. "Why," she mused, "do people travel across the country, too sick to even walk sometimes, to come to this group they know very little about, to be with people they don't know, to be away from all they know to be safe. Is it just idle curiosity?"[1]

Curiosity, perhaps, but no, not idle. Cancer seems to present everyone the opportunity to "learn so much about" this or that. Yourself. What really matters. How much you love your family. How beautiful the little things are. Mind-blowingly little in cancer's institutions allows for the recognition of grief and heartbreak.

And so we came together to discover community, to rediscover the selves that had been stolen by the cancer complex. A thirst emerged in the group, an unquenchable desire for new vocabulary, one that included suffering, but not victimhood; one that did not mimick conversations but rather reached for communication that mattered. We craved an alternative archive—a medical chart that included more than the scores on our pathology reports or the appeals to bicycle for a cure.

My journals remind me how much I wished, while I was undergoing treatment and attending retreats, that cancer were tangible. Not the actual tumors, exactly; rather, I wished that doctors, instead of responding to virtually any question with a shrug and a "We just don't know that yet," would take out an anvil and hit me over the head. Cancer's deepest discomfort lies not in the obvious physical pain, or in the surgeries, or the nausea, or the hair loss. It lies rather in the ways that things hurt so much more than they need to. Like when one had a drain removed after a surgery and the nurse, lacking a sharp pair of scissors, couldn't just cut the plastic tube and so ended up pulling and tearing the bloody mess of flesh and stitches around the implant as if yanking a lawnmower starter. Her oblivious cheer nailed the carnivalesque experience, as did the fact that she actually seemed like quite a nice person. Retreat offered a way to capture all the pain that had been too elusive to even think about, all the events that had no metric of comprehension.

At our first encounter, we sized each other up through the usual introductions while examining photos of our children, families, and friends that were laid out on the table. (Alice worried that the humungous framed photo of her ten-year-old son took too much space.) After dinner, we were introduced to "counsel," a ritual in which each of us had an opportunity to speak. Janie read a short piece, by the physician author Rachel Remen, on listening: "Perhaps the most important thing we ever give each other is our attention. And especially if it's given from the heart. When people are talking, there's no need to do anything but receive them. Just take them in. Listen to what they're saying. Care about it. Most times caring about it is even more important than understanding it. Most of us don't value ourselves or our love enough to know this. It has taken me a long time to believe in the power of simply saying, 'I'm so sorry,' when someone is in pain. And meaning it."[2] Listening in this way became our methodology, and a couple of times a day we each had a chance to share whatever we wanted this kind, fun, open, raw, grief-stricken crowd to know about us: our fears; our experiences; a joke or a song or a poem . . . anything.

In addition to encouraging trust, these sessions helped us explore the issue of self-representation. What did we want the group to know about us? We had the liberty, over the course of the week, to propose parts of ourselves, to create something that could only be completed in the witnessing of the process. Unlike academic work, which needs to be critiqued to gain credibility and meaning, this work needed only to be heard. Remen teaches that the process of expressing and witnessing is what matters. In "How to Tell a True War Story," Tim O'Brien writes it this way: "In a true war story, if there's a moral at all, it's like the thread that makes the cloth. You can't tease it out. You can't extract the meaning without unraveling the deeper meaning. And in the end, really, there's nothing much to say about a true war story, except maybe 'Oh.' True war stories do not generalize. They do not indulge in abstraction or analysis."[3]

Forms of expression change in the medical system. After my surgeries, nurses asked me to describe the pain level on a scale from one to ten. At first I had no way to gauge what that meant. Later I became adept at knowing what number to say to get the amount of medication I wanted. Pain ranking substituted for a dose request. Much of living in cancer requires this instrumental language: what to say to be seen as a person, not a statistic; how to request the things you need; when to know that saying something will be worse than grinning and bearing the next necessary invasion. At retreat these events and emotions—sometimes out of reach—could be hinted at, verbalized, gathered, with no summation or conclusion. Some of the vocabularies we learned inevitably relied on standard cultural narratives about illness; others sought to interpret or find meaning; others simply expressed sadness or fury or the losses borne as people shifted off the course of everyday life.

Despite how ungrounded it sometimes feels, illness happens in actual places—waiting areas with soft-rock radio, bathrooms, the holding center as one comes out of anesthesia, a good friend's couch, a prison on a Hawaiian island—and so it was fitting that this process of healing was also rooted in a physical space that reshaped the physical experiences of touch, taste, smell, architecture, and eye contact to undo the "othering" that cancer can be. It was as if the unfocused pleasures of retreat—the warm hands of a massage, as opposed to the icy hands of a busy IV nurse; the wholesome foods at dinner, versus hospital Jell-O; the behind-the-scenes organization, against the on-the-fly confusion of post-op—coalesced in comfort, which in turn allowed us to face the issues that cancer raised, the ones we were most uncomfortable to speak.

The detailed labor and experience of the Callanish organizers took us outside of the official cultures of illness, freeing people to speak of excruciating pain. Two women were on their third recurrences. Two people had been left by their partners; another's partner, unable to comprehend cancer, had told her that she should go on a golf trip to get over it, rather than on retreat. One man talked about how chemotherapy had dried out his tear ducts, taking away even his ability to cry. Another person wondered how she would come to terms with not seeing her son grow up, not hearing his voice deepen, not seeing whiskers grow on his chin, not attending his marriage. Everyone talked about how other people reacted to their diagnosis, how little friends and peers knew about cancer. People had lost careers, financial stability, family, friends, social networks, their belief in themselves and their bodies, notions of the future, possibilities for joy and pleasure—and the ability to take all these things for granted. In speaking aloud what we feared about death—pain, leaving friends and family behind, long illness, loss of independence—we could prepare to alleviate some of those concerns, try to free ourselves from fearing the future.

Typically, we only read about such details in accounts of the disarray of the medical system or overhear them in a shred of cafe gossip. Actually witnessing the sufferings of illness—to experience those sufferings as borne by real people, to hear with no other mission than to listen, to let all the mixed messages of cancer just be out there, to humanize the experience of disease and disclosure: that changed my life. The deep politics of retreat lay in the fact that nothing needed to be constructed from the suffering. It bore no message, no compensation, no rationalization, no call to get well soon, no pat on the knee.

For cancer to be recognized as a scourge and as a violent visitation, it has to be acknowledged. In some intense, really intense, way, retreat made me realize that real people get cancer and that even after they do, they remain real people. The fact that it took so long for me to acquire this small glint of knowledge made me realize the depth of my assumption that cancer is an exceptional state, not a phenomenon we all live with, all the time, with varying degrees of kinship and complicity. Throughout the subsequent events and retreats I attended, as I looked out over a group of people I'd realize full bore that they had all had to deal with cancer. This became a familiar sadness to me.

I have written this book as a statement of that sorrow and as a continuation of that first striving for communication and recognition. The betrayed child in me longs for a doctor-mommy who can take care of everything. The entitled first-worlder in me wants a clear cause: not just a test for carcinogens, but the abolishment of them (without having to give up my car). The activist in me wants angry mourning, not celebratory mourning. The scholar in me wants a pathology report with robust, not sketchy, information. And as a qualified mammal I want my dead friends back.

Long after diagnosis, I told as few people as possible that I was sick. *At least you aren't dead,* they'd say. Or, *I know so many people with cancer, everything from partial mastectomies to death.* Or, *My grandmother died of breast cancer; you are such a champ!* Or, *At least you didn't lose a leg.* Or, *You look so good!* Or, *My friend died of lymphoma last year.* It's not easy to be put in a conversational category filled with dead friends and family. For years after diagnosis I felt deflated by the tension between what I knew about myself—my fear and despair—and what others knew about me—my bravery, my good fortune. I felt kind of like that black pirate balloon at Kahlo's fifth-birthday party: one moment taut and full and shiny, and the next, popped and making a hasty journey around the ceiling until falling into a tiny, scrunchy pile in the corner of the room, forgotten about until swept into a dustpan with a few crumbs of stale pirate cake.

It's not just me who inhabits this quieted but unquiet space. At one of the many funerals I've attended over the last few years, I met a woman who never knew that her close friend from law school had been through cancer treatment—until the friend's death. The friend had not told her, wary, I'm sure, of the same deflation.

Even as a coconspirator in the silence, it was weird to have the mind-blowing and crazy-making alternate world I lived in for so many months just disappear. Cancer drowned under the surface of my person and now reels around like an unclaimed corpse, thudding against the banalities of everyday life. However cancer becomes invisible in one individual, that disappearance accrues to millions of people. The ways we disguise this thoroughly traumatic experience ensure, sometimes purposefully and other times as an unintended consequence, that we miss huge implications of this disease. Cancer can't be inside so many people and remain outside society.

My girlfriend and I have an agreement that if one of us dies indecorously, the other will make up a story. (That Alaskan fellow whose body was never found after he tried to swim down through one fishing hole under the ice and come up at another probably wished he'd such an agreement.) One website listing "the 50 most embarrassing ways to die" ranks "the cancer" fifth, right after "Looking down the barrel of a gun to see if it's loaded" and well before "Being killed by your kids." The stories my girlfriend and I have concocted include allusions to a smote dragon. Beating back a fire-breathing creature has a certain butch cachet that dying wrinkled and bloated with an IV in your arm and a wig slipping into your eyes just doesn't have.

Even without a dragon, you can still assure a good story for your finale. In the "real" death community, Dignity replaces drama. (If you don't believe me, just check out Dignity Memorial®, the brand that offers "assurance of quality, value, caring service, and exceptional customer satisfaction" through its network of over 1,600 funeral, cremation, and cemetery providers.)[4] People involved in the end of things like to think you can plan a dignified death—though the dead body leaks, though the dead body stiffens and starts to smell, though the dead body refuses to decompose because of all the preservatives in our diets. Doggedly untidy, death is the ultimate un-American activity.

Malignant has mapped out some of the cultural containment strategies for this crazy disease, its everywhere- and nowhereness, the emergence of powerful and rich experts in the context of uncertainty. I've traced how uncertainty can be reproduced as knowledge, particularly by gathering populations and then again by comparing the populations as they undergo different treatments. I'm not arguing that such an approach doesn't hold the potential for finding cures for cancer. However, this method comes with costs too often hidden behind the commonsensical notions of what data mean, how results should be understood and traded, and how comparisons should be made. If gathering statistics about populations offers one way to comprehend individuals who can no longer make sense of their own selves, the practice harbors dangers as well.

Living amid charts and statistics that both represent and occlude you leads to a spooky cognitive dissonance in which we think we know—but can't know for sure—that cancer is caused as much as it is lived with and died from, treated and ignored, and marched for. Every "survivor against the odds" comes at the expense of someone who has been beaten by the same odds. Every individual who receives a misdiagnosis or an exposure, every person who files a malpractice suit, everyone who has a screening (or doesn't), becomes compressed within a necessary collective logic that also leads to confusion. The more steps forward a cancer patient takes, the more completely—by data, by precedents (or the fear of them)—she is obscured.

Even more confusingly, in cases such as IVF and many chemicals and industrial pollutants, no one collects safety data. We suspect, but we don't know. And because we don't know, a logic that matches risk distribution to the Game Face asserts that there is no reason *not* to continue the exposures. Cancer appears and disappears through statistics, Social Security, prognoses, law, chemotherapy, diagnosis, and cliché. This shifting presence of the disease underlies huge questions: who can access insurance, how we perceive risk, who makes a profit, how communities are constituted, who dies and how.

The toggle between absent and present held open by survival-, cure-, and early detection–speak maintains a fantasy about what-might-have-been. The cancer might have been caught earlier, or under a different cancer funding structure, there might have already been a cure. A different government might have outlawed the chemical that caused this particular cancer. A warning sign might have been heeded, a particular carcinogen avoided. The counterfactuals hold within themselves sadness and death and cure and hope and mourning.

Each of the interactions that seeks to describe, discuss, cure, and treat cancer also nurtures it. As a labor issue, cancer requires physical work—by the drug manufacturers, by the nurses who administer the drugs, by the sick person and the person who drove her to the hospital. Cancer requires social labor, too: valuing people who may get sick and those who are sick; comparing cancer to other similar and dissimilar possibilities for cure; interpreting the statistics; tracking how money accumulates and dissipates. Cancer's inexplicably replicating cells sustain some of the most profitable industries and professions in the United States. Perhaps America needs cancer, in this sacrificial economics. But because cancer is a culture, it is also a changeable form—something that could be consciously worked on to produce a better society, one that is less polluted, less prone to moralizing disease, kinder in treatment and recovery; one that recognizes the cumulative toxic effects of industry. Sidestepping the well-intentioned sigh—"cancer must be *so hard*"—I've aimed to make it *more* difficult, to make it everywhere, to proliferate its meanings so that all those wrap-ups, all those nice columns and flowcharts and path reports and injunctions to hang in there don't get the last word.

Cancer is both okay—it has to be, because ultimately, for people who are dying, death has to be okay—and not okay. It is not okay that so many people are so ill from something so predictable. It is not okay that our languages are deceitful, that people with cancer are blamed or shamed or promised that they will survive or asked to disguise themselves in the very same lipstick and prostheses and plastic hair that are loaded with carcinogens. An elegiac politics—a stance that admits to the inevitability of these deaths given the environmental and economic landscape—helps make this contradiction (okay, but not okay) not only legible, but livable and dieable. An elegiac politics demands the recognition of both enormous economic profits and enormous cultural and personal losses. An elegiac politics stares down the Game Face with the private face of cancer. Whether considered statistics or the victims of a war, cancer's casualties are individual people.

There is much more to say—about race and class and sexuality, among other things—than I have said here, and those books, too, will become flags of peace or surrender. It matters, of course, that each of us is white, black, brown; single, partnered, married; low income, heirs; immigrants; handsome, intimidating, tubby. Where we are located in these social structures matters to our experience with cancer, to our survival chances, and to the ways we are treated. But rather than examining these in detail, I have aimed here to retrieve the individual—as a unit with specific features—from the aggregatated thinking that contemporary cancer knowledge forces us into.

I began this book in order to explore cancer-the-noun, but in writing about it I've come to realize again, as I did when living it, that cancer is also a verb, an adjective, an invective, a shout-out, indeed, a grammar all its own. I offer this book in an attempt to speak to—and from within—the cancer complex, to understand how the constituent parts of this experience spin the web that we call cancer and, unless we are vigilant, entrap us in it. I want a new version of accounting, a bigger, richer vocabulary, and a voice to speak it with.

If the term *survivor* offers a false identity formed around cancer, living in prognosis offers an uneasy alternative, one that inhabits contradiction, confusion, and betrayal. In elegiac politics, prognosis marks the moment one become someone who thinks differently about a future, a death, and a life. The term stands as a small monument to those who will not make it past the five- and ten-year marks.

One night while we were lying in bed, my partner said: "I like your watch."

And I said: "I'll leave it to you in my will."

And she said: "Okay, but don't specify the details of the watch."

And I said: "Why not?"

And she said: "Because in forty years when you die battling that dragon, you may not have the same watch."

Acknowledgments

An effect of community, friendship, family (defined in so many ways), loneliness, investigation, and discussion, *Malignant* offers more than anything the results of a several-year-long collaboration. I have more people to thank than I can possibly name here. Countless librarians, many of whom I haven't even met, made work on this sprawling yet specialized topic possible. Many more people—doctors, researchers, lawyers, patients—have spoken to me about their involvement in cancer worlds. A slew of reviewers, editors, students, mentors, friends, and colleagues have improved the text.

Particular gratitude goes out to: Vincanne Adams, Aneesh Aneesh, Bettina Aptheker, Jennifer Bajorek, Bay Area Young Survivors, Lauren Berlant, João Biehl, Anne Bloom, Erica Bornstein, Liz Bradfield, Barbara Brenner, Janie Brown, Mary Bryson, Victor Buchli, the Callanish Society, Kathy Chetko, Elizabeth Churchill, Jennifer Cohen, Lawrence Cohen, Jean Comaroff, Commonweal Cancer Help Program, Natalie Conforti, Anjali Dixit, Joseph Dumit, First Descents, Michael Fischer, Kim Fortun, Carla Freccero, Catherine Gallagher, Angelica Glass, Jody Greene, Brian Goldstone, Zeynep Gursel, Jane Guyer, Chenxing Hahn, Rebecca Hardin, Cori Hayden, Stefan Helmreich, Gail Hershatter, Seth Holmes, Sharon Kaufman, Ann Kim, Mary Kinzie, Anna Kirkland, Hannah Landecker, Simon Craddock Lee, Samara Marion, Sally Engle Merry, Michelle Murphy, Jackie Orr, Otter Bar, Damani Partridge, Adriana Petryna, Jo Plante, Sue Porter, Elizabeth Povinelli, Fabienne

Prior, Maria Puig de la Bellacasa, Louise Rafkin, Elizabeth Roberts, Teemu Ruskola, Austin Sarat, Lea Scarpelli, Dayna Scott, David Serlin, Sarah Snell, Susan Leigh Starr, Leah Stork, Marilyn Strathern, Lucy Suchman, Kathryn Takabvirwa, Charis Thompson, Miriam Ticktin, Fred Turner, Martha Merrill Umphrey, Nina Wakeford, Marina Welker, Susann Wilkinson, Kate Zaloom, Ceide Zapparoni, and Susan Zieff. I also thank all the members of the Anthropology Department at Stanford University, and in particular Ellen Christensen, Shelly Coughlan, Jim Ferguson, Jen Kidwell, T.M. Luhrmann, and Barbara Voss.

Jake Kosek's insatiable curiosity, cosmic store of energy, brilliance and gusto in sniffing out unpredictable intellectual passageways have ensured that my passion for this topic never waned, while his on-demand pep talks ensured a timely end to the work. In Derek Simons—willing to go to (and emerge from) dark places and search for the words to describe them, able to read pages and pages and offer gemlike glints of insight in detailed responses—I found the intellectual companion most scholars only dream of. As the book went to press, Shelley Wilcox burned the midnight oil with me, parsing lines of argument, organization, and wording. In the moments that the book threatened to take over our lives, she reminded me that Aristotle's rule of the Golden Mean is no cop-out to the median. Rather, she has shown me the route toward maximal bliss.

A special shout-out to those who read and offered thoughts on the entire manuscript in its final stages: Misha Bykowski, Christine Byl, Anne Canright, Cordelia Erickson-Davis, Alexa Hagerty, Jennifer Hsieh, Saree Kayne, Meriel Lindley, Yi Lu, Reed Malcolm, Joseph Masco, Diane Nelson, Cam Awkward-Rich, Philippe Rivière, Ellen Shapiro, and three anonymous reviewers.

Anyone who has had an extraordinary teacher knows how life-altering this can be. Many years ago, Donna Haraway laid the foundation for this book by teaching me how to be a critically engaged scholar in a world that often prefers things to be black and white. She taught me the solace of not forcing dismay into a box of chocolate and that contradiction is a profound aspect of resolution.

I would be no one, nowhere, without the hearts and blood of my incredible kin. My parents, Evelyn and Sudhir, have wavered in their implausibly profound support of me only once or twice, and have even then been good-naturedly quick in redoubling their efforts. My sisters Kamini and Anita are as resolute and tenacious in their patience and love as they are in all of their brainiac and Olympian endeavors. Kahlo and Asha have experienced far too much for people of their height, yet they remain enchantingly open to life's offerings. All of that makes all the difference.

Malignant has been supported with funding from the Stanford Center for the Advanced Study of Behavioral Sciences, the Stanford Humanities Center, the Ethics Program at Stanford University, a National Endowment for the Humanities Fellowship, a National Humanities Center Rockefeller Fellowship, and funding from the Clayman Center for Women and Gender. Any views, findings, conclusions, or recommendations expressed in this publication do not necessarily reflect those of NEH or any of these organizations. Despite my enormous cast of generous and brilliant readers from many desciplines, any errors in the text remain my own.

Notes

INTRODUCTION

1. "Find Frozen Sleep Aids in Cancer War," *New York Times*, Nov. 3, 1939.

2. Adjuvant! Online is a website for health professionals that presents mortality and relapse rates of "additional therapy (adjuvant therapy: usually chemotherapy, hormone therapy, or both) after surgery." One plugs in the various numbers listed on the pathology report to get prognostic data with and without treatment. As an example, Adjuvant! Online predicts that a male with Stage 3, Grade 2, colon cancer and four positive nodes will have a 29.9 percent chance of being alive in five years without chemotherapy. Add chemotherapy, and he will have a 53 percent chance. (Here is where the numbers can become complicated, and open to manipulation depending on the message desired. One could read these stats as saying either that [1] chemo will increase one's absolute chance of survival by 13.1 percent or [2] chemo will nearly double one's survival chance. That difference matters if a company is trying to sell chemotherapy.) Still, 50 percent of the population with that particular level of colon cancer will relapse in five years, even with the treatment. See www.adjuvantonline.com/colonstandard.jsp (accessed August 6, 2011). For more on how data remove the particular local conditions to enable comparison, see Bruno Latour, "Visualization and Cognition: Drawing Things Together," *Knowledge and Society: Studies in the Sociology of Culture and Present* 6 (1986): 1–40.

3. Susan Sontag, *Illness as Metaphor and AIDS and Its Metaphors* (New York: Picador, 2001).

4. See, e.g., James T. Patterson, *The Dread Disease: Cancer and Modern American Culture* (Cambridge, Mass.: Harvard University Press, 1989).

5. One physician traced cancer as a "biography": Siddhartha Mukherjee, *The Emperor of All Maladies: A Biography of Cancer* (New York: Scribner 2011).

6. Once the tissue was detached from me, I had no control over it or its fate. For all I know, I could be the next Henrietta Lacks, the woman whose tumor cells were used in 1951, without her permission or the knowledge of her family, to create the HeLa line of cells. These cells from an extremely rare glandular adenocarcinoma of the cervix, which killed her within eight months of the discovery of them in her body, became the first human material that could be used in the lab without the human attached. But this experiment in reproducing human material backfired. Between the 1950s and 1970s, HeLa cells colonized cell cultures across the globe. Of course, they had the help of post-WWII scientific infrastructure, which distributed thousands of free vials of the cells in the march against polio. Years later, scientists who thought they had been working with certain cell lines found that they were actually working with HeLa cells. Since there was no way to root out accurate from inaccurate science, most of the findings from work done with the wrong cell line still stand—and since there is still virtually no oversight of basic cancer research, many scientists believe that such errors remain rampant. See Hannah Landecker, *Culturing Life: How Cells Became Technologies* (Cambridge, Mass.: Harvard University Press, 2007); and Adam Curtis, *The Way of All Flesh,* BBC documentary available at http://topdocumentaryfilms.com/the-way-of-all-flesh/.

7. According to Elizabeth Toon, in initiating the Sloan-Kettering screening program "funder Alfred P. Sloane, President to GM, and board member Charles Ketting, GM's director of research, encouraged director [physician] Cornelius P. Rhoads to adopt the industrial research model . . . and Rhoads embraced this vision. Together with other facilities that adapted the industrial model to biomedical investigation, Sloane-Kettering promised that coordinating and directing the efforts of researchers from multiple disciplines would provide a scientific solution to the cancer problem" ("Does Bigger Mean Better? British Perspectives on American Cancer Treatment and Research, 1948," *Journal of Clinical Oncology* 25 [2007]: 5833). See also Ilana Löwy, *Between Bench and Bedside: Science, Healing, and Interleukin-2 in a Cancer Ward* (Cambridge, Mass.: Harvard University Press, 1996); R. F. Bud, "Strategy in American Cancer Research after WWII: A Case Study," *Social Studies of Science* 8 (1978): 425–459. Methods from the automotive industry are currently being adopted to improve hospital service delivery and decrease error rates.

As Ilana Löwy points out, "The wish to compare the efficacy of different treatments of cancer favored the homogenization of diagnosis and outcomes, while the use of expensive substances and instruments, such as radium and cobalt bombs or high voltage radiotherapy machines, promoted the centralization of cures. Cancer research, diagnosis, and treatment were at the forefront of the development of 'big medicine,' a multi-level, science-grounded endeavor" (*Preventive Strikes: Women, Precancer, and Prophylactic Surgery* [Baltimore: Johns Hopkins University Press, 2009], 233).

8. Dan Greenberg et al., "When Is Cancer Care Cost-Effective? A Systematic Overview of Cost-Utility Analyses in Oncology" *Journal of the National Cancer Institute* 102 (2010): 82–88. Pharmaceutical companies have been upfront about the fact that the prices charged for drugs are very often unrelated to the research, design, manufacturing, distribution, and advertising costs. While the

cost of AIDS drugs constituted a large part of early patient activism, drug prices have taken a back seat in most cancer advocacy. In many cases, the physician reimbursement fee structure adds an incentive to prescribe the most expensive treatments. This leads to two important ways in which the organization of drug research as a private endeavor, with its first responsibility to shareholders, affects cancer disease categorization. First, a company will need to maintain that disease categories be as large as possible, thus allowing larger numbers of people to be treated. One can see this with "at risk" populations that are targeted with blockbuster drugs such as statins and antidepressants. A desire for broad disease categories militates against running trials that break down cancers into subtypes. Second, companies can attain huge profits for small survival increases. Critics who blame the pharmacuetical companies for letting patients down misread the structural constraints on pharmacuetical research. It is a business, not a curative enterprise.

Pharma profits skyrocketed during the 1980s and 1990s, giving it unprecedented control over the FDA through its lobby efforts in Congress. By 1990, the top ten drug companies had profits of nearly 25 percent of sales, and by 2001 the ten U.S. pharma companies in the Fortune 500 list ranked far above all other industries on average net return (18.5 percent of sales, as opposed to the median net return of other industries, which was 3.3 percent of sales). R&D expenses hover at 10–15 percent of sales, whereas marketing is more like 36 percent. See Marcia Angell, *The Truth about the Drug Companies: How They Deceive Us and What to Do about it* (New York: Random House, 2004).

9. Figures based on 2012 reports from the National Cancer Institute and the American Association of Cancer Research: www.cancer.gov/aboutnci/serving-people/nci-budget-information; also www.aacr.org/home/public–media/science-policy–government-affairs/resources-for-policymakers/federal-cancer-research-funding.aspx. For information on cancer shams, see Lea Goldman, "The Big Business of Breast Cancer," *MarieClaire,* Sept. 14, 2011. She traces how, "All told, an estimated $6 billion is raised every year in the name of breast cancer, though millions of those dollars are made in sham fundraisers." On the rise in federal spending on cancer, see Maureen Hogan Casamayou, *The Politics of Breast Cancer* (Washington, D.C.: Georgetown University Press, 2001).

10. Board on Health Care Services, *Delivering Affordable Cancer Care in the 21st Century: Workshop Summary* (Washington, D.C.: National Academies Press, 2013), 9. The report indicates the numerous challenges in "estimating and projecting cancer costs, including a lack of complete data, especially the costs for uninsured patients, as well as unanticipated changes in treatment practices." As a result, "both current and projected estimates in cancer care costs are probably underestimates" (9). Still, the report predicts that total healthcare costs will likely account for 25 percent of the U.S. GDP, up from the current 18 percent (4). It also suggests that "because cancer is such a prevalent set of conditions and so costly, it magnifies what we know to be true about the totality of the health care system. It exposes all of its strengths and weaknesses" (3).

11. Reported in Livestrong and the American Cancer Society, *The Global Economic Cost of Cancer,* 2010 (available at www.cancer.org/acs/groups/content/@internationalaffairs/documents/document/acspc-026203.pdf).

12. For a version of this argument questioning the wisdom of such high expenses, see Steven Shapin, "Cancer World: The Making of a Modern Disease," *New Yorker*, Nov. 8, 2010, 78–83. Costs for drugs vary internationally, and that affects treatment decisions and ways in which toxic side-effects are weighed. See D. H. Smith et al., "A Comparative Economic Analysis of Pegylated Liposomal Doxorubicin versus Topotecan in Ovarian Cancer in the USA and the UK," *Annals of Oncology* 13 (2002): 1590–1597.

13. Whereas, for example, the Board on Health Care Services report suggests that to reduce health expenses would be to resolve a major fiscal crisis, it's critical to note as well that markets around health constitute their own kind of economy, such that reducing those expenses would also produce another type of fiscal crisis. Board on Health Care Services, *Delivering Affordable Cancer Care.*

14. The total annual healthcare tab in 2010 was $2.6 trillion, according to the Centers for Medicare and Medicaid Services, and healthcare is the fastest-growing industry in the United States (www.cms.gov/Research-Statistics-Data-and-Systems/Statistics-Trends-and-Reports/NationalHealthExpendData/downloads/proj2010.pdf).

15. David Goldhill, "How the Healthcare System Killed My Father," *Atlantic Monthly*, Sept. 2009.

16. See www.whitehouse.gov/sites/default/files/omb/budget/fy2013/assets/health.pdf; www.whitehouse.gov/omb/budget/Historicals). The "$2.6 trillion spent on health care in the United States is more than twice what the nation spends on food" (Board on Health Care Services, *Delivering Affordable Cancer Care in the 21st Century*, 5).

17. Monika L. Metzger, Amy Billett, and Michael Link, "The Impact of Drug Shortages on Children with Cancer—The Example of Mechlorethamine," *New England Journal of Medicine* 367 (2012): 2461–2463.

18. www.rare-cancer.org/rare-diseases.php (accessed Aug. 25, 2012).

19. See Anne Pollock, "Transforming the Critique of Big Pharma," *BioSocieties* 6 (2011): 106–118; and Joseph Dumit, *Drugs for Life* (Chapel Hill, N.C.: Duke University Press, 2012).

20. See David U. Himmelstein et al., "Medical Bankruptcy in the United States, 2007: Results of a National Study," *American Journal of Medicine* 122 (2009): 741–746. This is the most thorough and well cited of recent studies addressing medical debt in the United States.

21. The Supreme Court opinion offers a very clear example of economic health directly opposing public health; see *FDA v. Brown and Williamson Tobacco Corp.*, 529 U.S. 120 (2000): 98–1152.

22. Jim Hightower, *There's Nothing in the Middle of the Road but Yellow Stripes and Dead Armadillos* (New York: Harper Collins, 1998).

23. EPA, "Cumulative Risk Assessment for the Chloroacetanilids," March 29, 2006 (available at www.epa.gov/oppsrrd1/cumulative/chloro_cumulative_risk.pdf).

24. The company minimized the risks, some severe, of the drug in what anthropologist Jennifer Fosket calls "disease substitution"—i.e., emphasizing the potential of a lower risk of breast cancer while playing down the increased risk of stroke ("Constructing 'High-Risk Women': The Development and

Standardization of a Breast Cancer Risk Assessment Tool," *Science, Technology, and Human Values* 29 [2004]: 291–313). Fosket argues that whereas tamoxifen has been demonstrated to lower breast cancer incidence, it also increases endometrial cancer, incidence of pulmonory embolism (blood clotting in the lung), and deep vein thrombosis. She also finds that no tests have been developed to calculate the risks of those side-effects, risks that advertisements for the drug generally downplay.

25. Epstein is a vocal critic of the cancer industry, and this quote is widely cited. See, e.g., www.whale.to/cancer/breat6.html.

26. Information of price-fixing cases available at www.hbsslaw.com/resources/newsroom/appeals-court-denies-astrazeneca-in-awp-case. Global sales of tamoxifen in 2001, the last year of its patent, amounted to $1.024 billion. See www.news-medical.net/health/What-is-Tamoxifen.aspx (accessed April 4, 2012).

27. A searchable database of Superfund sites is available at www.epa.gov/superfund.

28. Susan Sontag wrote that "illness is *not* a metaphor, and the most truthful way of regarding illness—and the healthiest way of being ill—is one most purified of, most resistent to, metaphorical thinking" (*Illness as Metaphor,* 3).

29. Marcel Mauss, *The Gift: Forms and Functions of Exchange in Archaic Societies* (London: Cohen & West, 1966), 76–77.

30. As Edward Said described, certain issues present themselves as "something to be thought through, tried out, engaged with—in short, as a subject to be dealt with politically" (*The Question of Palestine* [New York: Vintage Books, 1992], xli). Miriam Ticktin defines politics as a "set of practices by which order is created and maintained," and the political as a "disruption of established order" (*Casualties of Care: Immigration and the Politics of Humanitarianism in France* [Berkeley: University of California Press, 2011], 19).

31. This question—what and where is cancer?—has been a key struggle for historians of the disease. In *The Breast Cancer Wars: Hope, Fear, and the Pursuit of a Cure in Twentieth-Century America* (Oxford: Oxford University Press, 2003), Barron Lerner writes of the "social construction" of cancer. Siddhartha Mukherjee, in *The Emperor of All Maladies,* configures his history of the disease as a "biography." Robert Aronowitz tells patient stories in his book *Unnatural History: Breast Cancer and American Society* (New York: Cambridge University Press, 2007).

In *Malignant,* I treat knowledge not so much as neutral and descriptive, as histories of cancer might do, but as a creative force: in discovering and treating phenomena known collectively as cancer, scientists, social scientists, and historians have also created what we recognize as the disease. Cancer may start as a series of dividing cells (just as carbon forms the basis of living matter), but it is more richly understood as a rhetorical term that can powerfully organize relationships and as a key player in the broader history of the United States and elsewhere.

32. Only recently have patient advocacy groups been allowed at oncology conferences, and their admission is strictly regulated and not genuinely participatory. At the San Antonio Breast Cancer Symposium (SABCS) meetings every December, for example, patient advocates each evening may listen to a panel of

medical experts who translate the events of the day into lay language. The week I attended, the tone was sometimes condescending and sometimes simply explanatory, but the forum was never taken as an open exchange among knowledgeable participants in the cancer complex.

33. Consider, for example, the statement that "the triumph of pediatric oncology today is a triumph of the multidisciplinary management concept" (Jerome M. Vaeth, ed., *Childhood Cancer: Triumph over Tragedy* [Basel: S. Karger, 1981], 7).

34. Rose Kushner, "Is Aggressive Adjuvant Chemotherapy the Halsted Radical of the '80s?" *CA: A Cancer Journal for Clinicians* 34 (1984): 345–351. Kushner underwent treatment for breast cancer in the 1970s before dying of metastatic disease (the recurrence was found seven years after her initial diagnosis) in 1990.

35. Barron H. Lerner, "Ill Patient, Public Activist: Rose Kushner's Attack on Breast Cancer Chemotherapy," *Bulletin of the History of Medicine* 81 (2007): 221–240.

36. Lerner, *Breast Cancer Wars.*

37. Lerner, "Ill Patient, Public Activist," 240.

38. Kushner, "Aggressive Adjuvant Chemotherapy," 345.

39. Science scholar Donna Haraway describes this divide and its errors well: "The modest witness [i.e., the one with no apparent stakes in a scientific procedure] is the legitimate and authorized ventriloquist for the object world, adding nothing from his mere opinions, from his biasing embodiment. And so he is endowed with the remarkable power to establish the facts. He bears witness: he is objective; he guarantees the clarity and purity of objects. His subjectivity is his objectivity. His narratives have a magical power—they lose all trace of their history as stories, as products of partisan projects, as contestable representations, or as constructed documents in their potent capacity to define the facts. The narratives become clear mirrors, fully magical mirrors, without once appealing to the transcendental or the magical" (*Modest_Witness@Second_Millennium. FemaleMan©_Meets_OncoMouse™: Feminism and Technoscience* [New York: Routledge, 1997], 24).

40. Richard W. Clapp, Geneveive K. Howe, and Molly M. Jacobs, "Environmental and Occupational Causes of Cancer: A Call to Act on What We Know," *Biomedicine and Pharmacotherapy* 61 (2007): 631–639. The authors write that by ignoring the scientific evidence, we enable "tens of thousands of unnecessary illnesses and deaths every year."

41. Derek Simons, "The Impressive City Cantos: Death and Life amid Urban Materiality," Ph.D. diss., Simon Fraser University, 2010.

42. James S. Olson, *Bathsheba's Breast: Women, Cancer, and History* (Baltimore: Johns Hopkins University Press, 2005), 84. For explanations of why therapeutic efficacy is neither the necessary outcome of biomedical research nor a prerequisite for the use of particular drugs, see, e.g., Joan Fujimura, *Crafting Science: A Sociohistory of the Quest for the Genetics of Cancer* (Cambridge, Mass.: Harvard University Press, 1996); and Robert Proctor, *The Cancer Wars: How Politics Shapes What We Know and Don't Know about Cancer* (New York: Basic Books, 1996).

43. Eileen Welsome (*The Plutonium Files* [New York: Dial Press, 1999]) and Gerald Kutcher ("Cancer Therapy and Military Cold War Research: Crossing Epistemological and Ethical Boundaries," *History Workshop Journal* 56 [2003]: 105–30) write about radiation experimentation that involves massive doses of radiation or the injection of radioactive elements, and Elizabeth Toon ("Does Bigger Mean Better?") traces how bodies with cancer have been caught in big professional shifts, such as the movement by radiologists to have radiation treatments added to the protocol despite major debates about their efficacy. See also Löwy, *Between Bench and Bedside;* and Bud, "Strategy in American Cancer Research after WWII." Such histories often leave a critical question open: Is the disease by definition more horrible than any potential—no matter how implausible—treatment, or are people with cancer somehow less than human and thus easier to use as experimental subjects for new discoveries?

44. Although I have spoken with many people across many disciplines, I by no means have gathered anything like what might be called a generalizable "cancer experience." Nor do I question the integrity of oncologists. Oncologists, like other experts, practice their profession for various reasons, both complementary and contradictory, with greater or lesser skill, within often difficult circumstances. I remain agnostic on questions of hope, survival, and treatment. I point no fingers at researchers, at people choosing among a sparse set of treatments, or at those raising money for more research, camps, awareness, or rides to the hospital. Many patients, caretakers, and doctors tell their stories sincerely and sympathetically, with a great deal of anger, frustration, resignation, and grief, and these emotions remain central to any possibility of understanding the cultural status of cancer.

CHAPTER 1

1. Maurice Blanchot, *The Instant of My Death,* and Jacques Derrida, *Demeure: Fiction and Testimony,* trans. Elizabeth Rottenberg (Stanford: Stanford University Press, 2000), 9.

2. The *Oxford English Dictionary* defines the word *prognosis* thus: "Med. A forecast of the probable course and termination of a case of disease; also, the action or art of making such a forecast."

3. Mary Dunlap, "Eureka! Everything I Know about Cancer I Learned from My Dog," ms. on file with author.

4. Post on the website *CancerBaby,* http://cancerbaby.typepad.com/cancerbaby/mother_may_i/index.html (accessed Oct. 17, 2006).

5. Prognostic logic continues to gain power and legibility through the creation of new groups of risk subjects: those encouraged to understand themselves as "at risk" for various diseases may take prophylactic drugs such as statins in the hope of countering their risky futures.

6. See "What Led Survivorship Care to Emerge as a Distinct Component of the Continuum of Care in Oncology?" *Supplement to Oncology Nurse Edition* 22, no. 4 (2008), for a medical history of the survivorship movement. For a genealogy of the "survivor" in cancer literature and medicine, see Emily Bartels, "Outside the Box: Surviving Survival," *Literature and Medicine* 28 (2009): 237–252.

7. *Survivor* takes the sting out of the stigma, but the rhetoric may also be understood as part of a broader cultural cancer-management technique. Recall, for example, sociologist Talcott Parsons's still-relevant description of the "sick role" from the 1950s. Parsons hypothesized that the break from responsibility required by illness was rendered legitimate when the ill person followed culturally determined conventions of being ill, such as seeking healthcare and trying to become healthy. See Parsons, "The Sick Role and the Role of the Physician Reconsidered," *Milbank Memorial Fund Quarterly: Health and Society* 53 (1975): 257–278.

8. Bernie S. Siegel, *Love, Medicine, and Miracles: Lessons Learned about Self-Healing from a Surgeon's Experience with Exceptional Patients* (New York: William Morrow, 1990).

9. Quoted in Douglas Steinberg, "Combination Therapy Tames Stage III," *CURE: Cancer Updates, Research, and Education* 2, no. 3 (2003): 41

10. Nicholas A. Christakis, *Death Foretold: Prophecy and Prognosis in Medical Care* (Chicago: University of Chicago Press, 2001).

11. The *OED* attributes the first use of the term to Donne, some 150 years after the appearance of the verb *to survive.*

12. John Donne, *Devotions upon Emergent Occasions, together with Death's Duel* (Ann Arbor: University of Michigan Press, 1959), 108–109. The modernist writer and Nobel Prize–winner Elias Canetti also wrote about the survivor. Different though they are, both Donne's and Canetti's versions of survival predate the rise in population statistics and the use of numbers to manage questions of political and economic power. According to the philosopher Michel Foucault, this shift toward numerical aggregation and explanation arose with a political shift away from God and the sovereign as the primary sources of governance and toward the state and corporation. Thus, Canetti could write that the "true subject" gives up his life for the ruler, that the ruler needs these deaths in order to maintain and demonstrate his power over death and life (*Crowds and Power* [New York: Farrar, Straus & Giroux, 1984], 232). In other words, in Canetti's view, the sovereign could pick out individuals who might live or die. The ability to let live or make die distinguished sovereign power and marked his position as sovereign.

Foucault, on the other hand, considered subjects in terms of populations. With the rise of population accounting, individuals are no longer of interest to political power. Thus, Foucault requires a different notion of death. According to Foucault, our present notion of death could not be more different from Donne's idea, in which death is necessarily a collective and political endeavor. In contrast, in the age of population statistics and aggregates, death is a limit on political power; death, rather, becomes "the moment when the individual escapes all power, falls back on himself and retreats, so to speak, into his own privacy. Power no longer recognizes death. Power literally ignores death" (*"Society Must Be Defended": Lectures at the Collège de France, 1975–1976* [New York: Picador, 2003], 248).

13. Survivorship can only ever be temporary. Donne's version of survival predates the change in power necessitated by a political shift away from God and the sovereign toward the state and corporation. Foucault writes that our notions of death differ from contemporaries of Donne.

14. Stephen J. Gould, "The Median Isn't the Message," *Discover* 6 (June 1985): 40–42.

15. Hilaire Belloc, "On Statistics," in *The Silence of the Sea and Other Essays* (London: Cassell, 1941), 173.

16. One could turn to many places to get at the uniqueness and historical specificity of this way of understanding time and death. Marcus Aurelius, for example, wrote in *Meditations:* "Always remember then these two things: one, that all things from everlasting are of the same kind, and are in rotation; and it matters nothing whether it be for a hundred years or for two hundred or for an infinite time that a man shall behold the same spectacle; the other, that the longest-lived and the soonest to die have an equal loss; for it is the present alone of which either will be deprived, since (as we saw) this is all he has and a man does not lose what he has not got" (*Meditations: Book II* [Oxford: Oxford University Press, 1989], 14). This idea underwrites a completely different notion of age and lifespan. Thanks to Derek Simons for the quote.

17. Juliet McMullin and Diane Weiner, "Introduction: An Anthropology of Cancer," in *Confronting Cancer: Metaphors, Advocacy, and Anthropology* (Santa Fe, N.M.: SAR Press, 2009), 16.

18. American Cancer Society [ACS], "Cancer Facts and Figures 2012," www.cancer.org/acs/groups/content/@epidemiologysurveilance/documents/document/acspc-031941.pdf (accessed Feb. 2013).

19. Janet Gray, *State of the Evidence 2010: The Connection between the Environment and Breast Cancer?* 6th ed. (San Francisco: Breast Cancer Fund and Breast Cancer Action, 2010), 10; Ahmedin Jemal, Rebecca Siegel, Elizabeth Ward, et al., "Cancer Statistics, 2008," *CA: A Cancer Journal for Clinicians* 58 (2009): 71–96 (available online at http://onlinelibrary.wiley.com/doi/10.3322/CA.2007.0010/pdf).

20. Jemal et al., "Cancer Statistics, 2008," 81.

21. See, for example, www.cancer.gov/newscenter/newsfromnci/2011/survivorshipMMWR2011

22. NCI Press Release, "Report to the Nation Finds Continuing Declines in Cancer Death Rates since the Early 1990s," March 28, 2012; available at www.cancer.gov/newscenter/pressreleases/2012/ReportNationRelease2012 (accessed July 28, 2012). Those who were diagnosed between 2001 and 2007 have a five-year survival rate of 67 percent, compared to 49 percent for those who were diagnosed in the mid-1970s. This statistic does not control for stage at diagnosis (ACS, "Cancer Facts and Figures 2012").

23. The statistics reported here and in what follows, unless otherwise noted, are from www.cancer.gov/cancertopics (accessed June 9, 2012).

24. Although sources vary in terms of the numbers they report, certain trends remain consistent. For women overall, the highest cancer incidence rates are of breast cancer, followed by lung cancer, while for men it is lung, followed by prostate. Death changes the rankings somewhat: for women and men combined, lung cancer has the highest mortality rates, followed by colon, breast, and prostate. See Jemal et al., "Cancer Statistics, 2008." Incidence and mortality rates vary substantially from state to state for some cancers. Lung cancer incidence rates, for example, are nearly four times as high in Kentucky as in Utah (74).

25. "The increase cannot be attributed to improved diagnosis and cancer registration": Richard W. Clapp, Genevieve K. Howe, and Molly M. Jacobs, "Environmental and Occupational Causes of Cancer: A Call to Act on What We Know," *Biomedicine and Pharmacotherapy* 61 (2007): 631–639. See also ACS, "Cancer Facts and Figures 2012."

26. National Cancer Institute, "Annual SEER Incidence and U.S. Death Rates, 1975–2003," http://seer.cancer.gov/csr/1975_2003/results_merged/topic/annualrates.pdf (accessed Feb. 2013).

27. Vinyl chloride propellants, for example, an ingredient of hair sprays, insecticides, deodorants, and spray paints, were used long after they were shown to be carcinogenic. Studies showed that average concentration of the chemical in hair sprays was five times the legal threshold, and "in some cases where the duration of spraying is long (3 minutes) the concentration may be as high as 1400 ppm, 28× recommended" (Gerald Markowitz and David Rosner, *Deceit and Denial: The Deadly Politics of Industrial Pollution* [Berkeley: University of California Press, 2002], 185). A carcinogeneity of this compound was known by government and industry at least fifteen years before it was banned as a propellant in 1974. A smear campaign launched by the chemical industry in response to *Deceit and Denial* was reported in Jon Wiener, "Cancer, Chemicals, and History," *The Nation*, Feb. 7, 2005 (available at www.thenation.com/article/cancer-chemicals-and-history).

28. Richard Doll and Richard Peto, *The Causes of Cancer: Quantitative Estimates of Avoidable Risks of Cancer in the United States Today* (Oxford: Oxford University Press, 1981), 1197.

29. The historian Juan A. del Regato wrote in 1995, after a century of the most minuscule funding of breast cancer research, that "the mortality rate from cancer of the breast, the most common malignant tumor in American women, has not improved an iota since 1927, when Hugh Auchincloss proposed self examination as a means of earlier diagnosis" ("One Hundred Years of Radiation Oncology, 1885 to 1995," in *Current Radiation Oncology*, vol. 2, ed. Jeffrey S. Tobias and Patrick R.M. Thomas [London: Arnold; New York: Oxford University Press, 1995], 1–35.

30. Incidence of cancer: 472.9/100,000 for African Americans, 456.5/100,000 for whites; death from cancer: 216.4/100,000 for African Americans, 177.6/100,000 for whites. Statistics are from the Center for Disease Control and Prevention's United States Cancer Statistics (USCS) for 2009.

31. See, for example, American Council on Science and Health, "The Mentholation of Cigarettes: A Position Statement of the American Council on Science and Health," spring 2010.

32. Steven Whitman, David Ansell, Jennifer Orsi, and Teena Francois, "The Racial Disparity in Breast Cancer Mortality," *Journal of Community Health*, published online Dec. 29, 2010 (accessible via www.suhichicago.org/reports-publications). They argue that the racial disparity in cancer mortality is "inconsistent with the notion that [it] is a function of differential biology." They show that lack of access to mammography, poorer quality of mammograms (in both machinery and reading of the results), lack of follow-up regarding results (black women are twice as likely not to be notified about an abnormal result), inability

to interpret information received, and lack of access to treatment are factors that tend not to be taken into account in studies that attribute mortality differences to race and tumor biology. Dionne J. Blackman and Christopher M. Masi, "Racial and Ethnic Disparities in Breast Cancer Mortality: Are We Doing Enough to Address Root Causes?" *Journal of Clinical Oncology* 24 (2006): 2170–2178, shows black women's mortality rate ratio relative to white women increasing over the last two decades. White women have a higher *incidence* of breast cancer, which may reflect "a combination of factors that affect diagnosis . . . [including] later age at first birth, and greater use of hormone replacement therapy" (Jemal et al., "Cancer Statistics, 2008," 82).

33. Linda Vona-Davis and David P. Rose, "The Influence of Socioeconomic Disparities on Breast Cancer Tumor Biology and Prognosis: A Review," *Journal of Women's Health* 18 (2009): 883–893.

34. K.H. Mayer, J.B. Bradford, H.J. Makadon, et al., "Sexual and Gender Minority Health: What We Know and What Needs to Be Done," *American Journal of Public Health* 98 (2008): 989–995. See also R.J. Wolitski, R. Stall, and R.O. Valdiserri, eds., *Unequal Opportunity: Health Disparities Affecting Gay and Bisexual Men in the United States* (New York: Oxford University Press, 2008).

35. Mautner Project, "Lesbian Health Risks: Factors Facing a Medically Underserved Population," available at www.mautnerproject.org (accessed July 29, 2007).

36. K.A. Schulman, J.A. Berlin, W. Harless, et al., "The Effect of Race and Sex on Physicians' Recommendations for Cardiac Catheterization," *New England Journal of Medicine* 340 (1999): 618–26. See also M. Loring and B. Powell, "Gender, Race, and DSM-III: A Study of the Objectivity of Psychiatric Diagnostic Behavior," *Journal of Health and Social Behavior* 29 (1988): 1–22.

Despite the huge role of African Americans in forwarding the cause of medicine—from slaves bought for the purposes of medical experimentation in the eighteenth century, to the Tuskegee Syphilis Experiment that tracked the progression of untreated syphilis in a group of black men for decades after a treatment was available, and including the fact that African Americans were the primary source of cadavers for medical schools in the nineteenth and twentieth centuries—African Americans continue to have dramatically higher rates of nearly every illness, preventable complication, and accidental death. See Harriet Washington, *Medical Apartheid: The Dark History of Medical Experimentation on Black Americans from Colonial Times to the Present* (New York: Harlem Moon, 2008).

37. Margaret Edson, *W;t: A Play* (New York: Faber & Faber, 1999), 14–15.

38. See Carla Freccero, "De-Idealizing the Body: Hannah Wilke, 1940–1993," in *Bodies in the Making: Transgressions and Transformations*, ed. Nancy Chen and Helene Moglen (Santa Cruz: New Pacific Press, 2006), 12–18.

39. Roland Barthes, *Camera Lucida: Reflections on Photography*, trans. Richard Howard (New York: Hill & Wang, 1981), 124.

40. Lucy Grealy, *Autobiography of a Face* (New York: HarperPerennial, 1995), 27–28.

41. These quotes are from my ongoing participant observations in survivor groups and interviews with people with cancer beginning in 2005.

CHAPTER 2

1. http://firstdescents.org.

2. Stephen Ohlemacher, "U.S. Slipping in Life Expectancy Rankings," *Washington Post,* Aug. 12, 2007 (available at www.washingtonpost.com/wp-dyn/content/article/2007/08/12/AR2007081200113_pf.html).

3. Peter J. Pronovost, "Re-Engineering Health Care to Keep Patients Safe" (Nov. 2, 2012), available at www.huffingtonpost.com/peter-j-pronovost/reengineering-health-care_b_2056543.html.

4. American Cancer Society, "Cancer Facts and Figures 2012," available at www.cancer.org/acs/groups/content/@epidemiologysurveilance/documents/document/acspc-031941.pdf (accessed Feb. 2013).

5. Interview, July 12, 2009.

6. One blogger diagnosed finally with metastatic disease in her thirties wrote, "I knew something was wrong by the look on his face. . . . He then reached for a prescription pad and ordered me to get a mammogram at a nearby radiologist's office. I was shocked by how easy it was for him to do that. If all he had to do was write my name at the top of a pre-printed prescription pad, why hadn't he done that the year before?" ("Karen's Breast Cancer Blog," entry of March 8, 2005: "It Started with a Delayed Diagnosis," available at http://fighting-breast-cancer.com/delayed-diagnosis-breast-cancer; accessed March 28, 2007).

7. A couple of things stand out among the stories I've gathered. First, in several cases of breast cancer, *only* the core biopsy (which takes out more tissue than a fine needle aspiration) gave a positive result, even though the other tests are often used alone as though they would rule out malignancy. Second, patients talk about their hesitancy and embarrassment to talk about symptoms, especially when doctors have already ruled out cancer and reassured them.

8. Archie Bleyer, "Latest Estimates of Survival Rates of the 24 Most Common Cancers in Adolescent and Young Adult Americans," *Journal of Adolescent and Young Adult Oncology* 1 (2011): 37–42.

9. David Chilton, *The Wealthy Barber: Everyone's Commonsense Guide to Becoming Financially Independent,* updated 3d ed. (New York: Three Rivers Press, 1997).

10. Personal correspondence, March 15, 2009.

11. Another friend organizing a fundraiser for her particular and rare cancer, when thinking about asking her doctors to attend her event, said: "They've made enough money off my cancer; they could pay some back" (personal correspondence, April 11, 2009). She omitted that sentiment from her welcoming speech.

12. Angela Pruitt, "Lance Armstrong Agrees to Peddle for a New Team; American Century Signs Tour de France Champion to Tout Its Life-Cycle Funds," *Wall Street Journal,* Feb. 13, 2006, C9.

13. www.americancentury.com/funds/livestrong.jsp; accessed June 16, 2011.

14. Lance Armstrong, *It's Not about the Bike: My Journey Back to Life* (New York: Putnam, 2000).

15. Miriam Engelberg, *Cancer Made Me a Shallower Person* (New York: Harper, 2006), unpaginated.

16. Caitlin Zaloom, "The Productive Life of Risk," *Cultural Anthropology* 19 (2004): 365.

17. David U. Himmelstein et al., "Medical Bankruptcy in the United States, 2007: Results of a National Study," *American Journal of Medicine* 122 (2009): 741–746.

18. These structures carry invisible costs even for straight people who believe themselves to be outside of these cycles. Think, for example, of the shooting of Harvey Milk and George Moscone. The short sentence Dan White received for the murders is usually ascribed to the fact that Milk was queer, and so the judge believed that his life was not worth much. Moscone was considered collateral damage. See *The Times of Harvey Milk,* dir. Rob Epstein, 90 min., Black Sand Productions, 1984.

19. Personal correspondence, April 10, 2008.

20. Walter Mischel and Ebbe B. Ebbesen, "Attention in Delay of Gratification," *Journal of Personality and Social Psychology* 16 (1970): 329–337; Walter Mischel, Ebbe B. Ebbesen, and Antonette Raskoff Zeiss, "Cognitive and Attentional Mechanisms in Delay of Gratification," *Journal of Personality and Social Psychology* 21 (1972): 204–218; and Yuichi Shoda, Walter Mischel, and Philip K. Peake, "Predicting Adolescent Cognitive and Self-Regulatory Competencies from Preschool Delay of Gratification: Identifying Diagnostic Conditions," *Developmental Psychology* 26 (1990): 978–986.

21. Susan Strange, *Casino Capitalism* (Manchester: Manchester University Press, 1997).

22. The ad also relies on a slippage between screening and treatment, for it is unclear what the initial $700 is for: if it is for treatment of an early-stage cancer, it will not be enough. If it is for screening, screening in itself does not keep anyone healthy—it just leads to the treatment of a potentially earlier stage cancer, which will have a higher chance of success.

23. The issue of whether the ACS is referring to prevention solely through early detection, or if it also means by industrial and military regulation and environmental cleanup, is totally elided in this ad.

24. Lee Edelman, *No Future: Queer Theory and the Death Drive* (Durham, N.C.: Duke University Press, 2004).

25. Edelman refers to the Child as the "repository of variously sentimentalized cultural identifications, the Child has come to embody for us the telos of the social order and come to be seen as the one for whom that order is held in perpetual trust" (ibid., 11). This use of the Child as the bearer of the future and of the ideals placed on that future maintains the cultural primacy of what Edelman calls "pro-procreation," or the cultural norms of procreation.

26. As Edelman (ibid., 15) writes, "This fatal embrace of a futurism so blindly committed to the figure of the Child . . . will justify refusing health care benefits to the adults that some children become."

CHAPTER 3

1. Although the sum is paltry compared to the self-reported figures of say, the $115 million raised by Ford for breast cancer, the $65 million raised by

Revlon, or the $780 million raised by Avon, it's still not exactly chump change. For more information, see www.fordcares.com, www.revloncares.com, and www.avonfoundation.org.

2. Postsurgery pamphlet referencing wall washing on file with author. The pink kitsch of breast cancer culture, claims Barbara Ehrenreich in "Welcome to Cancerland" (*Harper's,* Nov. 2001), is as much a cult as a culture—and one that is downright infantilizing. Her widely circulated article touched a nerve with the many women who chafe at the pink, at the tips on how to look better in the midst of treatments, and at the calls to be warriors and vixens. She writes that the pink allows women to take a stand without having to identify as "feminists," and that "cheerfulness is more or less mandatory, dissent is a kind of treason" (50).

3. Susan Sontag, *Illness as Metaphor and AIDS and Its Metaphors* (New York: Picador, 2001), 49.

4. Eve Kosofsky Sedgwick, "White Glasses," *Yale Journal of Criticism* 5 (1992): 202–203. Sedgwick liked to identify as a gay man even though she was also out as a woman married to a man.

5. Ibid., 204.

6. Lorde, *The Cancer Journals* (San Francisco: Aunt Lute Books, 1997), 61. Lorde goes on to say, "Nobody tells him to go get a glass eye, or that he is bad for the morale of the office."

7. Ibid., 60.

8. See Gerald Markowitz and David Rosner, *Deceit and Denial: The Deadly Politics of Industrial Pollution* (Berkeley: University of California Press, 2002). To be "grandfathered" through a regulation means that no new evidence of safety is required for some products already on the market.

9. See Kate Sheppard, "Republicans Attempt to Ax Program Monitoring Carcinogens," Aug. 24, 2012; available at www.motherjones.com/blue-marble/2012/08/republicans-attempt-ax-program-monitoring-carcinogens.

10. In her dissertation on scars and scarring, Carol. E. Henderson writes that "slaves in the ante-bellum era and African Americans in the post-bellum period manipulate and re-vision this site of abuse to their bodies as a sign of empowerment and self-ownership" ("The Body of Evidence: Reading the Scar as Text in Williams, Morrison, Baldwin, and Petry," Ph.D. diss., University of California, Riverside, 2007).

11. Lauren Berlant, in *Cruel Optimism* (Durham, N.C.: Duke University Press, 2011), theorizes the notion of slow death as a physical wearing away of the population.

12. Lynn Kohlman, "Inside Out," *Mamm* (Jan.–Feb. 1995): 14–19.

13. David Serlin, "Reconstructing the 'Hiroshima Maidens': Cosmetic Surgery and Cultural Imperialism after World War Two," paper presented at Stanford University, Seminar on Science, Technology, and Society, May 30, 2007.

14. Judith Halberstam writes about the link between the material body and sets of gendered expectations: "If adolescence for boys represents a rite of passage (much celebrated in Western literature . . .), and an ascension to some version (however attenuated) of social power, for girls, adolescence is a lesson in restraint, punishment, and repression. It is in the context of female adolescence

that the tomboy instincts of millions of girls are remodeled into compliant forms of femininity. . . . The image of the tomboy can be tolerated only within a narrative of blossoming womanhood; within such a narrative, tomboyism represents a resistance to adulthood itself" (*Female Masculinity* [Durham, N.C.: Duke University Press, 1998], 6).

15. Do not get me wrong here: I totally understand why someone would want reconstruction. I know how it feels to stand in front of a group of people at a professional event thinking one's body is screaming "breast cancer" or "Shame, Shame, Shaaaaammmme." My point is certainly not about judging how people respond to mastectomy.

16. When I published an early version of this essay in *Cultural Anthropology* 22 (2007): 501–538, the editors asked me write a short sidebar describing the term *butch*. Here is an abbreviated version:

> I explain my identity by the simple fact that I like nice deep pockets and hate carrying a bag for my wallet, keys, and phone. Aah, if only it were that simple. Not everyone feels so comfy when those people they want and expect to be girls and women choose a gender-neutral or masculine manner, whether through fashion or attitude. Although butches can be straight, queer historical associations position the butch in the more masculine-identified role of pursuer and protector. Oddly, given the multiple, banal, and exciting ways that men and women perform masculinity, butches tend to be stereotyped (yes, still!) by the culture as brawny, overbearing, and badly dressed. In other words, qualities of normative male identity—jocularity, physical strength, confidence, straight-talking, space-taking—seem often to be perceived, outside of a few key urban areas, as threatening when performed by women. Men have masculinity options that do not make this conflation: think computer geek.
>
> Butch phobia has been—and indeed, continues to be—used to diminish and ridicule personal strength for all women. Women athletes, for example, were dismissed as lesbians for using weights in their training well into the 1970s, and Martina Navratilova lost millions of dollars in sponsorship because she did not compensate for her physical strength by femming it up. Nevertheless, butch identities proliferate (aristocratic, soft, sissy, geek, indie, stone, etc.), many of which carry class and race inflections. The word *butch* has been joined recently by a plethora of words for gender nonconformity, such as boi and genderqueer, though it may also be included in a series of such terms to suggest conjoined identities, e.g. trans-gender-queer-butch-dyke-mommy.

17. Years ago, I submitted a paper analyzing the legal cases that resulted from silicone breast implants and the FDA request for evidence of their safety from the manufacturers. I was refused publication on the basis that I had not experienced mastectomy and, therefore, was not qualified to comment. By this allegorical unveiling, I do not mean to imply that only certain ones among us are qualified to speak of mastectomies, a point with which I emphatically disagree as much now as I did then. See Renato Rosaldo, "Grief and a Headhunter's Rage," in *Violence in War and Peace: An Anthology*, ed. Nancy Scheper-Hughes and Philippe Bourgois (London: Blackwell, 2003), 150–156.

18. Literary and gay scholar Michael Warner writes, "It is often thought, especially by outsiders, that the public display of private matters is a debased narcissism, a collapse of decorum, expressivity gone amok, the erosion of any

distinction between public and private" (*Publics and Counterpublics* [New York: Zone Books, 2000], 62).

19. Sandy M. Fernandez, "Pretty in Pink," *Mamm,* June/July 1998; available at http://thinkbeforeyoupink.org/?page_id=26 (accessed Dec. 20, 2012).

20. See Jo B. Paoletti and Carol Kregloh, "The Children's Department," in *Men and Women: Dressing the Part,* ed. Claudia Brush Kidwell and Valerie Steele (Washington, D.C.: Smithsonian Institution Press, 1989), 29–34.

21. Lizabeth Cohen, *A Consumers' Republic: The Politics of Mass Consumption in Postwar America* (New York: Vintage Books, 2003), 137. Similarly, Dodge introduced a car it called "La Femme" in 1955 to gain a foothold in a rising woman's market. The car was pink and included a matching purse (with lipstick and cigarette cases), umbrella, and raincoat.

22. Fernandez, "Pretty in Pink."

23. Personal correspondence, Feb. 8, 2007. And of course, nowhere have women been so useful in this enterprise than draped across car hoods in ads and car shows.

24. "Because the ideology of true feeling cannot admit the nonuniversality of pain . . . the ethical imperative toward social transformation is replaced by a civic-minded but passive ideal of empathy. The political as a place of acts oriented toward publicness becomes replaced by a world of private thoughts, leanings, and gestures. Suffering, in this personal-public context, becomes answered by survival, which is then recoded as freedom" (Lauren Berlant, "Poor Eliza," *American Literature* 70 [1998]: 641).

25. In critiquing that narrative, I do not mean that each person does not have to figure out the impact cancer will have in the design of their lives: those both with and without the disease will be called on to make fight-or-flight decisions, and some of those may or may not make one's life richer or shallower. The point, rather, is that if cancer is a private experience, it is also public, and so I want to maintain scars as more than public spectacles; I want them to come with an understanding of more than the "gift" of cancer.

26. Juanne Nancarrow Clarke, "A Comparison of Breast, Testicular, and Prostate Cancer in Mass Print Media (1996–2001)," *Social Science and Medicine* 59 (2004): 546. The tongue-in-cheek newspaper *The Onion* poked fun at the ridiculousness of such a claim as "cheating death" when it reported that Lance Armstrong held a press conference to announce that "he will be taking the next three months to prepare for a rematch against the opponent with whom he is most often identified: cancer" ("Over-Competitive Lance Armstrong Challenges Cancer to Rematch," *Onion,* Nov. 9, 2006, 16). The humor of this article works only if you assume that no one decides if they will live or die in a fight against cancer. Thanks to Diane Nelson for sending me this clipping.

27. See the American Cancer Society's "Cancer Facts and Figures 2011," www.cancer.org/acs/groups/content/@epidemiologysurveilance/documents/document/acspc-029771.pdf.

28. The U.S. Environmental Protection Agency's National Priorities List (NPL) lists over 130 contaminated military sites. In a 2009 study, doctors at Walter Reed Army Medical Center found that military women are 20 to 40 percent more likely to get cancer than civilian women in the same age groups,

possibly indicating cancers related to hazardous military exposures (Kangmin Zhu et al., "Cancer Incidence in the US Military Population: Comparison with Rates from the SEER Program," *Cancer Epidemiology, Biomarkers, and Prevention* 18 [2009]: 1740–1745).

29. The Safe Drinking Water Act was not passsed until 1984, and several of the chemicals at Camp Lejeune were not included in the regulated chemicals. On July 18, 2012, the U.S. Senate passed a bill—called the Janey Ensminger Act in honor of Jerry Ensminger and his daughter Janey, who died of cancer at age nine—authorizing medical care to military and family members who had resided at the base between 1957 and 1987 and developed conditions linked to the water contamination. The measure applies to up to 750,000 people. See Franco Ordonez, "Senate Passes Lejeune Water-Contamination Bill," *Raleigh News and Observer,* July 19, 2012. The House approved the bill on July 31, 2012, and President Obama signed the bill into law on August 6, 2012.

30. Each year, 232,620 Americans are diagnosed with breast cancer, with 39,520 women and 450 men dying annually (American Cancer Society, "Cancer Facts and Figures 2011"). For each car death there are some sixty-eight disabling car-related injuries (www-nrd.nhtsa.dot.gov/Pubs/811552.pdf). The risk of death in a car crash is gendered, too, with males accounting for 22,902 deaths, and females, 9,979. In 2010, according to the U.S. Department of Transportation, National Highway Traffic Safety Administration, an estimated 2.24 million people were injured in motor vehicle traffic crashes.

31. Centers for Disease Control, National Center for Injury Prevention and Control, "Leading Causes of Death Reports, 1999–2007," http://webapp.cdc.gov/sasweb/ncipc/leadcaus10.html; and "WISQARS Years of Potential Life Lost (YPLL) Reports, 1999–2010," http://webapp.cdc.gov/sasweb/ncipc/ypll10.html (both accessed Feb. 14, 2013).

32. It is canny also in the sense that both the car and the health industries seem to have gathered their own momentum and in their vastness have forgotten the very things that they purportedly grew up around: transportation and health.

33. Geoffrey Gorer, "The Pornography of Death," *Encounter* 5 (1955): 49–52.

34. For a reading of gendered automobile deaths and violence, see S. Lochlann Jain, "Violent Submission," *Cultural Critique* 61 (2005): 186–214; and idem, "Urban Violence: Luxury in Made Space," in *Mobile Technologies of the Future,* ed. Mimi Sheller and John Urry (London: Taylor & Francis, 2005), 86–99. I argue that the culture of the car (and its associated myths of death, violence, and skill) has had a structural organizing effect on American heterosexuality in the twentieth century, leading to a relentlessly physical production of heterosexuality.

35. For more on Pollock's death, see Stephen Jay Schneider, "Death as Art/The Car Crash as Statement: The Myth of Jackson Pollock," in *Car Crash Culture,* ed. Mikita Brottman (New York: Palgrave Macmillan, 2002), 267–284.

36. See, for example, "Dana Reeve Dies of Lung Cancer at 44; Widow Carried on Activism after Christopher Reeve's Death," March 8, 2006, available at http://www.cnn.com/2006/SHOWBIZ/03/07/reeve.obit (accessed March 2013).

37. Quoted in Elisabeth Bronfen's study of death and gender, *Over Her Dead Body: Death, Femininity, and the Aesthetic* (New York: Routledge, 1992). Berlant ("Poor Eliza," 664) notes that "sentimentality, unlike other revolutionary rhetorics, is after all the only vehicle for social change that neither produces more pain nor requires much courage."

38. Thanks to Vasile Stanescu for referring me to the ad, which can be viewed at www.video.ca/video.php?id=1880838688 (accessed June 4, 2007).

39. Erving Goffman, *Stigma: Notes on the Management of Spoiled Identity* (Englewood Cliffs, N.J.: Prentice-Hall, 1963), 121–122.

40. Ghost Bikes was a project of the activist group Visual Resistance; for more information, see http://ghostbikes.org (accessed Feb. 16, 2013).

41. Vito Russo, "Why We Fight" (1988), www.actupny.org/documents/whfight.html (accessed June 1, 2007).

42. For an analysis of the medical activism of ACT UP, see Steven Epstein, "The Construction of Lay Expertise: AIDS Activism and the Forging of Credibility in the Reform of Clinical Trials," *Science, Technology, and Human Values* 20 (1995): 408–437.

43. Lorde, *Cancer Journals*, 15.

CHAPTER 4

1. "There is . . . a central truth in medicine . . . : all doctors make terrible mistakes" (Atul Gawande, *Complications: A Surgeon's Notes on an Imperfect Science* [New York: Picador, 2003], 55–56).

2. For a study on the lack of "association between quality of care and publicly available characteristics of individual physicians," see Rachel O. Reid et al., "Associations between Physician Characteristics and Quality of Care," *Archive of Internal Medicine* 170 (2010): 1442–1449.

3. Julie Sevrens Lyons, "Medical Mistake May Have Killed Man," *San Jose Mercury News*, Nov. 2, 2005; E. Perry, "Kaiser Takes Corrective Action after Three Deaths," *Drug Topics*, Dec. 12, 2005 (available at http://drugtopics.modernmedicine.com/news/kaiser-takes-corrective-action-after-three-deaths; accessed Feb. 2013).

4. Eric G. Campbell, Genevieve Pham-Kanter, Christine Vogeli, and Lisa I. Iezzoni, "Physician Acquiescence to Patient Demands for Brand-Name Drugs: Results of a National Survey of Physicians," *JAMA Internal Medicine* 173 (2013): 237–239.

5. Personal interview, June 2008.

6. Institute of Medicine of the National Academies, *To Err is Human: Building a Safer Health System* (1999), 1, 3 (available at www.iom.edu/Reports/1999/To-Err-is-Human-Building-A-Safer-Health-System.aspx).

7. Institute of Medicine of the National Academies, *To Err is Human: Building a Safer Health System* (1999). Misdiagnoses most likely account for only a portion of overall injuries; many more are caused by insufficient protocols. For example, pulmonary embolisms cause 100,000–180,000 deaths a year. These would be reduced if hospitals adopted low-risk, yet nonstandard, postsurgery protocols, such as compression stockings and blood thinners. Similarly, the

Centers for Disease Control and Prevention has listed suggestions for reducing the 14,000 deaths from the common hospital bacterial infection *Clostridium difficile*. They recommend changes to hospital hygiene practices and antibiotic protocol. See Carolyn V. Gould and L. Clifford McDonald, "Bench-to-Bedside Review: *Clostridium difficile* colitis," *Critical Care* 12 (2008): 203 (available at http://ccforum.com/content/12/1/203).

8. Peter Pronovost, "Re-Engineering Health Care to Keep Patients Safe," available at www.huffingtonpost.com/peter-j-pronovost/reengineering-health-care_b_2056543.html (accessed Nov. 2, 2012).

9. David E. Newman-Toker and Peter J. Pronovost, "Diagnostic Errors—The Next Frontier for Patient Safety," *JAMA* 301 (2009): 1060–1062; available at www.aan.com/globals/axon/assets/7890.pdf.

10. Bradford Winters, Jason Custer, Samuel M. Galvagno, Jr., et al., "Diagnostic Errors in the Intensive Care Unit: A Systematic Review of Autopsy Studies," *BMJ Quality and Safety* (2012); abstract at http://qualitysafety.bmj.com/content/early/2012/07/23/bmjqs-2012–000803.abstract.

11. Tejal Gandhi et al., "Missed and Delayed Diagnoses in the Ambulatory Setting: A Study of Closed Malpractice Claims," *Annals of Internal Medicine* 145 (2006): 488–496.

12. Thomas Krizek, "Surgical Error: Ethical Issues and Adverse Events," *Archives of Surgery* 135 (2000): 1360.

13. See, e.g., T. A. Brennan, L. L. Leape, N. M. Laird et al., "Incidence of Adverse Events and Negligence in Hospitalized Patients: Results of the Harvard Medical Practice Study, I," *New England Journal of Medicine* 324 (1991): 370–376; and L. L. Leape, T. A. Brennan, N. M. Laird et al., "The Nature of Adverse Events in Hospital Patients: Results of the Harvard Medical Practice Study, II," *New England Journal of Medicine* 324 (1991): 377–384.

14. Krizek, "Surgical Error," 1360. Italics mine.

15. Gurney Williams III and Pamela Weintraub, "Mamm Special Report: The New Have-Nots—Are You One?" *Mamm,* Jan./Feb. 2006, 29–35. In the first six months of 2012, 45.1 million persons of all ages (14.6 percent) were uninsured (www.cdc.gov/nchs/data/nhis/earlyrelease/insur201212.pdf).

16. Ralph Nader, *Unsafe at Any Speed: The Designed-in Dangers of the American Automobile* (New York: Grossman, 1965). For more on the subject, see Lochlann Jain, "Dangerous Instrumentality: The Bystander as Subject in Automobility," *Cultural Anthropology* 19 (2004): 61–94.

17. Andrew A. Sandor, "The History of Professional Liability Suits in the United States," *JAMA* 163 (1957): 459–466, traces the earliest medical malpractice cases to the 1300s. For nineteenth-century history linking medical malpractice to increasingly flagrant promises and advertisements for medicine, and the lack of professional structures that might have premitted self-regulation and lack of controlled educational standards for physicians, see James Mohr, "The Emergence of Medical Malpractice in America," *Transactions and Studies of the College of Physicians of Philadelphia,* ser. 5, 14 (1992): 1–21. By the 1840s, antilawyer sentiments "became both common and blatant whenever physicians discussed malpractice," especially as lawyers began to sue not only for what physicians did but also for what they "did not do, thereby cashing in on an

implied responsibility to treat the public that popular newspapers of the 1850s also asserted" (ibid., 12).

18. J.V.C. Smith, editorial, *Boston Medical and Surgical Journal* 48 (1853): 506.

19. Walter Channing, "A Medico-Legal Treatise on Malpractice and Medical Evidence—Review," *Boston Medical and Surgical Journal* 62 (1860): 304.

20. Smith, *BMSJ* editorial, 506–507.

21. Jerome Groopman lays out in his book *How Doctors Think* (New York: Houghton Mifflin, 2007) that the process of diagnosis varies vastly, and in many, many cases there simply is no "standard of care." In any case, as Tom Baker reports in *The Medical Malpractice Myth,* patients have virtually no access to information on their treatments, what errors may have been made, or the standards of care in similar situations; occasionally this leads a patient to make a med-mal claim just to have access to the records and procedures.

22. Marc Franklin and Robert Rabin, *Tort Law and Alternatives: Cases and Materials,* 7th ed. (New York: Foundation Press, 2001), 106.

23. Karen Kelly, "Study Explores How Physicians Communicate Mistakes" (2005), http://web.archive.org/web/20060322154328/http://www.news.utoronto.ca/bin6/051117-1824.asp.

24. DavidHilfiker.com (accessed Dec. 2012).

25. David Hilfiker, "Facing Our Mistakes," *New England Journal of Medicine* 310 (1984): 118–122. For the classic sociological study on how physicians manage error internally, see Charles L. Bosk, *Forgive and Remember: Managing Medical Failure* (Chicago: University of Chicago Press, 1979). This illuminating study highlights the fact that "however lamentable the fact, the patient is an exogenous variable falling outside of the system of control" (25). Several recent studies also address the harm that doctors suffer for not being able to acknowledge errors: Lucian Leape, "Understanding the Power of Apology: How Saying 'I'm Sorry' Helps Heal Patients and Caregivers," *Focus on Patient Safety: A Newsletter from the Patient Safety Foundation* 8 (2005); Aaron Lazare, *On Apology* (New York: Oxford University Press, 2005) and "Apology in Medical Practice: An Emerging Clinical Skill," *JAMA* 296 (2006): 1401–1403; Thomas Gallagher et al., "Disclosing Harmful Medical Errors to Patients," *New England Journal of Medicine* 356 (2007): 2713–2717; and Nicholas Tuvachis, *Mea Culpa: A Sociology of Apology and Reconciliation* (Stanford: Stanford University Press, 1991).

26. Gary T. Schwartz, "Medical Malpractice, Tort, Contract, and Managed Care," *University of Illinois Law Review,* 1998, 886.

27. Personal communication, Jan. 15, 2013.

28. For the effects of MICRA, see Nicolas M. Pace, Daniela Golinelli, and Laura Zakaras, *Capping Non-Economic Awards in Medical Malpractice Trials: California Jury Verdicts under MICRA* (Santa Monica, Ca.: RAND Institute for Civil Justice, 2004); available at www.rand.org/pubs/monographs/2004/RAND_MG234.pdf. According to that study, the cap most affects those cases in which juries have found high losses due to pain and suffering (damages that were then limited, rather than being set by the jury as they were prior to the passage of MICRA).

29. For more on the politics of personal injury law, see S. Lochlann Jain, *Injury: The Politics of Product Design and Safety Law in the United States* (Princeton: Princeton University Press, 2006); and Tom Baker, *The Medical Malpractice Myth* (Chicago: University of Chicago Press, 2005).

30. Plaintiff win rate in med-mal is about 36 percent; by comparison, 69 percent of federal employers' liability cases find for plaintiffs and 57 percent of motor vehicle–related cases find for plaintiffs. Shirley Grace, "The Law: Trial Lawyers Tell All," *The Advocate* (newsletter of the Trial Lawyers Section of The Florida Bar) 38, no. 4 (spring 2009).

31. Todd S. Aagaard, "Identifying and Valuing the Injury in Lost Chance Cases," *Michigan Law Review* 96 (1998): 1335–1361.

32. This judge was clearly unaware that cancer treatment has progressed somewhat since the 1950s, and he brought an egregiously outdated version of medical ethics to the table. In 1961, a survey showed that 90 percent of physicians did not tell their patients a diagnosis of cancer, but by 1971 a similar survey indicated that 97 percent did inform their patients. See Dennis H. Novak et al., "Changes in Physicians' Attitudes toward Telling the Cancer Patient," *JAMA* 241 (1979): 897–900.

33. *Elaine Dumas v. David Cooney* (1991) 235 Cal. App. 3d 1593, 1609. Italics mine.

34. Despite the slipperiness of the concept—the confusion about what might be meant by cause, prognosis, and chance—the tort of "lost chance" does maintain that (1) early detection is important, (2) doctors should be accountable when their practice falls below the standard of care, and (3) patients should have a way to hold their doctors accountable to them.

35. Theodore M. Porter, *Trust in Numbers: The Pursuit of Objectivity in Science and Public Life* (Princeton: Princeton University Press, 1996), 48.

36. Atul Gawande, "When Doctors Make Mistakes," in *Complications,* 47–74. See also Sherwin B. Nuland, "Whoops!" *New York Review of Books,* July 18, 2002. Although Nuland celebrates this refreshing new voice of the surgeon willing to admit having made mistakes, he nevertheless collaborates in the erasure of the patient and fails to assign responsibility for mistakes. It is enough, for Nuland, that the mistakes are acknowledged—albeit not to the patients.

37. Gawande, *Complications,* 77.

38. For a debate about the merits and drawbacks of disclosure error, see Constantine D. Mavroudis, Keith Naunheim, and Robert Sade, "Should Surgical Errors Always Be Disclosed to the Patient?" *Annals of Thoracic Surgery* 80 (2005): 399–408.

39. See, e.g., Adrienne Pine, "From Healing to Witchcraft: On Ritual Speech and Roboticization in the Hospital," *Culture, Medicine, and Psychiatry* 35 (2011): 262–284.

40. J. B. Cooper et al., "Preventable Anesthesia Mishaps: A Study of Human Factors," *Anesthesiology* 49 (1978): 399–406. Also discussed in Gawande, *Complications,* 65–70.

41. Schwartz, "Medical Malpractice, Tort, Contract, and Managed Care," 890. Schwartz estimates that the actual number of claims is well below the rate of malpractice (893).

42. *Leonard v. Watsonville Community Hospital,* 47 Cal. 2d 509, 305 P. 2d 36 (1956). The court states: "It is a matter of common knowledge . . . that no special skill is required in counting instruments. Although under such circumstances proof of practice or custom is some evidence of what should be done and may assist in the determination of what constitutes due care, it does not conclusively establish the standard of care."

43. Anahad O'Connor, "When Surgeons Leave Objects Behind," Sept. 24, 2012, http://well.blogs.nytimes.com/2012/09/24/when-surgeons-leave-objects-behind.

44. *Merle Evers and Richard Evers v. Kenneth Dolliner, M.D., and Livingston Ob-Gyn Group, P.C.,* Supreme Court of New Jersey, 95 N.J. 399; 471 A. 2d 405; 1984 N.J. LEXIS 2395.

45. *Kennedy v. U.S.,* 750 F. Supp. 206 (1990).

46. The title of this concluding section is from an 1844 poem, "The Coming Event" by James Clarence Mangan (cited as the title of Stuart McLean's book *The Event and Its Terrors: Ireland, Famine, Modernity* [Stanford: Stanford University Press, 2004]). The last lines read: "So best shall ye bear to encounter alone/The Event and its terrors."

47. One person I spoke to says he sometimes regrets not having sued his doctors after a catheter broke and he nearly bled to death when the physician neglected for days to call a vascular surgeon. He thought about wanting to have something to leave to his children, "something to show for my suffering," he says. Ultimately, he didn't sue because a lawyer told him that he would, if he won, probably only clear about $10,000, and it would take him five years of struggle. This man told me he would rather just forget the whole thing.

48. Pronovost, "Re-Engineering Health Care."

CHAPTER 5

1. Patient Information Leaflet FINAL ver. 1.0, TroVax Renal Immunotherapy Survival Trial TRIST™, www.ackc.org/trovax (accessed August 12, 2007).

2. Action to Cure Kidney Cancer, www.ackc.org/trovax (accessed June 16, 2009).

3. Ilana Löwy, *Between Bench and Bedside: Science, Healing, and Interleukin-2 in a Cancer Ward* (Cambridge, Mass.: Harvard University Press, 1997), 65. She writes: "Randomization and the establishment of 'objective indicators' became tools to facilitate the articulation of tasks and the neutralization of conflicts between professional segments involved in trials of new therapies" (51).

4. Nicholas Christakis, *Death Foretold: Prophecy and Prognosis in Medical Care* (Chicago: University of Chicago Press, 2001), 11.

5. Mitchell Dowsett, "William L. McGuire Memorial Lecture: Biomarking the Estrogen Dependence of Breast Cancer," lecture presented at the San Antonio Breast Cancer Symposium (SABCS), San Antonio, Tex., Dec. 14, 2007. The SABCS is the main forum in which breast cancer study results and interim research findings are presented each year.

6. Another version of this cliché of self-abnegating nobility has been reported in the Canadian press in reference to a baby who will be a heart donor after her death: "She will leave behind more than just a heart-broken father and mother. Her parents will be the heroes behind her tragic sacrifice" (Don Martin, "Comment: Finding Good from Tragedy," *National Post,* April 9, 2009).

7. As Ann Oakley points out, researchers purposely elide humans, both patients and doctors, by not allowing either to decide which study arm the subject will belong to, treatment or placebo ("Who's Afraid of the Randomised Controlled Trial? Some Dilemmas of the Scientific Method and 'Good' Research Practice," in *The Ann Oakley Reader: Gender, Women, and Social Science,* ed. Ann Oakley [Bristol, U.K.: Policy, 2005], 233–244). In this sense, the RCT dispenses with several previous quandaries in human-subject research, such as who should receive new treatments (e.g., doctors' friends) and what pools subjects should be drawn from (e.g., prisoners).

8. A. Morabia, "Pierre-Charles-Alexandre Louis and the Evaluation of Bloodletting" (2004), James Lind Library, www.jameslindlibrary.org (accessed Oct. 5, 2006). Many other examples could be used here, for instance, [no author], "Says Tallest Humans Are Cancer's Victims," *New York Times,* July 21, 1928.

9. Theodore M. Porter, *Trust in Numbers: The Pursuit of Objectivity* (Princeton: Princeton University Press, 1995); Harry M. Marks, *The Progress of Experiment: Science and Therapeutic Reform in the United States, 1900–1990* (Cambridge: Cambridge University Press, 1997); Trudy DeHue, "Testing Treatments, Managing Life: On the History of Randomized Clinical Trials," *History of the Human Sciences* 12 (1999): 115–24; idem, "A Dutch Treat: Randomized Controlled Experimentation and the Case of Heroin-Maintenance in the Netherlands," *History of the Human Sciences* 15 (2002): 75–98. See also Vinceanne Adams, "Randomized Controlled Crime: Postcolonial Sciences in Alternative Medicine Research," *Social Studies of Science* 32 (2002): 659–90; and Adriana Petryna, *When Experiments Travel: Clinical Trials and the Global Search for Human Subjects* (Princeton: Princeton University Press, 2009). Others focus on the ethics of the trials and the treatment of subjects, and a burgeoning literature addresses the on-the-ground efficacy of trials in terms of the slippages between theory and practice, the value of different statistical models, and the politics of pharmaceutical funding. See Joseph Dumit, *Drugs for Life: How Pharmaceutical Companies Define Our Health* (Durham, N.C.: Duke University Press, 2012); and Jill A. Fisher, *Medical Research for Hire: The Political Economy of Pharmaceutical Clinical Trials* (New Brunswick, N.J.: Rutgers University Press, 2009). Fisher points out that 75 percent of trials are run privately by for-profit pharmaceutical companies, which fundamentally influences medical research. For a bioethics angle, see, e.g., Andrew Feenberg, "On Being a Human Subject: Interest and Obligation in the Experimental Treatment of Incurable Disease," *Philosophical Forum* 23 (1992): 213–30. For a more classically bioethical perspective, see George Weisz, ed., *Social Science Perspectives on Medical Ethics* (Dordrecht, Neth.: Kluwer, 1990).

10. It is easy enough to reiterate these elisions by skipping the grief and moving straight into an academic argument. Maybe it is unavoidable; maybe the elision is the requirement of the academic narrative form. No one who writes

about cancer can really escape the ways that language overwrites the helplessness and pain of mortality.

11. Löwy writes of patients' unrealistic hopes in *Between Bench and Bedside,* 78–79. See also Mary-Jo DelVecchio Good, "The Biotechnical Embrace," *Culture, Medicine, and Psychiatry* 25 (2001): 395–410; Helen Valier and Carsten Timmermann, "Clinical Trials and the Reorganization of Medical Research in Post–Second World War Britain," *Medical History* 52 (2008): 493–510. Cancer trials have often "delivered at best marginal benefits," with controversial endpoints and success difficult to assess. "Nevertheless, such controversy did not undermine the progress of the clinical trial as an increasingly essential feature of clinical bio-medical research" (Valier and Timmermann, "Clinical Trials," 501–502). These authors also comment on the changed cultural role of the trial: "Arguably this is a consequence of repeated reports on hopes associated with new experimental treatments since the 1960s (especially for childhood cancers) and the rigorous promotion of the randomized controlled trial as the gold standard of modern clinical research" (509).

Affective economies and RCT-based medical practice furthermore provide a basis on which to think through the recursive phenomenon of what medical historians refer to as the increasing alienation of medical care: treatment of and by strangers. Good finds that most people in America die under the direction of a physician who has known them for less than thirty-six hours ("The Biotechnical Embrace," 408). RCTs provide one place to see further how strangers, now as numbers, provide the grist for calculations that have created industries often quite separate from cancer survival and treatment.

12. Harry M. Marks, *The Progress of Experiment: Science and Therapeutic Reform in the United States, 1900–1990* (Cambridge: Cambridge University Press, 2000).

13. www.ClinicalTrials.gov, a service of the U.S. National Institutes of Health, presently holds a searchable database of 140,759 trials as of February 2013. Of the 44,853 open trials, 12,337 are related to cancer research.

14. Michel Foucault, "The Political Technology of Individuals," in *Power (The Essential Works of Michel Foucault, vol. 3: 1954–1984),* ed. James D. Faubion (New York: New Press, 1994), 405. Stuart Murray cites this quotation in a brilliant piece, "Thanatopolitics: On the Use of Death for Mobilizing Political Life," paper presented at the annual meeting of the American Political Science Association, Washington, D.C., Sept. 1, 2005.

15. Margaret Edson, *W;t: A Play* (New York: Faber & Faber, 1999). See also Catherine Belling, "The Death of the Narrator," in *Narrative Research in Health and Illness,* ed. Brian Hurwitz, Trisha Greenhalgh, and Vieda Skultans (Malden, Mass.: Blackwell, 2004), 146–155.

16. This is different, say, from azidothymidine, or AZT, a drug that was designed two decades before the AIDS epidemic and that had no disease to work against until then. The efficacy of a drug so soon after the rise of the disease it is used to treat colors the cultural formations related to AIDS activism in ways that are insufficiently acknowledged in comparisons between AIDS and cancer activism. See Steven Epstein's rigorous account of AIDS activism's

lasting effect on RCTs in *Impure Science: AIDS, Activism, and the Politics of Knowledge* (Berkeley: University of California Press, 1996).

17. Elaine Scarry, *The Body in Pain* (New York: Oxford University Press, 1985), 119.

18. Elias Canetti writes that the commander of an army can appropriate all the dead bodies that result from his decision: "He commands; he sends his men against the enemy, and to their death. If he is victorious, all the dead on the battlefield belong to him, both those who fought for him and those who fought against him. . . . The significance of his victories is measured by the number of the dead" (*Crowds and Power,* trans. Carol Stewart [New York: Farrar, Straus & Giroux, 1960], 230). The dead come to belong to the person who counts; otherwise deaths are dispersed and inexplicable. Canetti also writes of the autocrat's power over life and death. The autocrat "needs executions from time to time and, the more his fears increase, the more he needs them. His most dependable, one might say, his truest, subjects are those he has sent to their deaths" (232).

See also Drew Gilpin Faust's analysis of how the deaths related to the Civil War were understood: "The establishment of national and Confederate cemeteries created the Civil War Dead as a category, as a collective that represented something more and something different from the many thousands of individual deaths that it comprised. It also separated the Dead from the memories of living individuals mourning their own very particular losses. The Civil War Dead became both powerful and immortal, no longer individual men but instead a force that would shape American public life for at least a century to come. The reburial movement created a constituency of the slain, insistent in both its existence and its silence, men whose very absence from American life made them a presence that could not be ignored" (*This Republic of Suffering: Death and the American Civil War* [New York: Vintage, 2008], 249).

19. Here I quote Adrienne Rich, "A Woman Dead in Her Forties" (in *The Fact of a Doorframe: Selected Poems, 1950–2001* [New York: W.W. Norton, 2002]). This elegiac poem meditates on the public and private of breasts and mastectomy scars and mortality. The poem shifts among looking, touching, and speaking in remembering the story of a relationship with a childhood friend who dies of breast cancer as an adult. Rich writes: "I barely glance at you/as if my look could scald you." As adults they "kept in touch, untouching . . . fingering webs/of love and estrangement til the day/the gynecologist touched your breast/and found a palpable hardness." Rich reminds us that before cancer is about scars, it is about touch: the rituals of detection. The poem plays on the prohibition of intimate touching among women—"how can I reconcile this passion/with our modesty"—amid the impersonal medical touch of the physician and the "truths" told by the body "in its rush of cells," even as the women "never spoke at your deathbed of your death."

The following quote offers a classic explication of this trade-off: "Society . . . asks not only for good care today, but for better care tomorrow, and the medical profession has accepted this melioristic goal as legitimate and even obligatory. This has led to profound changes in a profession whose traditional commitment is to the individual patient. In order to give society the progress it demands for the future, we carry out clinical trials in which our patients of today become research subjects" (William J. MacKillop and Pauline A. Johnston, "Ethical Problems in Clinical Research: The Need for Empirical Studies of the Clinical Trials Process," *Journal of Chronic Diseases* 39, no. 3 [1986]: 178).

20. Quoted in "Barbara Brenner's Reflections on the 30th Annual San Antonio Breast Cancer Symposium—Day 2," http://archive.bcaction.org/index.php?page=2007-sabcs-day-2 (accessed March 6, 2008).

21. Anatole Broyard, "The Patient Examines the Doctor," in *Intoxicated by My Illness, and Other Writings on Life and Death* (New York: Clarkson Potter, 1992), 45.

22. See Robert Bazell, *HER2: The Making of Herceptin, a Revolutionary Treatment for Breast Cancer* (New York: Random House, 1998).

23. Canetti here writes of "the survivor" more generally, but the concept fits our subject as well. The quotation is preceded by this: "His calm and imperturbability in the midst of putrefaction [are] characteristic of the hero. All the people in the world could lie rotting on top of him and he would still remain, also in the midst of universal corruption, upright and intent on his goal" (*Crowds and Power,* 257).

24. "The highly asymmetric characterization of survival and complications," claims Gerald Kutcher, "typified the knowledge claims produced from clinical trials. On the one hand, the measure of success, the unit for comparing one treatment to another, was survival and its surrogate, disease-free survival. Almost the entire structure of the study, the whole of the statistical apparatus was designed to ensure that the reported survival differences were significant and not a consequence of hidden bias. Sophisticated statistical methods were developed to address pre-randomization, post-study stratification, and a host of other methodological difficulties, always with the goal of rooting out bias in reported survival. *On the other hand, the analysis of complications had no such elaborate statistical paraphernalia to support it.* Complications were presented as a stepchild of survival and characterized with qualitative terms like minimal and acceptable. This privileging of survival in the design and execution of clinical trials, however, . . . provided a limited measure for translating trial results into local practice" ("Cancer Clinical Trials and the Transfer of Medical Knowledge: Metrology, Contestation, and Local Practice," in *Devices and Designs: Medical Innovations in Historical Perspective,* ed. Carsten Timmermann and Julie Anderson [Basingstoke, U.K.: Palgrave, 2006], 217–218; italics mine).

25. See, for example, Kirsten Ball, "'If it almost kills you that means it's working!' Cultural Models of Chemotherapy Expressed in a Cancer Support Group," *Social Science and Medicine* 68 (2009): 169–176.

26. See Isabelle Baszanger, "One More Chemo or One Too Many? Defining the Limits of Treatment and Innovation in Medical Oncology," *Social Sciences and Medicine* 75 (2012): 864–872.

27. After a twenty-year follow-up study, some oncologists claim a marginal benefit of the CMF regime, while others claim that there was no survival benefit. Still others think that its success is contingent on the particular population of patients, depending on their pre- or postmenopausal status and on the kind and stage of cancer. "Statistics based on immature data are not necessarily significant," asserts Stuart G. Gilbert. "As an example, I cite the landmark 1976

report by Bonadonna and colleagues ['Combination Chemotherapy as an Adjuvant Treatment in Operable Breast Cancer,' *New England Journal of Medicine* 294 (1976): 405–410], which established adjuvant chemotherapy with cyclophosphamide, methotrexate, and fluorouracil (CMF) for node-positive breast cancer. They reported an extraordinary benefit in progression-free survival among postmenopausal patients at 27 months (P = 0.001). However, at 36 months, there was less benefit (P = 0.16), and at 20 years, there was no survival benefit from having received CMF" ("Trastuzumab in Breast Cancer," *Journal of the American Medical Association* 354 [2006]: 640).

The standard protocol for breast cancer chemotherapy treatment is as follows. For breast cancer patients between Stages I and III, more or less the same set of treatments are given: in a twenty-first-century ritual, after surgery and before radiation, about 100,000 Americans a year receive chemotherapy treatment, and 7,000 to 10,000 derive some benefit from it. (In other words, some people will survive for years longer, while the great majority will not.) Oncologists acknowledge this limited success of chemotherapy and bolster it with treatments such as radiation and pharmaceuticals. This is in part because treatments such as radiation and the use of hormones increase survival rates significantly over chemotherapy alone. Oncologists have accepted an ethics of giving everyone chemotherapy: it will kill a few, it will injure many, but it will save others. It is a trade-off at the level of population, and it is measured by the chance of a favorable prognosis.

28. Rose Kushner's papers (1953–1990) are stored at the Arthur and Elizabeth Schlesinger Library on the History of Women in America, Radcliffe College; see http://oasis.lib.harvard.edu/oasis/deliver/~sch00028. Kutcher, "Cancer Clinical Trials."

29. Dennis Slamon et al., "Role of Anthracycline-Based Therapy in the Adjuvant Treatment of Breast Cancer: Efficacy Analyses Determined by Molecular Subtypes of the Disease," paper presented at SABCS, San Antonio, Tex., Dec. 13, 2007. The indication is for HER2/neu-positive and topo-IIa-coamplified tumors; in 2008 the FDA approved a test for detecting the topo IIa amplification. The vast majority of patients will now receive the same treatments that were used then, albeit with the addition of new pharmaceuticals such as tamoxifen and aromatase inhibitors.

30. Charles Rosenberg, "The Tyranny of Diagnosis: Specific Entities and Individual Experience," *Milbank Quarterly* 80 (2002): 240. Discussing how physicians approach diagnosis, T. M. Luhrmann writes: "As they memorize the hyperdetails of bodily process, they . . . turn the emotional horror of disease into a scientific entity. That transformation leaves the person and the pain out of illness" (*Of Two Minds: The Growing Disorder in American Psychiatry* [New York: Knopf, 2000], 87).

31. James Holland of New York City's Mount Sinai Hospital asks: "Can it be more ethical to deny the possible good effects to most, by avoiding all toxicity in order to do no harm to one? The unmitigated disease must be calculated as a toxic cost of cancer. Underdosing, in an attempt to avoid toxicity, is far more deadly" (quoted in David J. Rothman and Harold Edgar, "Scientific Rigor and Medical Realities: Placebo Trials in Cancer and AIDS Research," in *AIDS:*

The Making of a Chronic Disease, ed. Elizabeth Fee and Daniel M. Fox [Berkeley: University of California Press, 1992], 196).

32. A study published in 2006—twenty years after the discovery of the HER2/neu gene—takes stock of developments in thirty years of chemotherapy: "The usual approach is to tailor the aggressiveness of the chemotherapy to the risk of recurrence. As compared with standard chemotherapy, aggressive chemotherapy is associated with a greater benefit, but also with more acute and long-term toxic effects. . . . Hence, patients at high risk for recurrence might be offered . . . an intensive anthracycline regimen" (Mark N. Levine and Timothy Whelan, "Adjuvant Chemotherapy for Breast Cancer—Thirty Years Later," *Journal of the American Medical Association* 355 [2006]: 1920). The equation presented here ignores the fact that aggressive treatments do not provide "greater benefit" across the board, but mostly for very specific disease. In other words, the term *aggressive* conceals the inability to predict the drug's efficacy.

33. For more on HDC, see Richard A. Rettig et al., *False Hope: Bone Marrow Transplantation for Breast Cancer* (New York: Oxford University Press, 2007).

34. Scarry, *Body in Pain,* 80, 114.

35. The term *outhealing* was coined by Elaine Scarry in a discussion in which I was trying out the following argument with her (Stanford, Calif., Feb. 26, 2008).

36. Moreover, treatments themselves may serve as shields for the uncertainty of oncology's knowledge of cancer. If expertise is often based on claims of certainty, it may be easy for treatment to become a sort of proxy for certainty, where doing something is perceived by patients and physicians alike as better than doing nothing.

37. One therapist who works exclusively with people with cancer told me, "People get treated for years, and the doctors are excited [that] people are 'living' longer with cancer. So they live longer on endless cycles of chemo, feeling sick and being tied to the cancer centers for years. I think there is a sacrifice of human dignity and a giving up of knowing what it is like to die without the horrendous effects of chemo, being bald, sick, etc., etc. The huge attachment to these treatments also forces communities to sacrifice caring for their members who are dying. Instead these people are trying to live and survive cancer and [are] dying in the process" (Janie Brown, founder of and therapist with the Callanish Society, Vancouver, B.C., pers. comm., Jan. 13, 2006).

CHAPTER 6

1. For a basic introduction to ART, see "What Is Assisted Reproductive Technology," www.cdc.gov/art/ (accessed March 12, 2011).

2. P. Lutjen et al., "The Establishment and Maintenance of Pregnancy Using In Vitro Fertilization and Embryo Donation in a Patient with Primary Ovarian Failure," *Nature* 307 (1984): 174–175; E.A. Kennard et al., "A Program for Matched, Anonymous, Oocyte Donation," *Fertility and Sterility* 51 (1989): 655–660.

3. Family Issue Fact Sheet No. 2010–03 (March 2010), S.B. 1306/H.B. 2651—Human Egg Provider Protection Act, Center for Arizona Policy.

4. In 2011, 7,494 births, over a quarter of all IVF births, involved donated eggs; see www.sartcorsonline.com/rptCSR_PublicMultYear.aspx?ClinicPKID=0. "Buying and selling human oocytes (eggs) is a $3 billion dollar industry" (Family Issue Fact Sheet No. 2010–03).

5. Physician Jennifer Schneider observes that "once a young woman walks out of an IVF clinic, she is of no interest to anyone. . . . In fact, the people who benefit from egg donations—IVF clinics and researchers—have every reason to avoid follow-up of egg donors and studies of their possible long-term risks" ("It's Time for an Egg Donor Registry and Long-Term Follow-Up," Testimony at Congressional Briefing on Human Egg Trafficking, Nov. 14, 2007 [available at www.geneticsandsociety.org/article.php?id=3820]). One study found that only 2.6 percent of donors were contacted by the clinic after their donation; see W. Kramer, J. Schneider, and N. Schultz, "U.S. Oocyte Donors: A Retrospective Study of Medical and Psychosocial Issues," *Human Reproduction* 24 (2009): 3144–3149. See also Nancy J. Kenny and Michelle McGowan, "Looking Back: Egg Donors' Retrospective Evaluations of Their Motivations, Expectations, and Experiences during Their First Donation Cycle," *Fertility and Sterility* 93 (2010): 455–466.

6. Canadian Royal Commission on the New Reproductive Technologies, "Proceed with Care: Final Report of the Royal Commission on New Reproductive Technologies" (1993), available at www.cwhn.ca/en/node/24428.

7. Archie Bleyer, "Latest Estimates of Survival Rates of the 24 Most Common Cancers in Adolescent and Young Adult Americans," *Journal of Adolescent and Young Adult Oncology* 1, no. 1 (2011). See also National Cancer Institute, "Adolescents and Young Adults with Cancer," www.cancer.gov/cancertopics/aya/types/quiz (accessed March 2013).

8. For a history of this story, see environmental historian Nancy Langston's *Toxic Bodies: Hormone Disruptors and the Legacy of DES* (New Haven, Conn.: Yale University Press, 2010).

9. Nelly Oudshoorn, *Beyond the Natural Body: An Archaeology of Sex Hormones* (New York: Routledge, 1994); Rebecca Jordan-Young, *Brain Storm: The Flaws in the Science of Sex Differences* (Cambridge, Mass.: Harvard University Press, 2010).

10. Elizabeth Roberts, "Abandonment and Accumulation: Embryonic Futures in the United States and Ecuador," *Medical Anthropology Quarterly* 25 (June 2011): 232–253.

11. See, e.g., Victoria Uroz and Lucia Guerra, "Donation of Eggs in Assisted Reproduction and Informed Consent," *Medicine and Law* 28 (2009): 565–575; and Francine Coeytaux, Testimony on Egg Retrieval to California Senate Committee, Joint Oversight Hearing on the Implementation of Proposition 71, the Stem Cell Research and Cures Act, March 9, 2005 (available at www.geneticsandsociety.org/article.php?id=180). Because of the difficulty in retreiving consent forms after the end of the procedure, it's difficult to know how well people are warned of the slim but very real risk of death. See David Magnus and Mildred K. Cho, "A Commentary on Oocyte Donation for Stem Cell Research in South Korea," *American Journal of Bioethics* 6 (2006): W23–W24.

12. Louise K. Stewart et al., "In Vitro Fertilization and Breast Cancer: Is There Cause for Worry?" *Fertility and Sterility* 98 (2012): 334–340. See also Helen Pearson, "Special Report: Health Effects of Egg Donation May Take Decades to Emerge," *Nature* 442 (2006): 607–608.

13. Dr. Linda Giudice, president-elect of the American Society of Reproductive Medicine; quoted in Andrew M. Seaman, "IVF in Young Women Tied to Later Breast Cancer," June 23, 2012, www.reuters.com/article/2012/06/22/us-ivf-breast-cancer-idUSBRE85L1DM20120622.

14. According to Dr. Suzanne Parisian, former chief medical officer of the FDA, "Pharmaceutical firms have not been required by either government or physicians to collect safety data for IVF drugs regarding risk of cancer or other serious health conditions, despite the drugs having been available in the United States for several decades" (Feb. 2005 memo, posted at www.ourbodiesourselves.org/book/companion.asp?id=25&compID=67&page=10).

15. See, e.g., Aaron Levine, "Self-Regulation, Compensation, and the Ethical Recruitment of Oocyte Donors," *Hastings Center Report,* March–Apr. 2010, 25–36. Based on advertisements aimed at potential egg sources, Levine finds that compensation to donors ranges from $3,000 to $50,000. No agency collects data on donor payment.

16. An FDA web page on xenotransplantation states, "Of public health concern is the potential for cross-species infection by retroviruses, which may be latent and lead to disease years after infection. Moreover, new infectious agents may not be readily identifiable with current techniques" (www.fda.gov/BiologicsBloodVaccines/Xenotransplantation/default.htm). In 2009, the FDA recommended against using nonhuman animal cells for the culture in which embryos are grown before implantation. Because of the dangers, they would allow the practice only by express permission. The FDA recommended that mothers and babies of embryos co-cultured with the Vero cell line (a contraction of the esperanto term *verda reno,* meaning "green kidney," in honor of the ancestral African green monkey cells from which it was created) be closely followed, since some viruses remain dormant for years. Embryos had been found to be more robust when co-cultured using the Vero cell line or other animal-derived cell lines or body parts, however, the FDA wrote that this "raises health concerns for the recipients of such embryos, the offspring resulting from such embryos, and the general public" ("Information and Recommendations for Physicians Involved in the Co-Culture of Human Embryos with Non-Human Animal Cells," available at www.fda.gov/BiologicsBloodVaccines/Xenotransplantation/ucm136532.htm). Rebecca Skloot reports on the use of a cow uterus to grow human embryos in "Sally Has 2 Mommies and 1 Daddy," *Popular Science,* Apr. 1, 2003, www.popsci.com/scitech/article/2003-04/sally-has-2-mommies-and-1-daddy.

17. Prospective parents can borrow and pay $120,000 for six cycles of treatment. If a woman gets pregnant on the first cycle, they get nothing back; however, if she doesn't get pregnant after six attmepts, she will get 20 percent of her money back (minus 20 percent interest). See, for example, Jessica Silver-Greenbert, "In Vitro a Fertile Niche for Lenders," *Wall Street Journal,* Feb. 24, 2012.

18. See www.pacificfertilitycenter.com/welcome/rates.php (accessed March 22, 2011). The median age of egg donors is 28.7. See L. R. Shover et al., "The Personality and Motivation of Semen Donors: A Comparison with Oocyte Donors," *Human Reproduction* 7 (1992): 575–576.

19. https://www.eggdonor.com (accessed April 4, 2011).

20. www.eggdonation.com/index.php (accessed April 4, 2011). Subsequent quotations in this paragraph are from the same web page.

21. www.thedonorsource.com/faq.htm.

22. Gaylene Becker, *Elusive Embryo: How Women and Men Approach New Reproductive Technologies* (Berkeley: University of California Press, 2000), 154.

23. Some donor recruitment ads do remind one of personals, such as this ad seeking an egg donor: "'Desperately Seeking Smart, Sensitive, Sunny Samaritan. We are [Yale] alumni looking for a donor match: A lovely light-eyed lady with a quick, sharp laugh. Wit and warmth a must" (quoted in Joseph Berger, "Our Towns: Yale Gene Pool Seen as Route to Better Baby," *New York Times*, Jan. 10, 1999).

24. The field of epigenetics (the study of heritable changes in gene expression or cellular phenotype) finds increasingly that what scientists took to be individual genetic expression immune to environmental factors over generations has in fact resulted from a complex interplay of genetic development and environment. Environmental factors such as chemical exposure to anything from tobacco to plastics and radiation, availability of food resources, and access to social networks or familial affection alter not just an individual's health and well-being, but also genetic messaging for generations. (Humans are becoming taller over generations because of better nutrition, and the grandchildren of mice that were licked by their mothers release fewer stress hormones even when they themselves are not licked—to name just two findings of epigeneticists.) Thus, the search for traits thought to be linked to genetic well-being, for example physical appearance and disease history—so carefully vetted through oocyte and sperm selection—may be completely misled.

25. Kinship confusions are still being worked out by parties as varied as potential grandparents, who feel they should get to meet the genetic children of their own children, and single mothers who introduce genetically related siblings to each other as "brothers" or "sisters" while steadfastly telling them they have "no dad." See, e.g., Peggy Orenstein, "Your Gamete, Myself," *New York Times Magazine*, July 15, 2007, 34–41, 53, 68.

26. See Pacific Fertility Center, www.donateyoureggs.com/egg-donor/egg-donor-testimonials (accessed April 4, 2011).

27. Ibid. Subsequent testimonials are from this same website, unless otherwise specified.

28. Ethics Committee of the American Society for Reproductive Medicine, "Financial Compensation of Oocyte Donors," *Fertility and Sterility* 88 (2007): 306; available at www.asrm.org/uploadedFiles/ASRM_Content/News_and_Publications/Ethics_Committee_Reports_and_Statements/financial_incentives.pdf.

29. Levine, "Self-Regulation, Compensation, and the Ethical Recruitment of Oocyte Donors." Not infrequently, people fly across the country to take IQ tests and interview for the job. It's impossible to gather information on average

or usual payments for oocytes. As Bonnie Steinbock puts it, "Donors should not be paid for their eggs, but rather should be compensated for the burdens of egg retrieval" ("Payment for Egg Donation and Surrogacy," *Mount Sinai Journal of Medicine* 71 [2004]: 255). See also Kenneth Baum, "Golden Eggs: Towards the Rational Regulation of Oocyte Donation," *Brigham Young University Law Review,* 2001, no. 1. No bright line separates reimbursement for the product of one's labor and the origin of one's labor; work by definition requires lending one's time, energy, and body in exchange for reimbursement. What difference does it make if that energy is expended on the courtroom floor, in a factory assembly line, or at the clinic? The framing of payment for a body part in opposition to reimbursement for the service maintains a false divide between the pay for one's services (spending time at the clinic, taking the drugs, undergoing surgery) and the actual thing that is being extracted and exchanged: the egg.

30. Ernlé Young, director of the Center for Biomedical Ethics at Stanford; quoted in Joan Hamilton, "What Are the Costs?" *Stanford Magazine,* Nov.–Dec. 2000 (available at http://alumni.stanford.edu/get/page/magazine/article/?article_id=39334).

31. On the other hand, one recent article suggests that because the reproductive industry artificially decreases the price of eggs through such recommendations, the industry should come under the rubric of antitrust laws, and at least one law firm has initiated such litigation. See Kimberly Krawiec, "Sunny Samaritans and Egomaniacs: Price-Fixing in the Gamete Market," *Law and Contemporary Problems,* 72 (2009): 59–90. David Magnus and Mildred K. Cho, "Issues in Oocyte Donation for Stem Cell Research," *Science* 308 (2005): 1747–1748 make the common mistake of assuming that oocyte donors who donate for research rather than reproduction should have different standards of informed consent.

32. Despite over $100,000 in medical bills that she was responsible for, she received only a "dropped cycle" fee of $650. See Hamilton, "What Are the Costs?" For these reasons, woman's health advocate Francine Coeytaux recommended that each woman should have her own doctor whose "only job is to look out for the well-being of the woman" (Testimony on Egg Retrieval . . . Hearing on the Implementation of [California] Proposition 71).

33. "Donor Source" website's FAQs claim that the risks of ovarian hyperstimulation syndrome (OHSS) occur in 1–3 percent of procedures. Although the difference between 1 percent and 3 percent leaves a whopping 300 percent margin of error, it still underestimates the available data by a significant degree, elides the lack of data on this point, and neglects to mention that the syndrome is on a continuum, with the 1–3 percent representing the most extreme, dangerous drug responses.

The American Society for Reproductive Medicine (ASRM) has consistently underrepresented the risks of OHSS for donors. In 2004, for example, before any studies had been done on fertile donors, its published practice guidelines quoted a 1 percent rate of OHSS experienced by women undergoing controlled ovarian hyperstimulation (COH) for IVF (that is, for infertile women, a population on which there is significant research) and speculated that the rate *may actually be lower in oocyte donors.* See Practice Committee of the American Society for Reproductive Medicine, "Repetitive Oocyte Donation," *Fertility and Sterility* 82, suppl. 1 (2004): S158–159.

A subsequent study of the donor population found, rather, that the rate of "complications severe enough to prompt the donor to seek medical attention after retrieval" was *8.5 percent,* and the rate of severe OHSS was *nearly 5 percent* (Kara N. Maxwell, Ina N. Cholst, and Zev Rosenwaks, "The Incidence of Both Serious and Minor Complications in Young Women Undergoing Oocyte Donation," *Fertility and Sterility* 90 [2008]: 2165). These researchers were not surprised that the results opposed the speculation of the ASRM, as "young donors often exhibit a high E_2 response to stimulation and thus are at increased risk for OHSS, compared with the larger pool of women undergoing IVF for infertility." These physicians note the problem of gaining informed consent when the information is not available and what is available is consistently underplayed. See also M.V. Sauer, R.J. Paulson, and R.A. Lobo, "Rare Occurrence of Ovarian Hyperstimulation Syndrome in Oocyte Donors," *International Journal of Gynecology and Obstetrics* 52 (1996): 259–262, who write: "The serious nature of OHSS warrants a judicious approach. This is especially true in young women." See also *Eggsploitation: The Infertility Industry Has a Dirty Little Secret,* a film by the Center for Bioethics and Culture, dir. Jennifer Lahl (Lines that Divide, 2009).

34. Robert Edwards, one of the scientists who developed the procedure, first with mice and then with Ms. Brown, was awarded the 2010 Nobel Prize in Medicine for his work on IVF.

35. "GnRH analogs are not like any other medication currently available for treatment of disease. As we continue to learn more about these analogs' mechanisms of action, it is increasingly apparent that they do not just affect the gonadal [sex] hormones, but are powerful modulators of autonomic neural function" (J.R. Mathias and M.H. Clench, "Placebo Controlled Study Randomizing Leuprolide Acetate," *Digestive Diseases and Sciences* 40 [1995]: 1405).

36. Judy Norsigian, a women's health advocate, writes that according to the Food and Drug Administration (FDA) Lupron has caused "asthenia gravis hypophyseogenea (severe weakness due to loss of pituitary function), amnesia, hypertension, rapid heart rate, muscular pain, bone pain, abdominal pain. . . . Although the FDA approved the drug for several specific uses, such as the treatment of endometriosis and fibroid-associated anemia, it has not approved Lupron for use in multiple egg extraction procedures—something that is not well understood by many women who undergo these procedures" ("Egg Donation Dangers," Council for Responsible Genetics, available at www.councilforresponsiblegenetics.org). The package inserts for Lupron discuss the testing of the drug on men regarding testosterone levels, but mention no testing on women. At the time that Lupron switched to being widely used, Andrew Friedman, the lead Lupron investigator, received numerous grants from Takeda Abbotts Pharmaceuticals and was found guilty of falsifying 80 percent of the data in Lupron studies, data that have been subsequently cited as credible (*Cloning: A Risk to Women?,* Proceedings of a Senate hearing: "Findings of Scientific Misconduct," *Federal Register* 61 [1996]: 19295–19296). During the 1990s, the NIH and OSHA placed Lupron on its list of hazardous drugs as a

known teratogen (an agent that increases the risk of abnormal fetal development). See T.H. Shepard, ed., *Catalogue of Teratogenic Agents,* 7th ed. (Baltimore: Johns Hopkins University Press, 1992), 233. Lupron was originally researched and indicated for the palliative care of prostate cancer (a disease that affects older men); when tested in rat studies, all rats at all doses developed pituitary adenomas (tumors) (Testimony of Lynne Millican before the Subcommittee of Science, Technology, and Space, Committee on Commerce, Science, and Transportation, U.S. Senate, March 27, 2003).

37. John Peterson Myers and Fred S. vom Saal, "Time to Update Environmental Regulations: Should Public Health Standards for Endocrine-Disrupting Compounds Be Based upon Sixteenth-Century Dogma or Modern Endocrinology?" *San Francisco Medicine* 81 (2008): 30–31. The cancer drug tamoxifen, aimed at blocking estrogen receptors to defer or prevent a cancer recurrence, has a similar effect, since it can sometimes activate tumor growth.

38. For a full explanation of the way different strains of mice have been bred to have different levels of susceptibility to hormones, and thus to derail attempts to measure the effects of hormones, see Langston, *Toxic Bodies.*

39. George Thomas Beatson, "On Treatment of Inoperable Cases of Carcinoma of the Mamma: Suggestions for a New Method of Treatment, with Illustrative Cases," paper presented to the Edinburgh Medico-Chirurgical Society, May 20, 1896; published in the *Lancet* 2 (1896): 104–107.

40. See also C.A. Bandera, "Advances in the Understanding of Risk Factors for Ovarian Cancer," *Journal of Reproductive Medicine* 50 (2005): 399–406; and J. Russo, R. Moral, G.A. Balogh et al., "The Protective Role of Pregnancy in Breast Cancer," *Breast Cancer Research* 7 (2005): 131–142.

41. Rowan T. Chlebowski et al., "Estrogen Plus Progestin and Breast Cancer Incidence and Mortality in Postmenopausal Women," *JAMA* 304 (2010): 1684–1692. Collaborative Group on Hormone Factors in Breast Cancer, "Breast Cancer and Hormonal Contraceptives: Collaborative Reanalysis of Individual Data on 53,297 Women with Breast Cancer and 100,239 Women without Breast Cancer for 54 Epidemiological Studies," *Lancet* 347 (1996): 1713–1727. One radiologist explained, based on years of reading mammograms, that the breast tissue of postmenopausal women who take hormones reacquires the density of younger women's breasts because of the hormone receptors in the tissue; interview with Dr. Fabienne Corlobe, March 10, 2012.

42. Brian L. Sprague et al., "The Contribution of Postmenopausal Hormone Use Cessation to the Declining Incidence of Breast Cancer," *Cancer Causes and Control* 22 (2011): 125–134.

43. See "Prempro Settlement Reached in Lawsuit over HRT Breast Cancer," Aug. 31, 2010, www.aboutlawsuits.com/prempro-settlement-reached-lawsuit-breast-cancer-12483 (accessed March 15, 2011); and Elizabeth Watkins, *The Estrogen Elixir: A History of Hormone Replacement Therapy in America* (Baltimore: Johns Hopkins University Press, 2007). See also Elizabeth Watkins, "'Educate Yourself': Consumer Information about Menopause and Hormone Replacement Therapy," in *Medicating Modern America: Prescription Drugs in History,* ed. Andrea Tone and Elizabeth Siegel Watkins (New York: New York University Press, 2007), 63–96.

44. Susan Bell, *DES Daughters, Embodied Knowledge, and the Transformation of Women's Health Politics in the Late Twentieth Century* (Philadelphia: Temple University Press, 2009).

45. *Sindell v. Abbott Laboratories,* 26 Cal. 3d 588, 163 Cal. Rptr. 132, 607 P. 2d 924 (1980). This decision, written by California Supreme Court justice Richard M. Mosk, is important in the history of product liability law. The court decided to have the producers of DES pay the damage award based on market share, since the defendant could not prove which manufacturer produced the drug she took. The FDA authorized the use of DES in 1947 as a miscarriage preventative on an experimental basis. Manufacturers did not test the drug for efficacy and safety, and the drug was removed from the market for miscarriage prevention in 1971.

46. Siddhartha Mukherjee, *The Emperor of All Maladies: A Biography of Cancer* (New York: Scribner, 2010), 456.

47. Despite the relative public silence, a robust academic debate exists around the issue. See, for example, Charis M. Thompson, "Fertile Ground: Feminists Theorize Infertility," in *Infertility Around the Globe,* ed. Marcia Claire Inhorn and Frank Van Balen (Berkeley: University of California Press, 2002), 52–78.

48. Attorney Dena S. Davis writes, "The continued hostility toward abortion, . . . coupled with the absence of attacks on IVF, can best be described as a relative indifference to the moral status of the embryo, but rather a great deal of hostility toward economic equality of women, sexual activity outside of marriage, and marriages that are not organized along traditional gender lines" ("The Puzzle of IVF," *Houston Journal of Health Law and Policy* 6 [2006]: 275).

49. Sharon R. Kaufman, Ann J. Russ, and Janet K. Shim, "Aged Bodies and Kinship Matters: The Ethical Field of Kidney Transplant," *American Ethnologist* 33 (2006): 81–89.

50. "Collecting immature oocytes from unstimulated ovaries for the purpose of oocyte donation is a simple procedure that totally avoids ovarian stimulation. With appropriate selection of women . . . the pregnancy rates of the recipients are comparable with those achieved through conventional IVF oocyte donor cycles" (Hananel Holzer et al., "In Vitro Maturation of Oocytes Collected from Unstimulated Ovaries for Oocyte Donation," *Fertility and Sterility* 88 [2007]: 62–67). See also R.C. Edwards, "IVF, IVM, Natural Cycle IVF, Minimal Stimulation IVF—Time for a Rethink," *Reproductive Medicine Online* 15 (2007): 106–219.

51. Because about 80 percent of infertility is age-related, David Fleming, director of the Center for Health Ethics at the University of Missouri, controversially asked: "With all due respect—is [IVF] a question of need or a question of want?" (quoted in Iva Skoch, "Should IVF Be Affordable for All?" *Newsweek,* July 21, 2010; available at www.thedailybeast.com/newsweek/2010/07/20/should-ivf-be-affordable-for-all.html [accessed March 15, 2011]).

52. Kristi Lew, *Egg Donation: The Reasons and the Risks* (New York: Rosen Publishing, 2010). In this book written for nine- to twelve-year-olds, Lew does not mention the lack of long-term studies on donation, other than to say that "most doctors" believe the procedure to be safe.

53. According to economist Nattavudh Powdthavee, "Using data sets from Europe and America, numerous scholars have found some evidence that, on aggregate, parents often report statistically significantly lower levels of happiness . . . , life satisfaction . . . , marital satisfaction . . . and mental well-being . . . compared with non-parents" ("Think Having Children Will Make You Happy?" *Psychologist* 22 [2009]: 308–310; available at www.thepsychologist.org.uk/archive/archive_home.cfm?volumeID=22&editionID=174&ArticleID=1493). It may be that parents most likely to have used IVF—wealthier, older people—are happier than the average family. However, health benefits are usually not calculated based on demographics.

54. Linda Giudice, Eileen Santa, and Robert Pool, eds., *Assessing the Medical Risks of Human Oocyte Donation for Stem Cell Research: Workshop Report* (Washington, D.C.: National Academic Press, 2007), 2.

55. See W. Kramer, J. Schneider, and N. Schultz, "U.S. Oocyte Donors: A Retrospective Study of Medical and Psychosocial Issues," *Human Reproduction* 24 (2009): 3144–3149; I. Pappo, L. Lerner-Geva, A. Halevy et al., "The Possible Association between IVF and Breast Cancer Incidence," *Annals of Surgical Oncology* 15 (2008): 1048–1055; K. Ahuja and E. G. Simons, "Cancer of the Colon in an Egg Donor: Policy Repercussions for Donor Recruitment," *Human Reproduction* 13 (1998): 227–231; J. Dor, L. Lerner-Geva, J. Rabinovici et al., "Cancer Incidence in a Cohort of Infertile Women Treated with In Vitro Fertilization," *52nd Annual Meeting of the American Society for Reproductive Medicine,* 1996, suppl., 147; F. Shenfield, "Cancer Risk and Fertility Treatments: A Question of Informed Consent," *Journal of Fertility Counseling,* 1996, 15–16; and B. J. Mosgaard, O. Lidegaard, S.K. Kjaer et al., "Ovarian Stimulation and Borderline Ovarian Tumours: A Case-Control Study," *Fertility and Sterility* 70 (1998): 1049–1055.

56. One of the early drugs has still not been studied: "Clomid is a drug of considerable pharmacologic potency. . . . Clomid is indicated only in patients with demonstrated ovulatory dysfunction. . . . Long-term toxicity studies in animals have not been performed to evaluate the carcinogenic or mutagenic potential of clomiphene citrate" (www.drugs.com/pro/clomid.html; accessed March 12, 2012). Since Clomid, newer fertility drugs have become standard, "but again, this standard has developed without any epidemiologically sound, long-term safety data. It is noteworthy that while Lupron has become 'standard' within superovulation regimes, it is administered at various doses for various times, varying even within the various patients, and has varying effects" (Testimony of Lynne Millican before the Subcommittee of Science, Technology, and Space, Committee on Commerce, Science, and Transportation, U.S. Senate, March 27, 2003).

57. R. Calderon-Margalit et al., "Cancer Risk after Exposure to Treatments for Ovulation Induction," *American Journal of Epidemiology* 169 (2009): 365–375.

58. Mary Anne Rossing, Janet R. Daling, Noel S. Weisset et al., "Ovarian Tumors in a Cohort of Infertile Women," *New England Journal of Medicine* 331 (1994): 771–776.

59. I. Pappo et al., "Possible Association between IVF and Breast Cancer Incidence."

60. F.E. van Leeuwen, H. Klip, T.M. Mooij et al., "Risk of Borderline and Invasive Ovarian Tumours after Ovarian Stimulation for In Vitro Fertilization in a Large Dutch Cohort," *Human Reproduction* online, Oct. 26, 2011, available at http://humrep.oxfordjournals.org/content/early/2011/10/19/humrep.der322.full.

61. "Correspondence: Risk of Ovarian Cancer after Treatment for Infertility," *New England Journal of Medicine* 332 (1995): 1300–1302.

62. "Overall, fertility-drug treatment was reported by 20 of 622 case patients with invasive ovarian cancer (3.2 percent), as compared with 11 of 1101 controls (1.0 percent)" (Daniel W. Cramer, Patricia Hartge, Philip C. Nasca, and Alice S. Whittemore, Letter to the editor, ibid.).

63. K.K. Ahuja and E.G. Simons, "Cancer of the Colon in an Egg Donor: Policy Repercussions for Donor Recruitment," *Human Reproduction* 13 (1998): 227–231.

64. See Schneider, "It's Time for an Egg Donor Registry and Long-Term Follow-Up."

65. Ahuja and Simons, "Cancer of the Colon in an Egg Donor," 228. Very rarely do studies on IVF children make note of the fertility drugs taken by their genetic and birth parents, and never do they refer to the co-cultures in which the embryos where developed. Some scientists question whether the petri dish medium affects the developing embryos, since IVF babies have been found to have significantly lower methylation rates (the process that switches genes on and off) in utero, and higher rates of cancers, ADHD, and other disabilities, including two severe syndromes, Beckwith-Wiedemann and Angelman. See the NOVA documentary *Ghost in Your Genes?*, www.pbs.org/wgbh/nova/genes.

University of Toronto geneticist Dr. Rosanna Weksberg found that rates of disabling genetic syndromes increase by over 1,000 percent for IVF babies, and yet she has been unable to find an IVF clinic willing to work with her to longitudinally collect data. For this reason, the increasing number of warnings about the health effects of IVF remain at the level of "association" rather than causal proof. See Tom Blackwell, "In-Vitro Fertilization Linked to Rare Genetic Disorders," *National Post,* Sept. 25, 2011.

There is some debate as to what damage the insertion of the needle does to the embryo, as well as about the lack of selection of the sperm. According to Marc Kirschner et al. ("Molecular Vitalism," *Cell* 100 [2000]: 86), "Part of the old misunderstanding of [cell] regulation, as even implied by the name, was the assumption that embryonic cells have a single path of development from a very early stage, and that regulation after surgery entails undoing that path and initiating another. Competence belies all this. The cells have a broad range of possibilities, all equally valid."

66. L. Brinton, "Long-Term Effects of Ovulation-Stimulating Drugs on Cancer Risk," *Reproductive BioMedicine Online* 15 (2007): 42; emphasis mine. Brinton finds that studies have short follow-up times (under ten years) and don't include newer drugs that have known links to cancer, nor do they consider how fertility drugs might affect women with genetic dispositions to cancer or who have used other hormones such as oral contraceptives. Going through the studies on fertility drugs and ovarian, breast, and endometrial cancers, she concludes

that it will be important to "fully resolve effects of exposures such as gonadotropins, used more recently with IVF" (38). She also notes the chemical similarity of tamoxifen, known to increase the risk of endometrial cancer, to clomiphene.

67. L. Brinton, conversation with author, March 11, 2011.

CHAPTER 7

1. One key factor among men is fear of intimacy, the other is "faecal/rectal embarrassment"; see Nathan S. Consedine, Inga Ladwig, Maike K. Reddig, and Elizabeth A. Broadbent, "The Many Faeces *[sic]* of Colorectal Cancer Screening Embarrassment: Preliminary Psychometric Development and Links to Screening Outcome," *British Journal of Health Psychology* 16 (2001): 559–579.

2. William Goodson III and Dan H. Moore II, "The Missing Clinical Breast Exam," poster session, San Antonio Breast Cancer Symposium, 2007; see also William Goodson III, Dan H. Moore II, and Ferris M. Hall, "Clinical Breast Examination for Detecting Cancer," *JAMA* 283 (2000): 1685–1691. According to Goodson and Moore, "When clinicians are encouraged to do at least a minimal 2-minute CBE [clinical breast exam], both men and women clinicians state, 'If I spend that much time doing a breast exam, the woman is going to wonder what I am up to.'"

3. [No author], "National Society to Fight Cancer," *New York Times,* Nov. 30, 1913.

4. See Hirshberg Foundation for Pancreatic Cancer Research, "Prognosis of Pancreatic Cancer," www.pancreatic.org/site/c.htJYJ8MPIwE/b.891917/k.5123/Prognosis_of_Pancreatic_Cancer.htm (accessed Feb. 28, 2012). Even still, nonmetastasized pancreatic cancer has a survival rate of only 20–25 percent, less than several other cancers over comparable time periods.

5. Opposition to the early-detection debate has been around since at least 1951, when Dr. I. MacDonald found that "biological type—the propensity of spread and development of remote metastasis—plays the predominant role in determining outcome" (quoted in Barron Lerner, "Fighting the War on Breast Cancer: Debates over Early Detection, 1945 to the Present," *Annals of Internal Medicine* 129 [1998]: 75). Even so, MacDonald argued that early detection of many cancers would improve survival.

6. The *New York Times* reported in 1921 that "cancer directs its terrific onslaught largely against mothers and fathers of families. . . . The immediate total of misery and suffering may well be considered greater [than the death of a child] when cancer removes, often with terrible agony, the parent who is the main source of support for the family" ("Prompt Action Will Cure Cancer, Lives Lost by Patients' Delay and Faulty Diagnosis, Declares Dr. Blake," *New York Times,* Nov. 3, 1921).

7. In 1948, Papanicolaou claimed that "the possibility of detecting early asymptomatic or hidden carcinomas by the smear technique has been convincingly proved . . . by a rather impressive number of reports" (quoted in Kirsten Gardner, *Early Detection: Women, Cancer, and Awareness Campaigns in the Twentieth-Century United States* [Chapel Hill: University of North Carolina Press, 2006], 123).

8. Devra Davis, *The Secret History of the War on Cancer* (New York: Basic Books, 2007), 132.

9. In 2007, 4,021 women died of cervical cancer in the United States (U.S. Cancer Statistics Working Group, *United States Cancer Statistics: 1999–2007 Incidence and Mortality Web-based Report* [Atlanta: Department of Health and Human Services, Centers for Disease Control and Prevention and National Cancer Institute, 2010]; available at http://apps.nccd.cdc.gov/uscs/). In 2005, the National Cancer Institute conducted a study of regions within the United States where cervical cancer incidence rates are high and found that cervical cancer rates reflected a larger problem of unequal access to healthcare. The resulting report, *Excess Cervical Cancer Mortality: A Marker for Low Access to Health Care in Poor Communities—An Analysis* (http://crchd.cancer.gov/attachments/excess-cervcanmort.pdf), supports reaching these medically underserved groups through trained, culturally sensitive care providers; increasing the number of female health providers, particularly those of the same race or ethnicity as their clients; and removing cultural and economic barriers to screening for cervical and other cancers.

10. Gardner, *Early Detection*, 93–123.

11. Monica J. Casper and Adele E. Clarke, "Making the Pap Smear into the 'Right Tool' for the Job: Cervical Cancer Screening in the USA, circa 1940–95," *Social Studies of Science* 28 (1998): 255–290.

12. Davis, *Secret History of the War on Cancer*, 123. For a reading of this history in relation to the recent Gardasil vaccination campaign targeting young women and their parents, see my essay "Survival Odds: Mortality in Corporate Time," *Current Anthropology* 52, no. S3 (2011): S45–S55 (available at www.jstor.org/stable/full/10.1086/656795).

13. I'm less interested here in screening itself—that is, whether it works as a means for early detection and mortality reduction—than in how the debates about it shift and travel among types of media and within expert and policy networks, on what bases they travel (the popularity or institution of the principal investgator? the use of certain kinds of evidence? the writing style?), and how these localized shifts in knowledge link with broader shifts in knowledge production.

14. According to political scientist Timothy Mitchell, "Between the 1930s and 1950s, economists, sociologists, national statistical agencies, international and corporate organizations, and government programs formulated the concept of the economy, meaning the totality of monetary exchanges within a defined space. . . . It occurred as the reorganization and tranformation of . . . processes, into an object that had not previously existed" (*The Rule of Experts: Egypt, Technopolitics, Modernity* [Berkeley: University of California Press, 2002], 4–5). Mitchell examines how new forms of calculability made the economy, as an object of study, possible. Similarly, I'm arguing, oncologists make cancer as we know it possible as an object of study, through methods of calculation.

15. See, e.g., Robert Aronowitz, *Unnatural History: Breast Cancer and American Society* (New York: Cambridge University Press, 2007); Baron Lerner, *The Breast Cancer Wars: Hope, Fear, and the Pursuit of a Cure in Twentieth-Century America* (New York: Oxford University Press, 2003); and

Peter C. Gotzsche, *Mammography Screening: Truth, Lies, and Controversy* (New York: Radcliffe Publishing, 2012).

16. See, e.g., "The Cancer Tests You Need—and Those You Don't," *Consumer Reports,* March 2013, available at www.consumerreports.org/cro/magazine/2013/03/the-cancer-tests-you-need-and-those-you-don-t/index.htm.

17. L. Esserman, Y. Shieh, and I. Thompson, "Rethinking Screening for Breast Cancer and Prostate Cancer," *JAMA* 302 (2009): 1685–1692. Other outspoken critics of screening state that "the proportion of screen-detected men who would not likely benefit from early diagnosis and treatment is much greater than for women with early breast cancer," a point not made by Esserman et al. See also Karsten Juhl Jørgensen and Peter C. Gøtzsche, "Overdiagnosis in Publicly Organised Mammography Screening Programmes: Systematic Review of Incidence Trends," *British Medical Journal* 339 (2009), available at www.bmj.com/content/339/bmj.b2587.

18. For more on the widespread reporting of the Esserman et al. paper, see, e.g., science journalist Gina Kolata's *New York Times* article "Cancer Group Has Concerns on Screenings" (Oct. 21, 2009), where she said that Esserman et al.'s study "finds that widespread adoption of regular breast and prostate cancer screening has . . . not substantially reduced the incidence of advanced and late-stage cancers" and, indeed, that screening often unearths "cancers that do not need to be found because they would never spread and kill or even be noticed if left alone" ("Cancer Society, in Shift, Has Concerns on Screenings," *New York Times,* Oct. 20, 2009). See also idem, "Cancers Vanish without Treatment, but How?" *New York Times,* Oct. 26, 2009. Implying both that Esserman et al. completed original research (which Esserman explained during a radio interview was not true; see KQED Forum—Michael Krasny interview with Laura Esserman, "Early Cancer Screening," Oct. 22, 2009, available at www.kqed.org/a/forum/R910220900) and that screening has no value, Kolata offers a misleading summary of the study. Neither Esserman nor Kolata clearly acknowledges that medical science cannot yet tell which cancers will spread and which will not, and neither article raises, let alone discusses, other ways of accounting for the continued existence of later-stage cancers.

19. The debate on the value of screening as raised by Esserman et al. reflects a recent manifestation of an older debate. Ilana Löwy cites a doctor in the 1950s who claimed that "if a cancer of the breast is growing slowly, a delay in its detection will not make much of a difference in terms of survival, and if it grows fast, it had already spread at the moment of detection" (*Preventive Strikes: Women, Precancer, and Prophylactic Surgery* [Baltimore: Johns Hopkins University Press, 2010], 144). Although there were big differences in treatment and virtually no screening then, such an attitude reflects a similar attempt to balance good for the population against good for individuals in that population.

20. Esserman et al., "Rethinking Screening," 1687.

21. Ibid., 1687. See also "SEER Stat Fact Sheets: Colon and Rectum," http://seer.cancer.gov/statfacts/html/colorect.html#incidence-mortality.

22. Esserman et al., "Rethinking Screening," 1685.

23. Ibid.

24. Isabelle Baszanger, "One More Chemo or One Too Many? Defining the Limits of Treatment and Innovation in Medical Oncology," *Social Sciences and Medicine* 75 (2012): 864–872.

25. Nigel Paneth, Letter to the editor, *JAMA* 303 (2010): 1032.

26. American Cancer Society, "Cancer Facts and Figures 2011," 2; available at www.cancer.org/acs/groups/content/@epidemiologysurveilance/documents/document/acspc-029771.pdf.

27. "The SEER Program is NCI's authoritative source for information about cancer incidence and survival. Over several decades, SEER has worked diligently to better represent racial, ethnic, and socioeconomic diversity and currently covers 23 percent of African Americans, 40 percent of Hispanics, 42 percent of American Indians and Alaska Natives, 53 percent of Asian Americans, and 70 percent of Pacific Islanders living in the United States." See www.cancer.gov/cancertopics/factsheet/disparities/cancer-health-disparities.

28. Langston, *Toxic Bodies: Hormone Disruptors and the Legacy of DES* (New Haven, Conn.: Yale University Press: 2011), 65–72.

29. Esserman et al., "Rethinking Screening," 1685.

30. Milayna Subar, Scott Lust, and Wenlong Lin, "Mammography Compliance Study," paper presented at the 33rd Annual San Antonio Breast Cancer Symposium, Dec. 9, 2010; available at www.medcoresearchinstitute.com/research-archive/post/mammography-compliance-study (accessed Apr. 27, 2011). Breaking the population down by those who are screened and those who are not, one finds that "among women aged 40 to 64 years, 73 percent of those with health insurance in 2005 had a mammogram within the past 2 years, compared with 38 percent of women who were uninsured at the time of survey interview" (U.S. Department of Health and Human Services, Office of Women's Health, *Healthy People 2010—Women's and Men's Health: A Comparison of Select Indicators* [Washington, D.C.: Government Printing Office, 2009]). See also "NBC Investigates Mammography Violations," April 24, 2008, www.nbc11.com/featurelinks/15981 8/detail.html?taf=bay (accessed Apr. 24, 2008), which lists "dozens of mammogram facilities in the Bay Area that have failed federal inspections year after year." The Mammogram Quality Standards Act became law in 1992.

31. For example, a well-done clinical breast exam can detect at least 50 percent of asymptomatic cancers. It's not clear in mammogram screening trials, more often than not, how these manual exams relate to data on mammography. See Mary B. Barton, Russell Harris, and Suzanne W. Fletcher, "Does This Patient Have Breast Cancer? The Screening Clinical Breast Examination: Should It Be Done? How?" *JAMA* 282 (1999): 1270–1280.

32. Y.N. Turner and I. Hadas-Halpern, "The Effects of Including a Patient's Photograph to the Patient's Radiographic Examination," paper presented to the Radiological Society of North America, Chicago, 2008.

33. On disease categorization and race, see Donna Armstrong, Steven Wind, and Herman Tyroler, "United States Mortality from Ill-Defined Causes, 1968–1988: Potential Effects on Heart Disease Mortality Trends," *International Journal of Epidemiology* 24 (1995), which finds that the underestimation of racial disparities in coronary heart disease may have affected the data used to "evaluate the efficacy of public health interventions."

34. O.S. Miettinen, "Screening for Cancer: Thinking before Rethinking," *European Journal of Epidemiology* 25 (2010): 368.

35. Retrospective comparisons are further complicated by the fact that cancers detected by screening generate diagnoses, on average, at younger ages. Epidemiologist O. Miettinen notes that with the introduction of screening, "age-specific rates of the cancer's detection increase; and they must be expected to remain increased so long as the screening continues" ("Screening for Cancer," 367). Once mapped onto age-adjusted graphs, this effect will be easy to interpret as higher rates of incidence rather than incidence at a younger age. This epidemiological insight corresponds with the breast cancer incidence data that show an increase of localized cancers in the first five years of screening and then a flattening out. Unfortunately, Esserman et al. did not compare the incidence population data to mortality data, which would have helped the reader to understand how they interpreted this issue.

36. Colin White, "Research on Smoking and Lung Cancer: A Landmark in the History of Chronic Disease Epidemiology," *Yale Journal of Biology and Medicine* 63 (1990): 29–46.

37. Marvin A. Kastenbaum, the head of the Stanford statistics department, took this latter view as late as 1987, writing on behalf of the industry-funded Tobacco Institute in "Diagnostic Errors and Their Impact on Disease Trends," *Theory and Application of Statistics,* 1987, 303–329. By this time, the causal relationship was well accepted, and such efforts were conscious attempts to muddy the data. (Thanks to Robert Proctor for passing this document along.)

38. Esserman et al., "Rethinking Screening," 1688.

39. "As it is not possible to distinguish between lethal and harmless cancers, all detected cancers are treated. Overdiagnosis and overtreatment are therefore inevitable" (Jørgensen and Gøtzsche, "Overdiagnosis in Publicly Organised Mammography Screening Programmes," 1). See also Steven Woloshin and Lisa Schwartz, "The Benefits and Harms of Mammography Screening: Understanding the Trade-Offs," *JAMA* 303 (2010): 164–165.

40. Several excellent studies of this experiment have been written; one of the best is Susan M. Reverby, *Examining Tuskegee: The Infamous Syphilis Study and Its Legacy* (Chapel Hill: University of North Carolina Press, 2009).

41. Esserman et al., "Rethinking Screening," 1690.

42. Historically, flowcharts stem from the field of scientific management, which aimed to regulate and improve workflow by charting increasingly efficient routes for work process. Without going into detail about this history, it's worth noting that the visual grammar developed in the history of flowcharts focuses attention on specific interactions through the placement of nodes, while naturalizing other elements of the flow. One notes similar elisions and focal points in this flowchart.

43. See, e.g., Dorothy Nelkin, "The Social Dynamics of Genetic Testing: The Case of Fragile-X," *Medical Anthropology Quarterly,* n.s., 10 (1996): 537–550, for an analysis of "the economic, entrepreneurial, and policy interests that are driving the development of genetic screening programs and the public support for genetic testing even when there are no effective therapuetic interventions." For a different perspective, see Donghui Li, Farzana L. Walcott, Ping

Chang et al., "Genetic and Environmental Determinants on Tissue Response to In Vitro Carcinogen Exposure and Risk of Breast Cancer," *Cancer Research* 62 (2002): 4566–4570.

44. In addition, a body of data addresses in more detail the difference in outcomes between screen detection and non-screen detected cancers that otherwise seem similar. See, for example, "Patients with screen-detected cancers had better survival than patients with nonscreening related tumors within each stratum of tumor size, with the most pronounced difference in tumors of 10mm or less in diameter" (*Journal of the National Cancer Institute* 103 [2011]).

45. Esserman et al., "Rethinking Screening," 1688.

46. See Sandra M. Gifford, "The Meaning of Lumps: A Case Study of the Ambiguities of Risk," in *Anthropology and Epidemiology: Culture, Illness, and Healing,* ed. Craig R. Janes, Ron Stall, and Sandra M. Gifford (Dordrecht, Neth.: D. Reidel, 1986), 213–246; and Margaret Lock, "Breast Cancer: Reading the Omens," *Anthropology Today* 14 (1998): 7–16, who writes: "In seeking to avoid misfortune we create new ambiguities and uncertainties" (7). The form of the debate reifies the use of population data and the creation of populations at risk. Esserman et al.'s suggestion that chemoprevention be used for those in high-risk categories is extremely problematic. As Jennifer Fosket has shown, the risk factors of these other diseases are often not taken into account when prescribing such chemical preventive measures ("Constructing 'High-Risk Women': The Development and Standardization of a Breast Cancer Risk Assemssment Tool," *Science, Technology, and Human Values* 29 [2004]: 291–313). Fosket analyzes the data, the risk models used in various interpretations of the data, and a direct-to-consumer ad campaign launched by AstraZeneca. She writes that no corresponding "model has emerged to assess the risks, and thus no devices of advertising campaigns have widely disseminated the idea that it is necessary to take a woman's risk of endometrial cancer, stroke, or pulmonary embolism into consideration" (309).

47. Statistics from SEER factsheets, using data from 2004–2008. See also Ahmedin Jemal, Rebecca Siegel, Elizabeth Ward et al., "Cancer Statistics, 2008," *CA: A Cancer Journal for Clinicians* 58 (2008): 71–96. A "new method for projecting incident cancer cases beginning with the 2007 estimates substantially affected the estimates for a number of cancers, particularly luekemia and female breast" (92–93). And see L.W. Pickle, Y. Hao, A. Jemal et al., "A New Method of Estimating United States and State-Level Cancer Incidence Counts for the Current Calendar Year," *CA* 57 (2007): 30–42.

48. American Cancer Society, "Cancer Facts and Figures 2012," www.cancer.org/acs/groups/content/@epidemiologysurveilance/documents/document/acspc-031941.pdf (accessed Feb. 2013). See also D.U. Ekwueme, H.W. Chesson, K.B. Zhang, and A. Balamurugan, "Years of Potential Life Lost and Productivity Costs because of Cancer Mortality and for Specific Cancer Sites Where Human Papillomavirus May Be a Risk Factor for Carcinogenesis—United States," *Cancer* 113, no. 10 suppl. (2008): 2936–2945.

49. R.H. Johnson, F.L. Chien, and A. Bleyer, "Incidence of Breast Cancer with Distant Involvement among Women in the United States, 1976 to 2009," *JAMA* 309 (2013): 800–805; B.L. Fowble, D.J. Schultz, B. Overmoyer et al.,

"The Influence of Young Age on Outcome in Early Stage Breast Cancer," *International Journal of Radiation, Biology, Physics* 30 (1994): 23–33.

50. Esserman et al., "Rethinking Screening," 1686, 1688.

51. Ibid., 1686.

52. Ibid., 1688.

53. Esserman et al. cite meta-analyses of the trial data (that is, studies that collate the data from original trials) which find a 0–20 percent reduction in cancer mortality. On the face of it, this difference between the data (20–30%) and the metadata (0–20%) is large and central to their argument. Yet it inexplicably goes unmentioned and unexplained in the article.

54. Esserman et al., "Rethinking Screening, 1686.

55. Ibid.

56. See, e.g., Xi-Xi Cao, Jing-Da Xu, Xiao-Li Liu et al., "RACK 1: A Superior Independent Predictor for Poor Clinical Outcome in Breast Cancer," *International Journal of Cancer* 127 (2010): 1172–1179.

57. See, e.g., S. Whitman, D. Ansell, J. Orsi, and T. Francois, "The Racial Disparity in Breast Cancer Mortality," *Journal of Community Health*, 2010. By treating the population as a whole, Esserman et al. do not take the opportunity to understand how screening might have a bearing in these so-called interval cancers. A more open-ended question, such as how access to screening affects stage-at-diagnosis and then mortality, may have enabled a more complex insight.

58. Nancy Krieger, "Is Breast Cancer a Disease of Affluence, Poverty, or Both? The Case of African American Women," *American Journal of Public Health* 92 (2002): 611–613. See also Susan A. Hall and Beverly Rockhill, "Race, Poverty, Affluence, and Breast Cancer," *American Journal of Public Health* 92 (2002): 1559.

59. United States Government Accountability Office, "Mammography: Current Nationwide Capacity Is Adequate, but Access Problems May Exist in Certain Locations," Report to Congressional Requesters GAO-06–724, Washington D.C., 2006.

60. J. S. Haas, E. F. Cook, A. L. Puopolo et al., "Differences in the Quality of Care for Women with Abnormal Mammogram or Breast Complaint," *Journal of General Internal Medicine* 15 (2000): 321–328.

61. Tejal K. Gandhi, Allen Kachalia, Eric J. Thomas et al., "Missed and Delayed Diagnoses in the Ambulatory Setting: A Study of Closed Malpractice Claims," *Annals of Internal Medicine* 145 (2006): 489.

62. See chapter 1 for more on cancer in this age group.

63. Interview, June 11, 2008.

64. Email communication, June 2008.

65. Barton et al., "Does This Patient Have Breast Cancer?"

66. Interview, June 11, 2008.

67. Per-Henrik Zahl, Jan Moehlen, and Gilbert Welch, "The Natural History of Invasive Breast Cancers Detected by Screening Mammography," *Archives of Internal Medicine* 168 (2008): 2311–2316.

68. Ibid., 2315.

69. Letter from Mette Kalager, M.D., and Michael Bretthauer, M.D., Ph.D., *Archives of Internal Medicine* 169 (2009): 997.

70. Letters to the editor, *Archives of Internal Medicine* (169) 2009: 996–997. See also S. Hofvind, B. Moller, S. Thoresen, and G. Ursin, "Use of Hormone Therapy and Risk of Breast Cancer Detected at Screening and between Mammographic Screens," *International Journal of Cancer* 118 (2006): 3112–3117.

71. See Editor's Correspondence, *JAMA Internal Medicine* 169, no. 10 (2009). See also Peter Ravdin et al., "The Decrease in Breast-Cancer Incidence in 2003 in the United States," *New England Journal of Medicine* 356 (2007): 1670–1673.

72. Comments and opinions, *Archives of Internal Medicine* (169) 2009: 996–997.

73. Interview and email communication with Esserman's coauthor Yiwey Shieh, June 1, 2011.

74. Personal correspondence, 2011. In her *New York Times* article, Gina Kolata cites Kramer as saying that the idea that some cancers will spontaneously regress is "so counterintuitive that it raises debate every time it comes up and every time it has been observed." ("Cancer Society, in Shift, Has Concerns").

75. Esserman et al., "Rethinking Screening," 1688. These numbers and their seeming exactitude travel widely (though with some variation). For example, the *UC Berkeley Wellness Letter* advises women to have mamograms once every two years after the age of 50 because, "according to the Task Force, to save one life in the 50-to-59 age group, 1,339 women must be screened for 10 years (337 women in the 60-to-69 group)" ("Mammograms: Still a Good Idea?" Feb. 2010, http://wellnessletter.com/html/wl/2008/wlFeatured0210.html; accessed June 15, 2011).

Esserman et al.'s sudden burst of precision (838 women as opposed to "many" biopsies) necessarily relies on knowledge of how many deaths have been prevented by screening. Yet the authors claim earlier in the article that mortality might have been reduced by anywhere from 0 to 30 percent, a range that is not precise enough to produce the number 838. Their cost-benefit calculation also premises that 22 percent of cancers will spontaneously regress. This accounting is by no means straightforward, even if one accepts their numbers. Elsewhere, H. Gilbert Welch and Peter C. Albertsen discuss prostate cancer statistics, estimating "that approximately 56,500 prostate cancer deaths had been averted and that approximately 23 men had to be diagnosed and approximately 18 treated for each man experiencing the presumed benefit" (www.medscape.com/viewarticle/708206; accessed March 9, 2011).

76. Esserman et al., "Rethinking Screening," 1688. According to Adjuvant! Online—a model for risk assessment into which one can enter variables including age, overall health, receptor status, grade, and tumor size—of 100 forty-year-olds diagnosed with an ER-positive, 2-cm, grade-II tumor, 90.5 will be alive in ten years with no therapy, 92.9 will be alive with hormonal therapy, 92.3 will be alive with chemotherapy, and with combined therapy, 94 will be alive. If a tumor with the same characteristics has grown to 5 cm, only 70.7 of the women will be alive after ten years (84 with combination treatment). The tricky thing, though, with such statistics and treatments is that it is impossible to tell which individuals will gain from the therapies, and so if all one hundred are given the treatments,

90.5 will have been "overtreated" in the first instance, and 70.7 in the second instance (if we accept the ten-year mark as a "cure"). (Adjuvant! Online charts are available at www.adjuvantonline.com. Anyone can register and insert variables for a variety of cancers, and the site will chart survival prognoses with and without treatment. The site also provides background on how its estimates are derived.)

77. Because Esserman et al.'s 22 percent spontaneous remission rate lacks credible evidence, I use here instead the standard reading of the statistics, which posits a 25 percent mortality rate of those treated for breast cancer (on average, across all stages). From Esserman et al.'s perspective, at least two of these people will have been overtreated.

78. Seth Borenstein writes, "The value of a 'statistical life' is $6.9 million in today's dollars, the EPA reckoned in May—a drop of nearly $1 million from just five years ago." Bureaucrats base these calculations not on earnings, family dependants, or social contribution, but on what people will pay to avoid certain risks, information that is garnered from from payroll statistics and opinion polls. See Borenstein, "AP Impact: An American Life Worth Less Today," July 10, 2008, available at http://usatoday30.usatoday/com/news/topstories/2008-07-10-796349025_x.htm. Typically, with breast cancer, the "precancerous" DCIS or LCIS (ductal or lobular carcinoma in situ) appears as a few blobs on a mammogram, signaling calcifications that have not yet become palpable masses or "infiltrated" into surrounding tissues. (The Latin *in situ* means "in its original place," "in its appropriate place," or simply "in its place.")

79. Aronowitz, *Unnatural History,* 261. In situ diagnoses account for 50,000 breast cancer occurrences in the United States each year (nearly 25 percent of total incidence). How they are categorized—as cancer incidence or not—has a potent impact on statistics, given that these "cancers" are largely responsible for the increased rate of breast cancer since the introduction of mammographic screening. Nevertheless, in Esserman et al.'s article, it is usually unclear whether they include DCIS/LCIS in the argument, since on the one hand they say "we shouldn't call these cancer" and on the other they argue that increased cancer rates are due solely to screening, which by definition includes the DCIS/LCIS. Although in one instance they claim that they are *not* talking about DCIS, later they cite the dangers of biopsying "a few calcifications," which must refer to in situ cancers. Never do they state outright that DCIS is being overtreated. In 1974, 4 percent of breast cancers were found at DCIS or stage I; today that figure is 30 percent. Correspondingly, death rates have dropped from 70 percent to 30 percent (these statistics from the SEER database). At the same time, incidence rates have increased dramatically, with a lifetime chance of being diagnosed with breast cancer rising from one in 20 to one in 7.5, while overall mortality has remained a more or less constant 40,000 annually.

80. Löwy, *Preventive Strikes,* 233.

81. Rose Kushner describes her effort to be diagnosed for a recurrence as follows: the lump seemed "slowly to grow as the months went by. While I wanted to get it removed the surgeon was sure it was getting larger only in my imagination and would go away if only I would keep my wandering fingers off

it" ("Is Aggressive Adjuvant Chemotherapy the Halsted Radical of the '80s?," *CA: A Cancer Journal for Clinicians* 34 [1984]: 347).

82. In 1992, the head of the FDA, David Kessler, made a similar distinction when he allowed the use of silicone breast implants for reconstruction following cancer surgery but not for cosmetic uses during a moratorium in which the industry was charged with gathering evidence to prove the safety of the device.

83. Ann Kim, "Dr. Me: Cancer Patients Want a Say, But Do We Have to Be the Doctor, Too?," www.zocalopublicsquare.org/2012/05/16/dr-me/ideas/nexus.

84. Florence Williams, *Breasts: A Natural and Unnatural History* (New York: W.W. Norton, 2012), 75–80.

85. For men, a whole different array of serious side-effects can accompany treatment. About 25 percent of men who have a prostate biopsy due to an elevated PSA level actually have prostate cancer, treatment for which includes surgery and radiation with the chance of significant long-term side-effects, including erectile dysfunctional and urinary incontinence. Again, a completely different array of details arises with the two types of cancer. M.J. Barry, "Clinical Practice. Prostate-Specific-Antigen Testing for Early Diagnosis of Prostate Cancer," *New England Journal of Medicine* 34 (2001): 1373–1377. G.L. Andriole, E.D. Crawford, R.L. Grubb et al., "Prostate Cancer Screening in the Randomized Prostate, Lung, Colorectal, and Ovarian Cancer Screening Trial: Mortality Results after 13 Years of Follow-up," *Journal of the National Cancer Institute* 104 (2012): 125–132; F.H. Schröder, J. Hugosson, M.J. Roobol et al., Prostate-Cancer Mortality at 11 Years of Follow-up," *New England Journal of Medicine* 366 (2012): 981–990.

86. Gardiner Harris, "Cigarette Company Paid for Lung Cancer Study," *New York Times*, March 26, 2008; available at www.nytimes.com/2008/03/26/health/research/26lung.html.

87. See, e.g., Robert Proctor, *Golden Holocaust: Origins of the Cigarette Catastrophe and the Case for Abolition* (Berkeley: University of California Press, 2012).

88. Löwy, *Preventive Strikes*, 46.

CHAPTER 8

1. For a brief history of the Bikini Atoll—including the nuclear tests and the fate of its inhabitants—see http://whc.unesco.org/en/list/1339.

2. Images of destroyed buildings in Hiroshima and Nagasaki were made available just after the war, but firsthand accounts, along with anything portraying the effects of the bomb on the human body, were strictly censored. See *White Light, Black Rain: The Destruction of Hiroshima and Nagasaki*, dir. Steve Okazaki (2006). In her analysis of America's response to Hiroshima directly after the bomb, historian Susan Lindee writes: "The bomb's peculiar form of terror, ionizing radiation, was known to cause biological changes in both humans and experimental organisms" (*Suffering Made Real: American Science and the Survivors at Hiroshima* [Chicago: University of Chicago Press, 1994], 10).

3. Joseph Masco, "Survival Is Your Business: Engineering Ruins and Affect in Nuclear America," *Cultural Anthropology* 23 (2008): 374.

4. See, e.g., www.cdc.gov/nceh/radiation/fallout/RF-GWT_home.htm and www.cancer.gov/cancertopics/causes/i131; and *Exposure of the American People to Iodine-131 from Nevada Nuclear-Bomb Tests: Review of the National Cancer Institute Report and Public Health Implications* (Washington, D.C.: National Academies Press, 1999) (available at www.ncbi.nlm.nih.gov/books/NBK100842). Radioactive iodine (I-131) has a short half-life and quickly decomposes in food and milk. Other radioactive substances have much longer half-lives and are more difficult to trace.

5. A "Manual of Protective Action Guides for Nuclear Incidents" by the Office of Radiation Programs is published at: www.epa.gov/rpdweboo/docs/er/400-r-92–001.pdf. The document includes a cost-benefit calculation for the recommendation of removing milk from the food chain. In 1983, Congress asked the National Cancer Institute (NCI) to study the consequences of the radioactive iodine release; in 1990, it finalized its report, "Estimated Exposures and Thyroid Doses Received by the American People from Iodine-131 in Fallout Following Nevada Atmospheric Nuclear Bomb Tests," though it did not publish it until 1997. The NCI admitted in testimony before the U.S. Congress in 1998, after an investigation by the U.S. Senate Governmental Affairs Committee, that it suppressed this study for five years. See www.hsgac.senate.gov/subcommittees/investigations/hearings/national-cancer-institutes-management-of-radiation-studies.

Nuclear technologies cause cancer as a direct result of bomb construction, testing, and detonation in war, as well as uranium mining, cleanup, and disposal; consequently, the project of tempering nuclear terror can be seen as directly underwriting ideologies of cancer. The National Cancer Insitute estimates that iodine-131, one element of toxic fallout from bomb testing, caused up to 212,000 thyroid cancers in the United States. The five-year survival rate is 95 percent for thyroid cancer, so it's easy to dismiss it as not serious, even though we are looking at about 11,000 deaths. See *Exposure of the America People to Iodine-131*. If one thinks more closely about the government injuring and killing citizens in this way, subjecting people to surgeries, radiation treatments, fear of recurrence, and torturous deaths, one can easily see how a few strategies might be in order for managing not only the violence itself but also the potential lack of trust resulting from the misrepresentations.

6. Stephen I. Schwartz, *Atomic Audit: The Costs and Consequences of U.S. Nuclear Weapons since 1940* (Washington, D.C.: Brookings Institution Press, 1998).

7. Gerald Kutcher, *Contested Medicine: Cancer Research and the Military* (Chicago: University of Chicago Press, 2009); David Cantor, "Cancer," in *Dictionnaire de la Pensée Médicale,* ed. Dominique Lecourt, François Delaporte, Patrice Pinell, and Christiane Sinding (Paris: Presses Universitaires de France, 2004), 195–201; Alison Kraft, "Between Medicine and Industry: Medical Physics and the Rise of the Radioisotope 1945–65," *Contemporary British History* 20 (2006): 1–35.

8. Eilene Zimmerman, "Career Couch: Continuing to Heal after Returning to Work," *New York Times,* June 1, 2008. The article, however, neglected to mention some of the reasons that people return to work while still undergoing treatment: the need for medical insurance; the high costs of co-pays and help; the need to support children.

9. Masco, "Survival Is Your Business," 368. On the one hand, we are asked to accept the most astonishing gaps in knowledge about the links between military waste and cancer. The Farallon Islands just off the coast of San Francisco host one of the largest nuclear dump sites in the world. Nearly 50,000 barrels, many of which are now corroding, containing nuclear waste were dumped between 1946 and 1970 (http://walrus.wr.usgs.gov/farallon/radwaste.html). Former military personnel report taking barrels of nuclear waste to the site during and after World War II, and if the barrels didn't sink, they would shoot holes in them until they submerged (Ayaz Ahmed Khan, "Disposal of Radioactive Nuclear Waste," Media Monitors Network, www.mediamonitors.net/ayazahmedkhan2.html; accessed Feb. 25, 2013). Marin County, twenty-seven miles across the sea from the dumpsite, now has one of the highest breast cancer incidence rates in the country. While research has traced these high cancer rates to nearly everything one can imagine—including a purported high consumption of nonorganic white wine—not one study has attempted to correlate the radioactive waste dumped at the Farallon Islands with the rates of cancer. In fact, the nuclear pollution at the islands is not tracked at all, nor is information on the amount and type of dumping that took place publicly available.

10. "ACS, Behind the Science—Mammography," www.youtube.com/watch?v=mjdUgmUvzjM, uploaded Oct. 8, 2010.

11. For example, discussing the costs of early detection in terms of the number of biopsies performed on benign disease, Laura Esserman and Ian Thompson worry about the emotional costs of continued testing. They write, "All diagnostic procedures have costs, direct (financial, opportunity cost) and indirect (time off from work, away from families), and are associated with risk of complications and negative emotional consequences" ("Solving the Overdiagnosis Dilemma," *Journal of the National Cancer Institute* 102 [2010]: 583–583). Here again, this anecdote is presented to make the case that screening should be pared back, whereas I suggest that the negative emotional consequences need to be better understood before policy implications can be drawn out.

12. Steven Shapin, "Cancer World, the Making of a Modern Disease," *New Yorker,* Nov. 8, 2010, 78–83.

13. At one of the retreats I attended, the group leader asked us to think very concretely about fear as a logistical, manageable problem. What was it, exactly, we feared? Was it being in pain? If so, maybe we could contact a pain specialist and find out about available medications. Was it that our children would not have access to certain things after we died? If so, maybe we could ask friends to assume specific roles in their lives. This valuable exercise served to tranform a generalized fear into specific fears about which, in many cases, action could be taken.

14. David Rieff, *Swimming in a Sea of Death: A Son's Memoir* (New York: Simon & Schuster, 2008), 58.

15. Miriam Engelberg, *Cancer Made Me a Shallower Person* (New York: Harper, 2006). For an especially bizarre example of the smiling patient phemonemon, showing people in Southwestern Native American garb sitting around a table smiling, see "Radioactive Iodine (I-131) and Thyroid Cancer: An Education Resource," published by the National Cancer Institute, National Institutes of Health, and the U.S. Dept. of Health and Human Services; available at www.cancer.gov/images/Documents/9967bda0–5059–4a3f-8d5e-ff5a70194221/NA_Flip_Chart_v_7_0.pdf (accessed Oct. 25, 2012).

16. Suzanne H. Reuben, "President's Cancer Panel 2008–2009 Report on Reducing Environmental Cancer Risk: What We Can Do Now," Department of Health and Human Services, 2010, ii; available at http://deainfo.nci.nih.gov/advisory/pcp/annualreports/pcp08–09rpt/PCP_Report_08–09_508.pdf. See also W.C. Hueper and W.D. Conway, *Chemical Carcinogenesis and Cancers* (Springfield, Ill.: Charles C. Thomas, 1964), 638: "Through a continued, unrestrained, needless, avoidable, and in part reckless increasing contamination of the human environment with chemical and physical carcinogens and with chemicals supporting and potentiating their action, the stage is being set indeed for a future occurrence of an acute, catastrophic epidemic, which once present cannot effectively be checked for several decades with the means available nor can its course appreciably be altered once it has been set in motion."

17. Reuben, "President's Cancer Panel Report," i–vi.

18. Ibid., 1.

19. Ibid., ix.

20. See, e.g., Robert Proctor, *Cancer Wars: How Politics Shapes What We Know and Don't Know About Cancer* (New York: Basic Books, 1995); Gideon Haigh, *Asbestos House: The Secret History of James Hardie Industries* (Melbourne: Scribe Publications, 2008); and Gerald Markowitz and David Rosner, *Lead Wars: The Politics of Science and the Fate of America's Children* (Berkeley: University of California Press, 2013).

21. Reuben, "President's Cancer Panel Report," ii.

22. Ann G. Grimaldi, "California Goes Green(er) through New Chemical Initiative," *Legal Backgrounder*, Aug. 14, 2009, 1.

23. Reuben, "President's Cancer Panel Report," 22–23.

24. Ibid., 46. See also Frank Ackerman, "The Economics of Atrazine," *International Journal of Occupational and Environmental Health* 13 (2007): 441.

25. Rachel Carson, *Silent Spring* (New York: Houghton Mifflin, 1962).

26. Reuben, "President's Cancer Panel Report," 47.

27. Barbara A. Cohn, Mary S. Wolff, Piera M. Cirillo, and Robert I. Sholtz, "Cancer in Young Women: New Data on the Significance of Age at Exposure," *Environmental Health Perspectives* 115 (2007): 1406–1414; available at www.ncbi.nlm.nih.gov/pmc/articles/PMC2022666 (accessed March 2012).

28. Reuben, "President's Cancer Panel Report," 30.

29. See www.epa.gov/pesticides/factsheets/index.htm.

30. Reuben, "President's Cancer Panel Report," 46.

31. Ibid., 18. See also Patricia A. Hunt et al., "The Bisphenol A Experience: A Primer for the Analysis of Environmental Effects on Mammalian Reproduction," *Biology of Reproduction* 81 (2009): 807–813. This article notes (809) that 90 percent of governmental studies (several times more studies than those with industry sponsors) find that BPA exposure during fetal development increases the risk of prostate cancer for the male children, whereas 0 percent of the industry studies find this correlation (in a review of articles published through December 2004).

32. See Norman B. Anderson, Rodolfo A. Bulatao, and Barney Cohen, eds., *Critical Perspectives on Racial and Ethnic Differences in Health in Late Life* (Washington, D.C.: National Academies Press, 2004); available at www.ncbi.nlm.nih.gov/books/NBK25526.

33. See, e.g., Environmental Working Group, "Body Burden—The Pollution in Newborns," July 14, 2005, www.ewg.org/reports/bodyburden2/execsumm.php.

34. Reuben, "President's Cancer Panel Report," 38.

35. Ibid., 45. See also http://epa.gov/pesticides/health/risk-benefit.htm.

36. Throughout the 1900s, tort law placed responsibility on the design and manufacturing processes as a way to protect consumers from predictable injuries and, where such injuries were impossible to avoid, to spread their costs. See S. Lochlann Jain, *Injury: The Politics of Product Design and Safety Law in the United States* (Princeton, N.J.: Princeton University Press, 2006).

37. In theory, a plaintiff could claim that a certain chemical should hold to strict liability; that is, wherever it causes damages, the manufacturer and/or user should be held responsible for those damages regardless of fault or intent.

38. See, generally, Michael D. Hultquist, "Fear of Cancer as a Compensable Cause of Action," *Brief* 30, no. 3 (2001): 8; and Keith J. Klein, "Fear of Cancer—A Legitimate Claim in Toxic Tort Cases?" *Air Force Law Review* 33 (1990): 193, 198. Courts have varied widely on the requisite level of actual risk of cancer and the standard of proof for the physical likelihood and evidence of potential cancer (such as precancerous lesions or pleural thickening). Generally, all courts agree that the fear of cancer must be both reasonable and causally related to the defendant's negligence. See ibid.; also Jay E. Znaniecki, "Cancerphobia Damages in Medical Malpractice Claims," *University of Illinois Law Review* 1997, no. 2 (1997): 639ff.

39. *Potter v. Firestone Tire & Rubber Co.* (1993), 6 Cal. 4th 965 [25 Cal. Rptr. 2d 550, 863 P. 2d 795]. The following account is based on this court case, esp. pp. 801–803.

40. "National Service Center for Environmental Publications Simple Search," U.S. Environmental Protection Agency, Sept. 29, 2010, http://nepis.epa.gov (check "1986–1990" and search Salinas; follow "Descriptions of 187 Sites Proposed for the National Priorities List," scroll down to thirteenth site; accessed July 2010).

41. *Potter v. Firestone*, 827.

42. Email communication with Gordon Stemple, plaintiffs' attorney, Oct. 29, 2012.

43. *Potter v. Firestone*, 811.

44. Gerald Markowitz and David Rosner, *Deceit and Denial: The Deadly Politics of Industrial Pollution* (Berkeley: University of California Press, 2003), 173–178.

45. Website of Robert L. Willmore, partner, Crowell & Moring ("Strong Beyond Measure"), www.crowell.com/Professionals/Robert-Willmore; accessed Aug. 31, 2010. Willmore's influential article is "In Fear of Cancerphobia," *Defense Counsel Journal* 50 (1989).

46. Willmore, "In Fear of Cancerphobia," 53.

47. Ibid., 56, 54.

48. J. Nonnemaker, M. Farrelly, K. Kamyab et al., "Experimental Study of Graphic Cigarette Warning Labels Final Results Report," prepared for the Center for Tobacco Products, Food and Drug Administration, Rockville, Md., Dec. 2010.

49. D. Hammond, G.T. Fong, A. McNeill et al., "Effectiveness of Cigarette Warning Labels in Informing Smokers about the Risks of Smoking: Findings from the International Tobacco Control (ITC) Four Country Survey," *Tobacco Control* 15, suppl. 3 (2006): iii19–iii25; G. Leshner, P. Bolls, and E. Thomas, "Scare 'Em or Disgust 'Em: The Effects of Graphic Health Promotion Messages," *Health Communication* 24 (2009): 447–458.

50. For an incredible analysis of the many components of cigarette design, see Robert N. Proctor, *Golden Holocaust: Origins of the Cigarette Catastrophe and the Case for Abolition* (Berkeley: University of California Press, 2012).

51. Jake Kosek, *Understories: The Political Life of Forests in Northern New Mexico* (Durham, N.C.: Duke University Press, 2006), 234.

52. Even in the Department of Labor's compensation program for nuclear workers set up in 1990, three out of four cases of cancer are denied compensation for radiation-based injuries. Recently, the head physician resigned in disgust at the out-of-hand dismissals of so many cases, despite the vast literature on the links between radiation and cancer. Furthermore, that program doesn't cover uranium miners (disproportionately Native Americans); instead, that industry is guided by the Department of the Interior. In other words, even when regulatory recognition of radiation injury exists, it is spread among many different organizations. For more detail on the nuclear workers compensation program, see www.dol.gov/owcp/energy (accessed July 2012). For a recent critique of the implementation of the program (which requires perfect documentation of exposures unless they correspond to a limited set of cancers), see www.propublica.org/article/plan-to-pay-sick-nuclear-workers-unfairly-rejects-many-doctor-says-731 (accessed July 2012). See also www.whistleblower.org/storage/documents/SystemicInjustice.pdf (accessed July 2012).

53. These were some of the systematic challenges to survivors noted in "Living Beyond Cancer: Finding a New Balance," National Cancer Panel 2003–2004 Annual Report, U.S. Department of Health and Human Services, National Institutes of Health, National Cancer Institute.

54. Masco, "Survival Is Your Business."

55. J. Honeybun, M. Johnston, and A. Tookman, "The Impact of a Death on Fellow Hospice Patients," *British Journal of Medical Psychology* 65 (1992): 67.

CHAPTER 9

1. Italo Calvino, "La Poubelle Agréée," in *The Road to San Giovanni*, trans. Tim Parks (New York: Vintage, 1994), 110.

2. Mary Douglas, *Purity and Danger: An Analysis of Concepts of Pollution and Taboo* (New York: Routledge, 1992).

3. http://lookgoodfeelbetter.org/about-lgfb/program-description (accessed April 13, 2011).

4. See Karen Dion, Ellen Berscheid, and Elaine Walster, "What Is Beautiful Is Good," *Journal of Personality and Social Psychology* 24 (1972): 285–290; and Murray Webster and James E. Driskell, "Beauty as Status," *American Journal of Sociology* 89 (1983): 140–165.

5. See, e.g., Deborah L. Rhode, *The Beauty Bias: The Injustice of Appearance in Life and Law* (Oxford: Oxford University Press, 2010). Appearance also influences judgments about competence and job performance, which in turn affect income and status. Résumés get a less favorable assessment when they are thought to belong to unattractive individuals. These individuals are also less likely to get hired and promoted, and they earn lower salaries, even in professions such as law where appearance has no demonstrable relationship to ability.

6. *Jespersen v. Harrah's Operating Co.*, 444 F. 3d 1104 (9th Cir. 2006), affirming 392 F. 3d 1076 (9th Cir. 2005).

7. Rhode, *Beauty Bias*, 11–13.

8. P.F. Infante, S.E. Petty, D.H. Groth et al., "Vinyl Chloride Propellant in Hair Spray and Angiosarcoma of the Liver among Hairdressers and Barbers: Case Reports," *International Journal of Occupational and Environmental Health* 15 (2009): 36–42.

9. Rhode, *Beauty Bias*, 36.

10. Environmental Working Group's Skin Deep® Cosmetics Database, "Myths on Cosmetic Safety," www.ewg.org/skindeep/myths-on-cosmetics-safety (accessed March 31, 2013).

11. Surgeons often don't hesitate to offer the opportunity of having a better body than one had before. Insurance will pay for two reconstructions, and surgeons will sometimes even throw in a tummy tuck or use a method of reconstruction that requires the redistribution of one's tummy fat. One person I interviewed said that three plastic surgeons encouraged her to have the reconstruction in both breasts, claiming they couldn't make an implant "small enough" to match the breast that remained. She was extremely happy with the results.

12. Calvino, "La Poubelle Agréée,"104.

CONCLUSION

1. In discussing the mechanics of retreat, Janie once wrote to me, "Would any group of people willing to show up fully have the same impact? Any group of people, each person sharing unique personal suffering . . . ? I am not convinced. I have a sense that having the experience of a diagnosis of cancer loosens the armoring so that real, authentic conversations are more likely to happen. I don't think people open that fully unless something has brought them to their knees."

2. Rachel Remen, "Just Listen," in *Kitchen Table Wisdom: Stories That Heal* (New York: Riverhead, 2006).

3. Tim O'Brien, "How to Tell a True War Story," in *The Things They Carried* (New York: Houghton Mifflin Harcourt, 1990), 84.

4. www.dignitymemorial.com/dm20/en_US/main/dm/index.page.

Index

Italic page numbers refer to illustrations.